Keys to Running Successful Research Projects: All the Things They Never Teach You

Keys to Running Successful Research Projects: All the Things They Never Teach You

Katherine Christian
Strategic Research and Alumni Program Manager
Cure Cancer Australia
Sydney, Australia

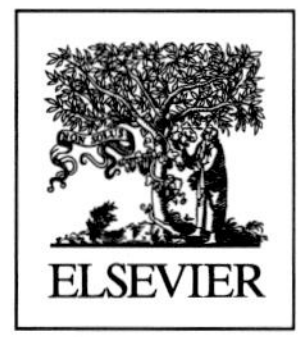
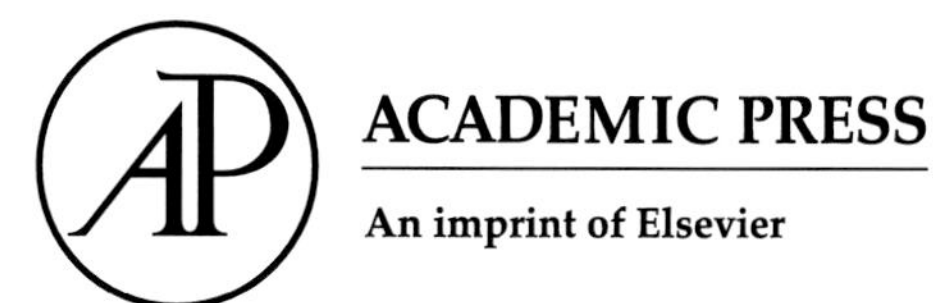
ACADEMIC PRESS
An imprint of Elsevier

Academic Press is an imprint of Elsevier
125 London Wall, London EC2Y 5AS, United Kingdom
525 B Street, Suite 1800, San Diego, CA 92101-4495, United States
50 Hampshire Street, 5th Floor, Cambridge, MA 02139, United States
The Boulevard, Langford Lane, Kidlington, Oxford OX5 1GB, United Kingdom

Library of Congress Cataloging-in-Publication Data
A catalog record for this book is available from the Library of Congress

British Library Cataloguing-in-Publication Data
A catalogue record for this book is available from the British Library

ISBN: 978-0-12-813134-3

For information on all Academic Press publications visit our website at https://www.elsevier.com/books-and-journals

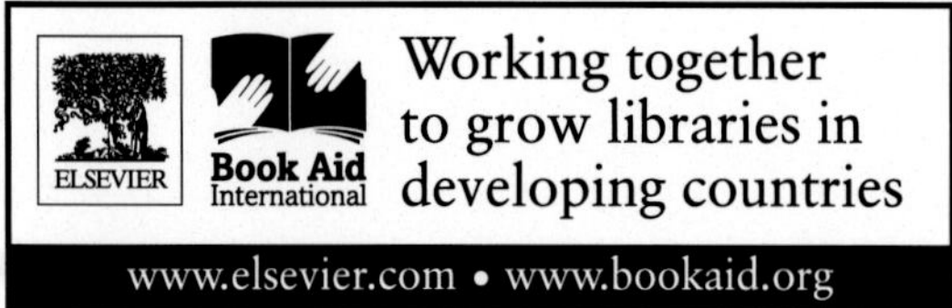

Publisher: Mica Haley
Acquisition Editor: Mary Preap
Editorial Project Manager: Mary Preap
Production Project Manager: Poulouse Joseph
Designer: Matthew Limbert

Typeset by TNQ Books and Journals

Contents

Preface

This book is about research management, not about how to actually *do* research. It is about how to manage yourself, your projects, and your team. It is aimed particularly at early career researchers, PhD students, and their supervisors. It is for the people who are good at, and understand, their specific subject matter, who know how to do the research that supports it—but who are finding out that there is more to a successful research career than just doing research.

Although most of the information could be aimed at anyone working in academia, this book is particularly for people in the sciences. Scientists are good at science but are often not much good at concentrating on broader management. It seems that it is the scientists who are most reluctant to attend research training sessions. It is certain that many scientists find themselves in trouble with their overall management skills.

Good research management takes time, but it saves much more time and a great deal of money. Funders and research institutes have hard-fought-for money and need to know it is being spent wisely and well. And the audiences for the projects need to know that the work is valuable and trustworthy. This guide will explain how to successfully achieve all this.

This resource provides a simple, plain language, step-by-step guide for managing a successful research project or program from start to finish and includes illustrative case studies. It will highlight all those aspects of management, which perhaps should be included during the researcher's training—but are not. References throughout will provide more detailed information from "gold standard" sources on every topic.

This book is designed to answer any question that may arise in these situations and to provide simple solutions or guides to those solutions.

Its high-level approach addresses most of the many hurdles a researcher will encounter. There is much similar advice available elsewhere, but until now it has not been brought together in one book as "Research Management 101."

Rather than using gender-neutral pronouns throughout this book, I have elected to use "she." No disrespect to men is intended!

There are many references to practices in Australian universities or other institutions. This is not parochialism, but simply because I am Australian and familiar with the institutions that display good practices. Australian science prides itself on being representative of world's best practice, so I am sticking with what I know, in the confidence that it is.

Endorsements for *Keys to Running Successful Research Projects: All the Things They Never Teach You*

Congratulations to Katherine Christian for a truly valuable book.

Research workers are notoriously reluctant to admit their defects, and one of the worst ones is their absence of management skills.

Yet in the modern world, a significant research enterprise takes a whole heap of management!

In this clear, practical, comprehensive and authoritative work, Christian provides a guide on how to manage research, covering all the bases.

Having been thrown in the deep end myself without any training, I would have gained enormously from a resource like this.

It deserves a wide and devoted readership.

Sir Gustav Nossal, AC, CBE, FRS, Australian of the Year 2000, The University of Melbourne

The book sounds amazing. And really important as no one ever teaches you that stuff.

Professor Andrew Biankin, Regius Chair of Surgery, University of Glasgow

I wish someone had given me your book 10 years ago! Would have made many things much easier.

Anne Holland PhD, Professor of Physiotherapy, Alfred Health and La Trobe University

Congrats on your much needed book

Professor Maria Kavallaris, Head of the Tumour Biology and Targeting Program, Children's Cancer Institute Director, Australian Centre for NanoMedicine at University of NSW Sydney

This is a dream Kate

A/Prof Tamera Corte, Sydney Medical School, University of Sydney

I GETTING STARTED

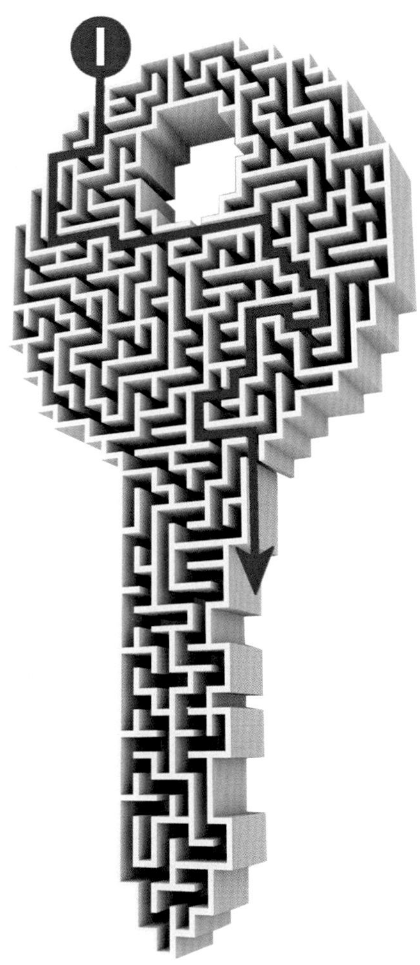

1.1 Introduction to Using This Book

- *If only I had understood that they wouldn't let me publish…*
- *I didn't know I had to get ethics approval for that…*
- *No one told me I should have asked for…*
- *If only I had backed up my data…*
- *Why didn't I write it down?*

This is not a book for reading cover to cover, like a novel. Instead, it is recommended that you dip in and out of the sections as you need to, each time you come up with an unfamiliar problem.

Follow all these instructions all the way through the book, and you'll be in line for a Nobel Prize. All you need to add is some good science!

The Checklists

Let's start with the checklists. Following the now well-established methodology proposed by Gawande [1], which has dramatically improved surgical outcomes and patient care across the world, there is a checklist at the beginning of every chapter. If you can manage to tick off each of the items listed for whichever topic is the focus of the moment, you will have managed the essentials. It will be even better if you go on to read and understand more detail. Some lists are longer than others, but in every case they are the must dos.

> If, at the very least, you can manage to think about and follow up on each thing on the checklist for every topic, you will be managing your research really well.

Trust me, it will make a difference.

The lists below represent a summary of the big picture, the multitude of points you need to think about early—preferably today—as part of your management of yourself, your projects and your team as you progress though your career. They are all covered, to a greater or lesser extent, in this book. Arranged in roughly chronological order, they are a list of things you must do on your way. The trouble is that you probably need to do all the things in these Getting Started chapters at once!

Checklist

(The Imperative Checklist for Managing Yourself)

- ☐ Try to map out an overall career plan. Set your direction and make a development plan.
- ☐ Learn to make a project plan and write a good grant application.

Then

- ☐ Don't leave working on your reputation until later. Start by building a social media presence and a personal web profile.
- ☐ Build a web profile for your project
- ☐ Find a mentor
- ☐ Book some training

Then

- ☐ Apply that project plan to actual project management. Learn about managing budgets as soon as (if not before) you have money to manage

Then start on the list for managing your team.

Checklist

(The Imperative Checklist for Managing Your Team)

- ☐ Help them understand your shared objectives
- ☐ Remember you're a mentor as well as a supervisor - mentor them well
- ☐ Be available to talk and listen to your team
- ☐ Practice and expect work life balance
- ☐ Celebrate success

Your research career path is like paths through a maze. Each section in this book illustrates a piece of the pathway - and provides a key to your project's success.

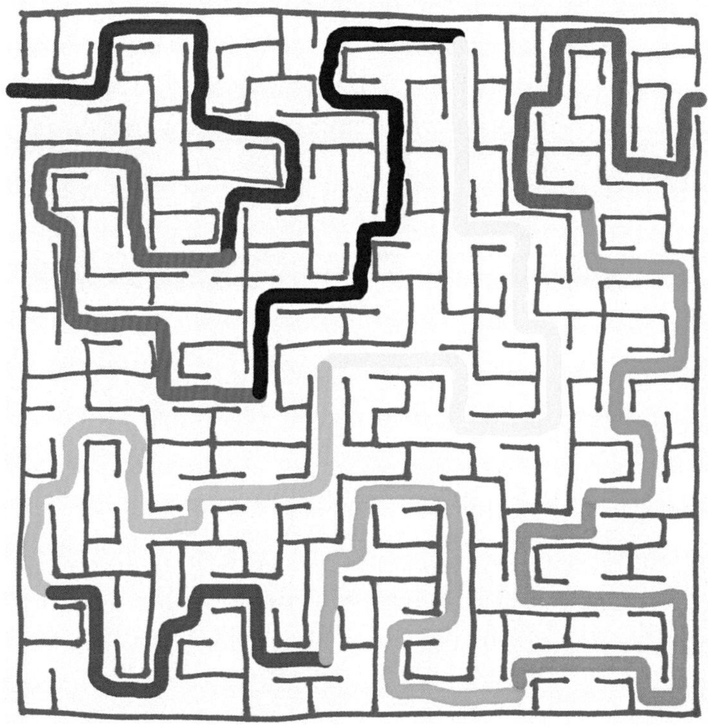

Reference—Introduction to the Checklists

[1] Gawande, A., 2011. The Checklist Manifesto, How to Get Things Right. Profile Books.

1.2 Career Planning—Managing Yourself

You have reached the ultimate dream and, at last, you are head of your own small lab or your own, discrete project. At the same time, you have suddenly discovered that there is more to being in charge than you had expected. Being the head of the team is more than just making big discoveries; it is about managing a small business. You have to worry about all sorts of management concepts you've never dealt with before.

Read on. This book is for you.

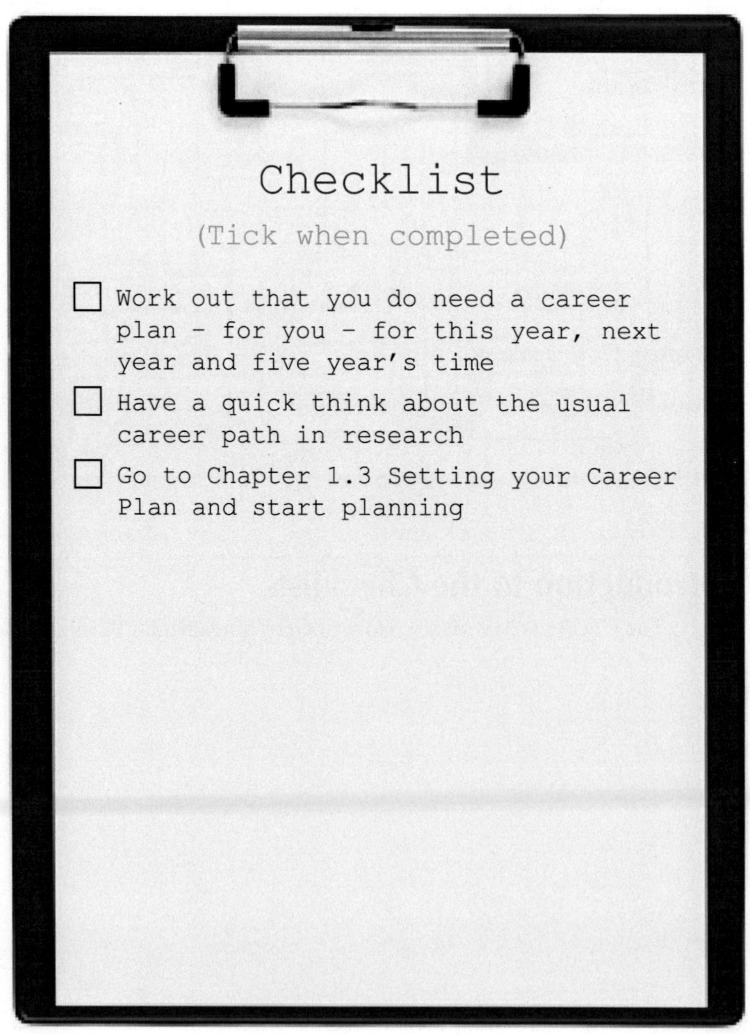

Your independence comes suddenly when you start your research career, and with it you can find yourself floundering unexpectedly. During your PhD, you will have learned analytical skills and critical thinking skills, clearly part of any research activity. You will have learned to generate innovative ideas. Now, around the edges of your research skills, you need to add strong project management skills. Your new projects will need careful planning, management, and evaluation, and you will have to learn to successfully manage the time, people, funds, relationships, and risks, which come with them. You will also need to come to grips with budgeting and contract management and will have to comply with your funding body's and institution's requirements. As your career progresses, you also need to learn how to manage staff and to develop strong leadership skills. There is much to be done and many balls to be juggled at once!

Your initial career aim must be to develop a strong track record. Without a strong track record, you will have difficulty attracting further funding. As you almost certainly know, you will build your track record by publishing in high-quality journals, presenting refereed papers at international conferences, and building a profile within your research community. Successful supervision of Honors and PhD students through to completion will also help.

The biggest challenge you will face as an early-career researcher is likely to be managing the many different calls on your time as you balance doing your research along with the development of skills you need to enhance it. It will all become easier over time, as you gain experience, but in the first year or two of your independent life, it is likely that managing your time will feel particularly overwhelming.

You need to start with planning. 48% of respondents to a UK Research Career Survey [1] admitted to not having a career plan. The reasons were many and varied, but none of them much good. You mightn't like to take the time to pause and reflect on your career ahead, but there is evidence that career planning does have positive effects, including on career decision-making, perceived competence, and career satisfaction. Ball [2] recommends that you have at least two career plans, each incorporating a life plan. She hypothesizes that life is unpredictable, especially in research, so there always should be a plan B to back up plan A. It is good advice.

So the moral of the story is to have a plan and to start on it right at the beginning of your career.

What to Do First?

Three main strategies can assist with managing yourself in your early years.

- First, work out what you need to achieve to further your career; this will help you clarify your priorities.
- Second, seek mentors and also help from your colleagues who can provide you with quick tips and assistance.
- Third, take up developmental opportunities that can help you to acquire the necessary skills.

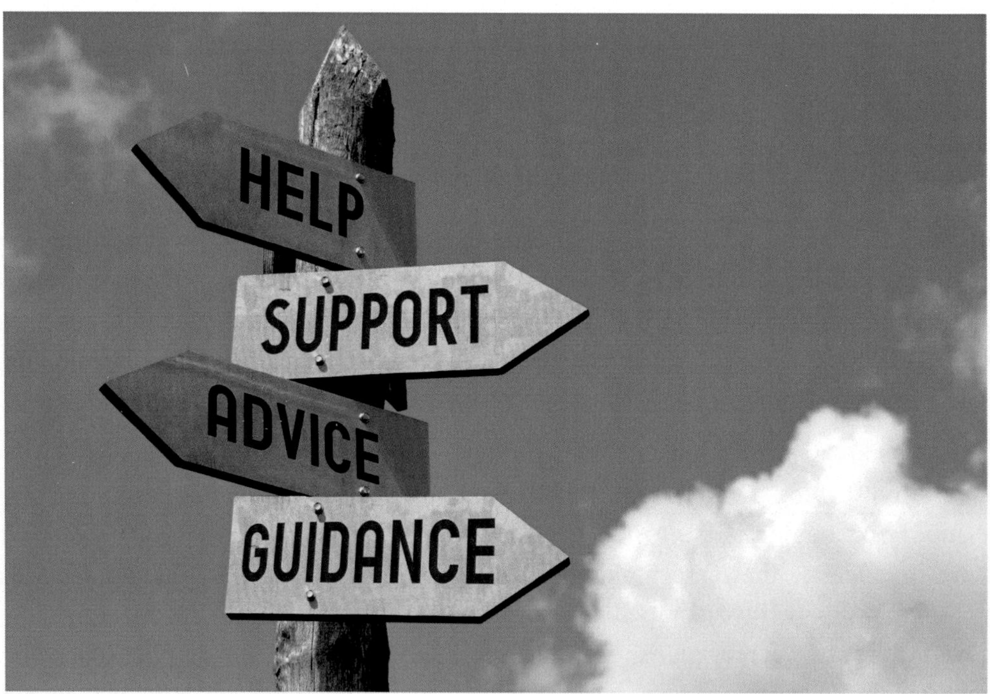

Image Credit: Help, support, advice, guidance signpost by 3D_generator/iStock

It is well known that early-career researchers, and particularly those in the sciences, are reluctant to look for opportunities for career development. You, too, probably feel you can't (or don't want to) take time away from your work. Please don't fall into this trap. Many people who have gone before you have reflected that this approach was a mistake which held back their career progression! A few hours away from your laboratory or research desk will be made up for very quickly when you practice your new skills.

Good time management, career management, media skills, interpersonal skills, budgeting, contract management, collaborations, project management, and understanding university processes are vital in a research career. They simply can't wait until later.

The Research Career Path

Scientists are particularly likely to think of their research on a project-by-project basis. A better approach, though, is to think about your current research project as a step in your career path. At the same time, think about the steps you need to take to travel from one stage to the next.

Most of these steps are in fact steps in management and personal development, not steps in research. If you haven't completed all the steps in one stage, you really won't be able to progress to the next.

PhD students are mostly able to exist in their own private research world. Conducting their research and writing up their thesis is a very personal journey, about "their" subject. They have to do it by themselves, as of course it has to be original work and their supervisors can only help so much. On the way, the PhD student needs to develop research skills, writing skills, and time management skills. She also needs to learn to communicate with their supervisors and articulate her findings or concerns. Apart from that she will find she is mostly able to follow instructions and will learn to generate data, which will be used to write the thesis. If she is lucky, she will be taken in as part of a larger team and will come to understand some of the management processes of a project and the culture of being part of a team.

In the next stage, *early-career researcher*s suddenly need to manage one or more staff, and perhaps supervise a PhD student. They might find themselves managing a lab or part of a lab. They may need to manage a budget or, horror of horrors, write a grant application because they are suddenly responsible for sourcing funding.

The project is bigger than the PhD topic. They don't know how to do everything themselves—so they need to find others to help. They need mentors and collaborators. Where should they look? What should they say?

As well as all this, they need to publish—but where is the time to do the actual work? By now they should also be focusing on their research pathway, their vision. What do they want their career to look like? What are their areas of particular interest? What are they *doing* here?

The *mid-career researcher* has all this and more. More staff, more students, more budgets, more worries. More people skills required. More pressure to attract grants. A greater need to publish so that their track record makes people want to give them grants. They need to be developing a reputation in a particular field. To build that reputation, the team needs to be on the same track as them, and that means there must be a shared vision. By now the mid-career researcher must have clarified their vision and learned to express it.

The last stage, the *research leader*, is the researcher who has made it. The leader might now be the Director of Research or the Dean. The leader probably has many staff, and many of them have students. There is so much administration to do there is hardly time for research, and life is terribly busy keeping everyone else afloat. The leader has to have the clearest vision of all and is the one who sets the culture for the whole organization. By now the leader may also have a big reputation to manage. People want to involve the leader in *their* research, which can lead to distraction from the planned track. They want the leader's name on their papers, and there are many requests for supervision. The leader has to be very careful with setting priorities and sticking to them.

That isn't really the last stage. That is for the emeritus professor, the senior researcher who sees the light, abandons the top position and probably a salary, and continues just doing research. With no one to tell them what to do any more, no forms to read or sign, they can just get on with what they started doing all those years ago during their PhD!

Research and researcher development go hand in hand—as the researcher develops so does the research, as described by Benner [3].

References—Managing Yourself

[1] Vitae Careers in Research Online Survey. https://www.vitae.ac.uk/impact-and-evaluation/cros.
[2] Happy Academic, 2017. Why You Should Not Have a Career Plan. https://happyacademic.wordpress.com/2017/03/01/why-you-should-not-have-a-career-plan/#more-116.
[3] Benner, P., March 1982. From novice to expert. American Journal of Nursing 402–407.

1.3 Setting the Career Plan—and Your Research Priorities

Now that you are a post-doc and have an element of independence it is tempting to bury yourself in your own world, just getting on with your research. This would be fun, but the real world is not like that. Unless you are in a very unusual environment, you are going to need to sing for your supper. This will require delivering research outcomes and providing return on investment. There are more people than just you who have a vested interest in your success. Step One is setting your career plan and then your research priorities.

Checklist

(Tick when completed)

- ☐ Decide you are going to have a career plan(compulsory)
- ☐ Work out that personal career plan, asking:
    - ☐ Where am I now? Think about what you can do now, then about your skill gaps - and plan for training to fill them
    - ☐ Where do I want to be? Identify your priorities - to help you build your track record
    - ☐ How can I get there?
- ☐ Follow your star

> *The future depends on what you do today.*
> Mahatma Gandhi

First Thoughts—Check the Priorities You Need to Comply With

When you are setting your research priorities, you should start with those of your institution. And take the time to think out how you fit within your institution's goals. If the focus for your organization is the productivity of agricultural crops, it is obvious that you would be unwise to start a course toward astronomy. This is an extreme example, but make sure you are aligned with the objectives of your host body. Look at the strategic plan on the website make sure you understand the institution's overall priorities.

The same thinking applies for the priorities of your funding agency, if you are fortunate enough to have a level of independence with your choice of research direction. They will not be pleased if you have been engaged to do research on heart health and you end up working on measles.

Having ensured that you are heading in the correct direction, find out what sort of resources will be offered to you as you progress. Check if any extra funding might be available for you and your team, and see if there are opportunities for career development on the way.

You will need to balance your short-term priorities with your long-term aims. If these are wildly different, your career progress will take a lot of planning.

Build Your Personal Development Plan

Dudovskiy [1] suggests you will need to answer the three basic questions in the checklist: (1) where am I now, (2) where do I want to be, and (3) how can I get there? When you have answered those questions, you'll have your plan.

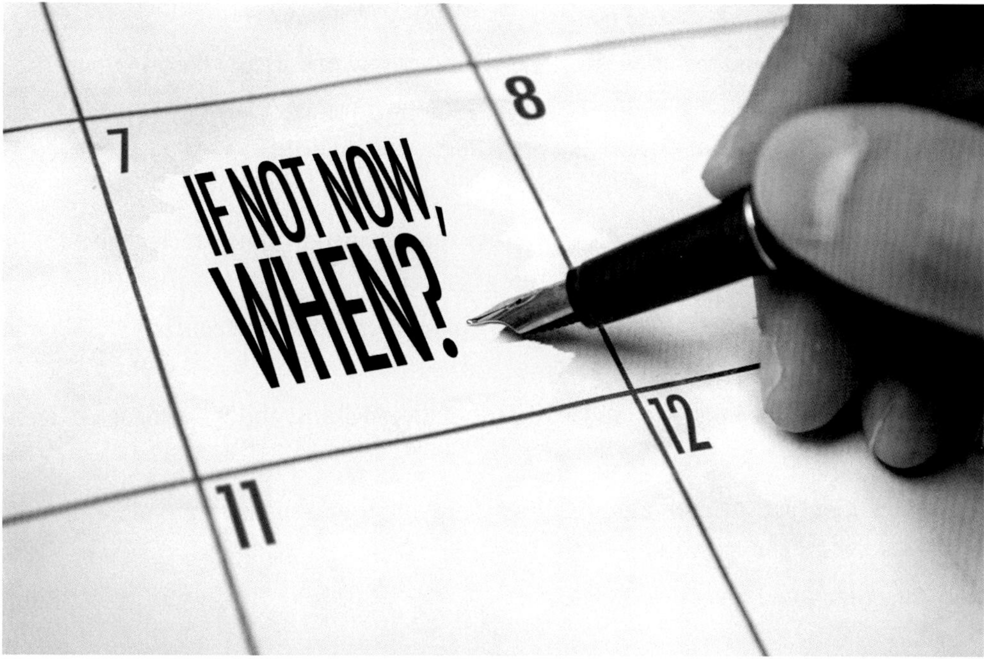

Image Credit: If Not Now, When? By gustavofrazao/iStock

1. Where Am I Now?

The first step is to work out *where you are now* and why you are there. Think about what has *pushed* you into research? Is it determination, ambition, curiosity/passion, or expectation of great things? Are you being pulled into it by your mentors, by your successes, or by the feeling that you are helping to make a difference? Any of these factors might be contributing to why you are doing what you are doing—and to what you might do next.

It is incredibly important to head in a direction that is going to make you, and keep you, satisfied. You spend a long time at work, so it might as well be fun. Follow your star!

Think out the answers to these questions put by Mitchell [2]:

- Assuming you want to become a "successful" researcher, what does this person look like to you?
- What criteria would you use to assess this success?
- What benchmarks would you use to measure it?
- How important is a "competitive track record" to you?

Now think about what *you need to be good at:*

- Research skills and techniques—understanding how research is done in your discipline (cutting edge questions, methodologies, techniques)
- Understanding research environment practices—responsible conduct of research, ethics requirements
- Research management skills—project management, time management, budget management
- Personal effectiveness—self-awareness, initiative, work independently, self-reliance, identification of own training needs
- Communication skills—writing skills, presentation skills, ability to engage others
- Managing staff
- Networking and team-working skills—developing and maintaining effective working relationships and networks
- Managing your career development

Completion of the answers for Activity 1, following, will help you work out what you are good at, what you can be better at and what you need to be good at to be successful.

Activity 1 Where am I now?

Strengths	Areas for Development	Opportunities	Barriers
What are you good at doing now?	What do you need to work on, develop, or improve?	What are your opportunities to improve? Who might help you?	What are the obstacles/ barriers that might prevent this improvement?

Take a close look at your research profile on your website (see Chapter 1.9), and think about how your track record might look to a pair of outside eyes. What are your areas of strength and weakness? What can you do about it? What should be your immediate priorities for the next couple of years?

2. Where Do I Want to Be?

Dudovskiy's second step helps you understand your motivations and to work out where you want to be with respect to those benchmarks for success you identified in Activity 1.

- How far away are you from the "successful" benchmarks now?
- What would you need to do to become competitive?

- Do you actually want to be competitive—or just left alone?
- What do you want from the research part of your work?
- Where do you want to be, research-wise, in 6 months, 12 months, and then 3–5 years?

Activity 2 Where do I want to be?

6 months	12 months	3–5 years
Employing a research assistant Supervising a student	Applying for my next grant Ready to write up	Presenting at meeting x Publishing y Funded by z

3. How Can I Get There?

Finally, in Step 3, the last part of your plan, you must work out what you are going to do to achieve your aims. Here, you are:

- Setting objectives—not just papers you want to write, not just grants you want to apply for, but learning skills, broadening knowledge, changing behaviors and habits, becoming more mature in attitudes and beliefs (including self-belief):
  - You want to write *better* papers—not just more of the same
  - You want to be able to target *better* journals—not just those that will accept your work
  - You want to be *more* competitive for grants—not just increase your number of publications unless they enhance your esteem and reputation
- Planning activities, resources, and opportunities to achieve these objectives;
- Setting a time frame—where do you want to be in 6 months, 12 months, 3–5 years?
- Able to provide evidence of achievements—how will you measure this?
- Reflecting on your learning—how will you know your work is *better*?

In Activity 3, you consider your specific goals for the next 6 months, then for a year and five years. What do you have to achieve in years one, three, and five to get there? What steps do you have to take?

Activity 3 How Can I get there?

6 months	12 months	3–5 years
Specific Objectives	**Specific Objectives**	**Specific Objectives**
1. Find out HR processes	1	1
2. Understand budgeting	2	2
3. Find a mentor	3	3
4	4	4
Specific Actions to Achieve Objectives	**Specific Actions to Achieve Objectives**	**Specific Actions to Achieve Objectives**
1. Visit HR department	1	1
2. Do budget training	2	2
3. Talk to supervisor about mentors	3	3
4	4	4

So now you have thought through the whole process. When you combine the answers to the questions in Activities 1, 2, and 3, there's your personal research development plan!

So what does it look like?

- Does it look like something you can achieve?
- Does it look like something that will help?
- Does it look like something you haven't had before?

What could be simpler?

Another Approach to the Same End

The University of Sussex Individual Research Plan [3] takes a slightly different approach to the planning process. They suggest that you think about your motivation and work out what you are most passionate about. As a next step, consider funding opportunities, and which avenues available to you are most fundable, or are likely to make you most competitive. They advise that when you are considering your plans for publications, you assess which avenues might lead you to the highest quality outputs, and suggest you also think about any unfinished publications which would be worthwhile to finish as a first priority, while at the same time working out what has been preventing you from completing them.

With regard to personal management, the University of Sussex approach recommends that you think about how you have been managing your time and your networking. Are you trying to accomplish too much at once and thus spreading yourself too thin? You might be better off doing fewer projects and managing them more effectively. Last, the plan asks that you outline the support you will require from others (your colleagues, line manager, Head of School, and any other relevant person) to achieve your aims, create your projected profile, and mitigate any obstacles.

You can still use the table for Activity 3, above, when using this approach to plan your next steps.

Next Step—Share Your Ideas

Having identified the path or paths, however, sketchy they may be, discuss them with your supervisor. Make sure your mutual goals align. If they do, you have a valuable ally. If they don't, there is work to do, possibly on both sides. Discuss your priorities with your mentor as well, in case they offer a different perspective.

Next, if you have one, talk to your team. Having these sorts of conversations ensures that everyone is quite clear about where they stand. When you can all head in the same direction you are in a much stronger position than if you are pursuing different goals and on a different trajectory.

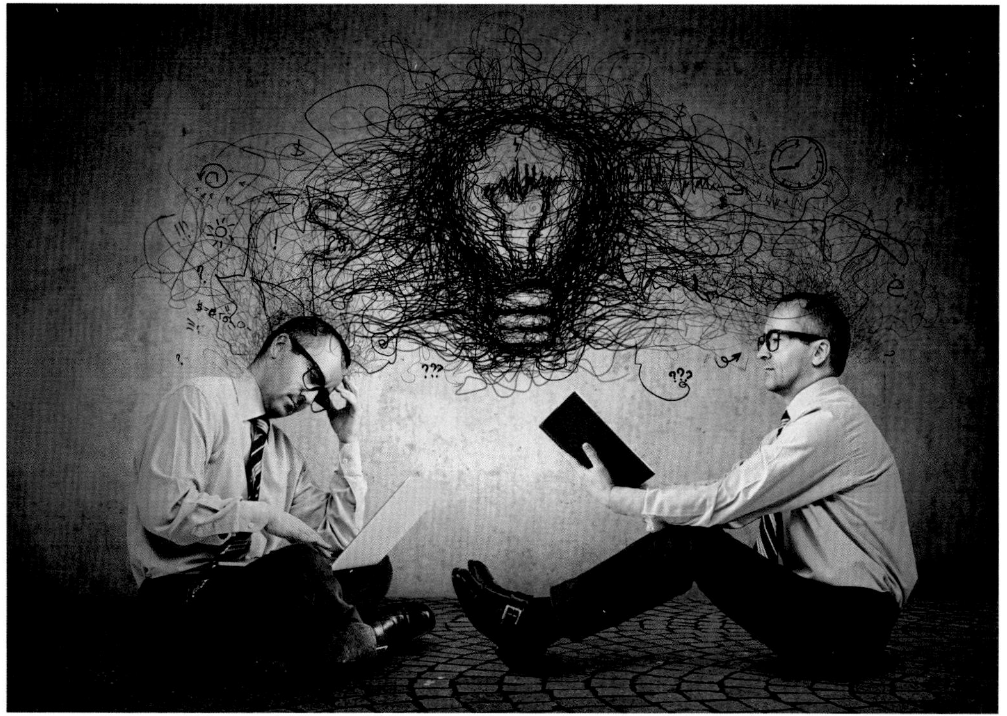

Image Credit: Men sitting on a floor by Siphotography/iStock

Integrate Your Research and Publication Plans

We have already established that you are aiming to publish to build your track record, and a vital part of that will be your publications. There is a balance to be struck between trying to produce the "dream papers," which may never happen, and trying to publish a set of fragmentary observations (which should definitely be avoided). One way to find the right balance is to integrate your plans for your research into your plans for publication.

Barker [4] suggests strategies for doing this. She recommends that, as you work out your long-term research goals, deciding on the experiments or calculations you want to do, you should imagine those experiments or calculations as parts of a published paper, or series of papers. While you are doing this, you can try to think graphically, and imagine how each set of results will look in a figure, graph, or table. If you write out your ideas, including your hypotheses, your planned methodology, and the results you hope for as part of your planning, you are already making progress with the project's work and its writing up.

Having started your project, the questions that come up as you analyze and then write up your results for each section of your research should suggest additional experiments, which further clarify your ideas. Make graphs or tables for these, too. As you write, you will uncover gaps in information and any questionable conclusions. Eventually, you should be able to see that you have a set of conclusions that are ready for you to work on for publication.

Continue Working on Your Career Plan and Objectives

Developing a research career is a long-term venture and will not happen overnight. It takes time to build your profile. In the early days, it helps if you can take a "building blocks" approach. You might find it possible to start with small projects in areas you may not have originally thought about. Keep an eye out for small value grants for which there might be many funding sources. You may be able to finish these small projects in a relatively short time, which will help you demonstrate your skills and show that you can deliver. You should aim to add to your track record during this time by presenting, supervising students and publishing where you can.

Keep a list of prospective project ideas and whenever you come up with a new idea, add it to the bottom. As a next step, expand the idea to a brief outline and think it over quietly. Your plan can be improved on as the idea develops. You can use Project Planning Form 1 (See Document 1.4.1 in Chapter 1.4) to capture this plan.

Re-visit your list of ideas when you have team planning meetings or when a grant round or sponsor becomes available. Your colleagues might come up with some valuable extra ideas to improve the project, so it can be useful to include them from the early planning stages.

Keep an Eye on Your Goals

It is all too easy to be permanently caught up with your current project for your whole career. You must train yourself to develop a longer view, of say five or so years, and you must monitor the success of your strategy in moving toward that goal. Keep a record of your goals so that you can monitor your progress towards them—or away from them. As always, seek advice from mentors, your supervisor, and successful researchers.

If, as is most likely, you're on a short-term grant, start work toward your next grant in plenty of time. You should be doing something about new grants around the mid-point of a three-year grant.

When you are planning your new project, you may need to build a new research team in order to have the necessary skills and expertise. Bringing the potential team into the project at the early conceptual stage will allow you to draw on their creative ideas and expertise. These new team members will bolster the track record of the project's research team. Planning ahead will also allow you to work out how the collaboration will be managed if the funding application is successful. At this point you can use Project Planning Form 2 (See Document 1.4.2 in Chapter 1.4).

You should not underestimate the time needed to refine an idea.

When you are languishing, and can't quite get your plans underway, read Messenger [5] on the "Biggest mistake any budding entrepreneur can make." She will get you moving.

References—Setting Your Career Plan and Research Priorities

[1] Dudovskiy, J., October 12, 2014. Career Planning and Personal Development. http://research-methodology.net/career-planning-and-personal-development-plan-sample/.

[2] Mitchell, B., November 8, 2016. In: Researcher Development Workshop. Impact Ecology Group, Federation University Australia.

[3] University of Sussex Research Plan Template. www.sussex.ac.uk/esw/internal/documents/individual-research-plan-template.docx.

[4] Barker, K., 2002. At the Helm: A Laboratory Navigator. Cold Spring Harbor Laboratory Press, Cold Spring Harbor, NY.

[5] Messenger, L., LinkedIn, 2017. Biggest Mistake Any Budding Entrepreneur Can Make. https://www.linkedin.com/pulse/biggest-mistake-any-budding-entrepreneur-can-make-lisa-messenger.

Further Reading

If you are able to access it via your university, the Vitae Research Development Framework provides extensive information for professional development for researchers.

Vitae has four aims:

- Influence the development and implementation of effective policy relating to researcher development
- Enhance higher education provision to train and develop researchers
- Empower researchers to make an impact in their careers
- Evidence the impact of professional and career development support for researchers

https://www.vitae.ac.uk/researchers-professional-development.

1.4 Project Planning

Born planners are easily recognizable: They are constantly on top of progress, what gets done when, and fiercely goal-oriented. But others are more likely to grab a pipettor with one hand and start sketching on a piece of paper towel with the other—just to get started—even if they're not exactly sure of their plan.

Price [1]

Checklist

(Tick when completed)

- ☐ Draft the project concept
- ☐ Make a more detailed project plan
  - ☐ Define your objectives
  - ☐ Map your milestones
  - ☐ Think about potential causes for delay
  - ☐ Define your deliverables
  - ☐ Check the availability of funding
  - ☐ Think about training
  - ☐ Do a SWOT Analysis
  - ☐ Draw up your Comprehensive Project Plan

Introduction to Project Planning and Project Management

> *Projects go wrong for the same reasons all the time.*
> *There are no new sins.*
> Haughty quoting Dean [2]

In a scientific setting, your goals may include publishing a paper, obtaining a research grant, completing a set of experiments, or even developing an actual product. Project planning and then project management can help you minimize wasted effort, track your progress (or lack of it), and help you respond quickly when you have drifted off track.

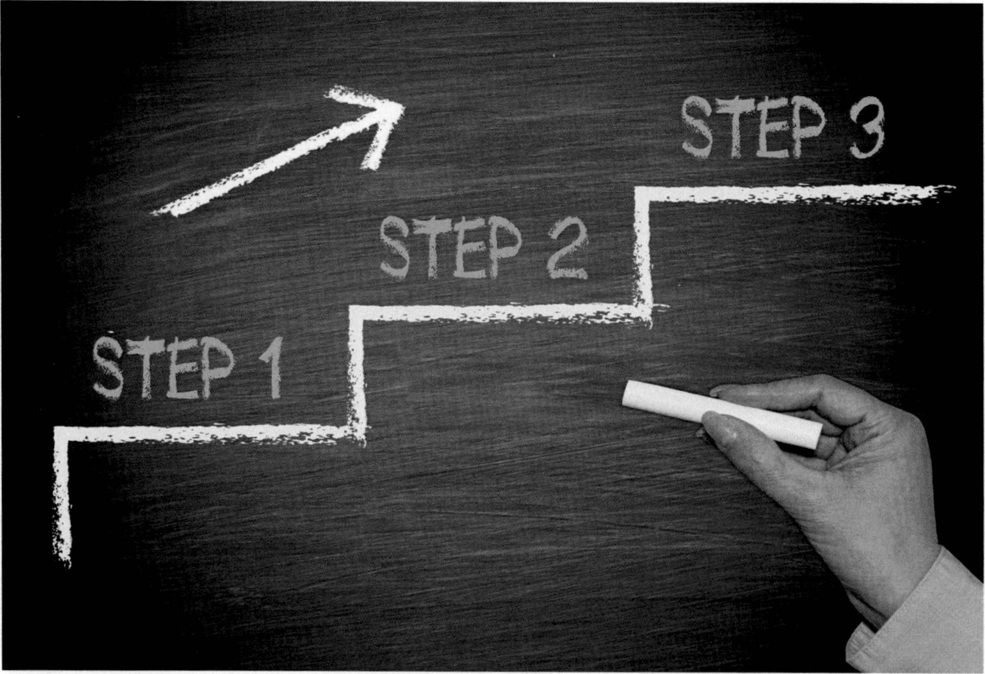

Image Credit: Step 1-Step 2-Step 3 by docstockmedia/Shutterstock

Once you have defined your overall objectives, how to achieve them, and who or what you will need to help you, you can start the detailed process of planning your project, working backward from your desired objectives.

Project management is a series of flexible but defined steps through which you identify where you want to go and a reasonable way to get there; it includes specifics of who will do what and when. The steps of project management are similar to the steps for preparation of a grant proposal. With a grant proposal, your probability of success is proportional to the thought that has gone into each part of the proposal. The reviewers, as well as the funding agency, want to see that you have thought things through properly. The same theory applies to running your projects and, indeed, to planning your career.

One of the most important benefits of project management is that it helps you accurately work out how much time a project will take and what resources you will need. Even when your "back-of-the-envelope" thinking convinces you that a project is worth pursuing, and that you will be able to generate an initial set of publishable results for your grant in a defined time, you will need to go on to plan each step.

A detailed, well-designed project plan is one of the sharpest tools you have for convincing a funder to give you the resources you require.

Thinking Out Your Project Plan

The best thing to do is to think out all the steps of your project right at the beginning. You might have had to do this as part of the grant application for the project; though occasionally, you can find yourself just landed with a project and money to spend on it. However, you got there, it is important to know where you are trying to get to next, and why. The checklist below lists thought processes for a new project.

It may be useful to complete 1.4.1 Project Planning Form 1 (at the end of this chapter) to help you cover all the steps.

Standard steps, whatever the discipline, should be the following:

- What is the starting point, i.e., what am I building on?
- What is the possible outcome? What do I hope to achieve?
- Why will it matter?
- Where might things go wrong?
- Is there any organizational risk? How will I mitigate that risk?
- Who will I need to help me? Consider both internal and external collaborators.
- What sort of people will I need in the team?
- What sort of equipment do I need?
- How much time is required?

> *Planning is an unnatural process; it is much more fun to do something. The nicest thing about not planning is that failure comes as a complete surprise, rather than being preceded by a period of worry and depression.*
> Sir John Harvey Jones, economist and businessman

Next Steps—A More Detailed Project Plan

As you work up toward a more detailed plan, using 1.4.2 Project Plan Form 2, at the end of this chapter, you can think in a little more detail and work up the project outline with the next steps:

- Write up the background (including relevant literature review).
- Prepare a needs assessment or a study rationale.
- Refine your research question.
- Work out your statement for the potential significance of the project (e.g., gap in the literature being addressed or particular workplace application).
- Plan your methodology and method (and your justification for their appropriateness).
- Develop a data collection plan.
- Plan the data analysis.
- Consider how much this project might cost and where you can source funding.
- Consider the ethical considerations.
- Map out the project timeline.

When mapping out your project into further detail, you need to consider the items below.

Objectives

What is it that you actually want—and expect to be able—to achieve with this project?

Objectives should be "SMART": specific, measurable, achievable, realistic, and time bound. There may be numerous objectives for any one project.

Remember to consider and make a note of further objectives that the project might achieve later, if further funding is obtained. Do not include unrealistic goals within a short-term funding application, and don't lose sight of them for later.

Milestones

Plan for when you expect to be able to complete specific tasks. Remember that some cannot be started until others have finished; some will be able to overlap. Consider the possibility of delays and the impact they will have on milestones and individual outcomes.

Potential Causes for Delay

There are some common causes of delay in research projects. Think about whether any of these might apply to you. Common causes include the following:

- Delays in obtaining ethics approval
- Lack of access to essential equipment, either because you are sharing or because it is not available for purchase
- Unavailability of project staff (due to inability to find staff; maternity leave)
- Slow recruitment

External Requirements

Consider requirements that may have been set by your institute or funding body. These could include the following:

- Accomplishment of a particular objective, e.g., appointment of a PhD student or application for ethics approval
- Project reporting
- Externally motivated deadlines

Deliverables

A project deliverable is the outcome or product that you will have created with your project funding by the end of the funding period. Define it. Is it a new technique, completion of a pilot study, a result of a series of experiments?

Availability of Funding

You might be fortunate to have funding from a successful grant application that covers all your requirements, but this is a rare situation. It is likely that you will need to add more to your project kitty to fund a PhD student or you might need a small pot of funding to supply essential equipment or a travel grant. Your institution might well have some discretionary funds available for this type of allocation.

Training

It is likely that members of the team will require training in techniques or use of equipment. Factor in the cost and/or time for this training—and remember to arrange it before the need arises.

SWOT Analysis and Risk Assessment

Once you have thought your way through all these steps, it is wise to conduct a SWOT analysis (see below) and then a risk assessment for your project.

As you almost certainly know, a SWOT analysis is a tool for examining the internal Strengths and Weaknesses and external Opportunities and Threats (SWOT) related to achieving the desired objective—in this case a successful research outcome.

Taking the time to conduct a SWOT analysis can help you decide whether the project is likely to succeed or whether, in spite of it being a good idea, it might have overwhelming difficulties.

There is further detail about risk management and SWOT analysis in Chapter 4.15.

Earlier it was suggested that you capture an initial project concept by completing Project Planning Form 1. By now, you should be ready to complete Project Planning Form 2. Once your project planning is finished, you should have covered—and included in your final documentation—all the elements of a comprehensive project plan shown in Table 1.4.1.

Once completed, your detailed project plan will provide guidance to all stakeholders regarding the project scope and activities, and ensure that there is clarity about what should be achieved. It will contain sufficient detail to provide the basis for grant proposals, accountability, reports, and quality assurance.

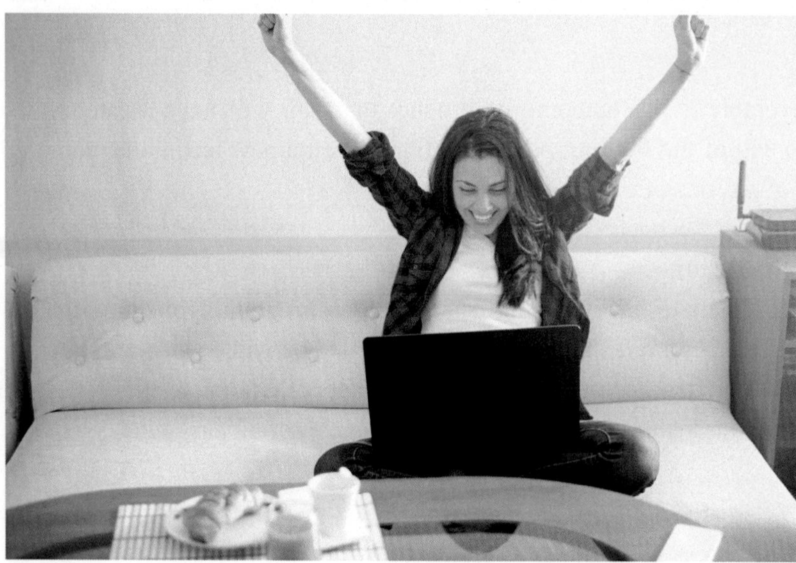

Image Credit: Happy woman with laptop by marrio31/iStock

TABLE 1.4.1 Elements of a Comprehensive Project Plan

1. Name of research project
2. Lead institution (and other partners)
3. Funder's name, if applicable
4. Research leader's name
5. Stakeholders (i.e., those who may need to have their issues addressed or who are otherwise involved in the research project background or outcomes)
6. Location of research project, if focused on a geographic place(s)
7. Project lay summary (100 words or less)
8. Research scope
9. Research aims
10. Objectives of the research
11. Potential benefits of the research
12. Deliverables
13. Context of the research project and any relevant background (including related research projects)
14. Research constraints
15. Potential research topics that are beyond scope
16. Work breakdown structure (see Chapter 4.2)
17. Projected timelines, milestones, and activity schedule
18. Project budget
19. Planned roles and responsibilities
20. Risk and contingency planning
21. Quality assurance mechanisms
22. Communication strategy
23. Procurement plans

References—Project Planning

[1] Price, R., 2002. Take your worst estimate and double it: project management for postdocs. Science. http://www.sciencemag.org/careers/2002/03/take-your-worst-estimate-and-double-it-project-management-postdocs.
[2] Haughty, D., 2014. Avoiding project failure: it's not rocket science. Project Smart. https://www.projectsmart.co.uk/avoiding-project-failure-its-not-rocket-science.php.

For more detailed information about Project Planning see:.

A Guide to the Project Management Body of Knowledge, fifth ed.2013. Project Management Institute (PMBOK Guide).

Associated Documents—Project Planning

1.4.1 Project Planning Form One

Project Overview

Project Owner	Click here to enter text.
Project Name	Click here to enter text.
Project Type	Click here to enter text.
Tick all that apply ☐ New study involving data collection ☐ New analysis of existing data. Name of dataset*: Click here to enter text. ☐ Requires biospecimens ☐ Other. Please specify: Click here to enter text.	
Has this Project Evolved from a Current or Past Project or Program? If yes, which?	
Click here to enter text.	
Which Issue is the Project Addressing?	
Click here to enter text.	
Project Description and Aims:	
Click here to enter text.	
Research Hypothesis	
Click here to enter text.	
What is the Relevance/Significance/Novelty of the Project and What is its Potential Impact?	
Click here to enter text.	
Alignment with Strategic Plan Objectives?	
Click here to enter text.	
Does this Project have any Internal Stakeholders from other Areas? Please specify:	
Click here to enter text.	
Does this project have any external stakeholders/collaborators? Please specify:	
Click here to enter text.	
What is the Potential Impact if Project is not Approved?	
Click here to enter text.	

Resource Requirements

Project Role/Area of expertise	Staff Member (if known)	Time Commitment (% FTE)	Duration
e.g. Research Assistant		80	2 years

Equipment and IT Requirements

Please specify any equipment or IT requirements for the project

Click here to enter text.
Click here to enter text.
Click here to enter text.

Budget

Estimated Project Budget	Click here to enter text.
Potential Funding Source:	Click here to enter text.

Risk Analysis

Please specify any known or potential risk for this project

Financial Risk	Click here to enter text.
Risk of Delay	Click here to enter text.
Reputational Risk	Click here to enter text.
Work, Health and Safety Risk	Click here to enter text.
Community Engagement Risk	Click here to enter text.
No Potential Risk	Click here to enter text.

Ethics Status

Is there an existing ethics application which will apply?	Click here to enter text.
Name of IRB/Ethics Committee	Click here to enter text.
Ethics Approval ID	Click here to enter text.
Date of Approval	Click here to enter text.

Approval of Concept ____
(Signature of Manager)

Date ______________________

1.4.2 Project Planning Form Two

Project Title: Click here to enter text.

<table>
<tr><td colspan="3">Background, and literature review</td></tr>
<tr><td colspan="3">Click here to enter text.</td></tr>
<tr><td colspan="3">Developments to Date: i.e. Early Investigation or Analysis. (please attach other documents if applicable)</td></tr>
<tr><td colspan="3">Click here to enter text.</td></tr>
<tr><td colspan="3">Needs Assessment or Study Rationale</td></tr>
<tr><td colspan="3">Click here to enter text.</td></tr>
<tr><td colspan="3">Refined Research Question/Project Aims</td></tr>
<tr><td colspan="3">Click here to enter text.</td></tr>
<tr><td colspan="3">Proposed Methodology</td></tr>
<tr><td colspan="3">Click here to enter text.</td></tr>
<tr><td colspan="3">Data Collection Plan</td></tr>
<tr><td colspan="3">Click here to enter text.</td></tr>
<tr><td colspan="3">Personnel Resources Required (insert name if possible, and time allocation for each position)</td></tr>
<tr><td>Position Name</td><td>Time Allocation</td><td>Duration</td></tr>
<tr><td>Click here to enter text.</td><td>Click here to enter text.</td><td>Click here to enter text.</td></tr>
<tr><td></td><td></td><td></td></tr>
<tr><td></td><td></td><td></td></tr>
<tr><td colspan="3">Equipment Resources Required (detail requirements)</td></tr>
<tr><td colspan="3">Click here to enter text.</td></tr>
<tr><td colspan="3">Click here to enter text.</td></tr>
<tr><td colspan="3">Click here to enter text.</td></tr>
<tr><td colspan="3">Ethics Requirements</td></tr>
<tr><td colspan="3">Click here to enter text.</td></tr>
<tr><td colspan="3">Expected Outputs (include timelines and contents)</td></tr>
<tr><td colspan="3">Click here to enter text.</td></tr>
<tr><td colspan="3">Dissemination Strategy (include potential audiences, desired outcomes, target journal)</td></tr>
<tr><td colspan="3">Click here to enter text.</td></tr>
<tr><td colspan="3">What will be the consequences if this project is not approved?</td></tr>
<tr><td colspan="3">Click here to enter text.</td></tr>
</table>

Risk Analysis

Please specify any known or potential risk for this project

Financial Risk	Click here to enter text.
Risk of Delay	Click here to enter text.
Reputational Risk	Click here to enter text.
Work, Health and Safety Risk	Click here to enter text.
Community Engagement Risk	Click here to enter text.
No Potential Risk	Click here to enter text.

Funding

Funding potentially available	Click here to enter text.
Funding definitely available:	Click here to enter text.

Budget

Please attach document

Project Timeline

Please attach document

Approval of Project ____________________________________
(Signature of Manager)

Date ______________________

1.5 Applying for Your Grant

Joe spent lots of time and energy cramming the full allowance of text into his grant application, but he failed to actually address why he was the one who most deserved to be offered this funding. Instead he wrote big picture statements about "heart disease kills" (they already knew that), too many people are obese (they knew that too) and "we have to do something about it." What he should have done was write clearly and concisely about his plans, and about how he would go about solving the problem. Then he should have provided some hard evidence to back up his claims. The granting body would have listened with interest.

Checklist

(Tick when completed)

- ☐ Start early
- ☐ Read the guidelines
- ☐ Define your objectives
- ☐ Think of this as a sales exercise; you need to persuade
- ☐ Take the advice of your reviewers
- ☐ See if there is special funding for early-career investigators in your field

Give Yourself Enough Time

There are a few vital commonsense rules when applying for a grant. You may notice a common theme.

- Start early with your application.
- Start early—talking to your co-investigators.
- Start early—talking to your research office.
- Start early—talking to your group leader.
- Allow plenty of time for both writing and reviewing.
- Allow plenty of time for collecting information from the team.
- Re-read and revise, again and again.

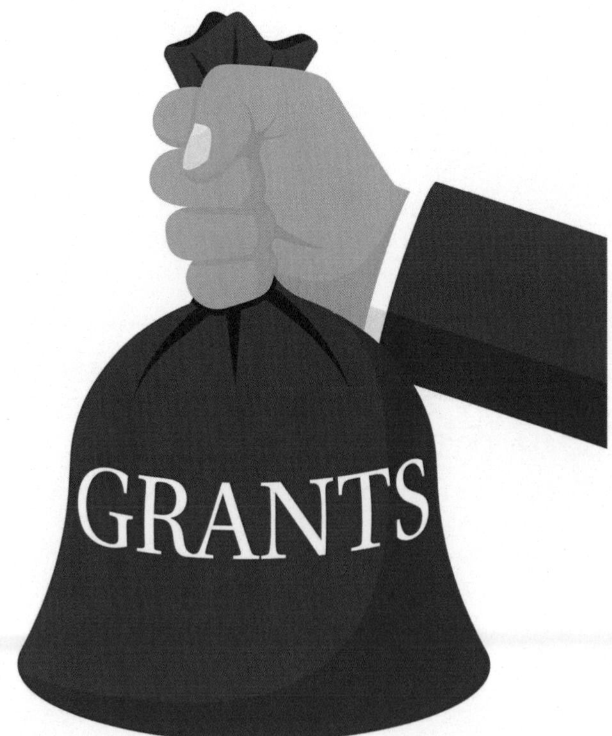

Image Credit: Grant funding by Hvostik/Shutterstock

You will probably know for at least six months ahead, if not for longer, that you are going to put in a funding request. There is absolutely no reason to ignore it for five of those six months.

Applying for a grant is very complex. It takes a long time to do it well.

As a first step, take the trouble to find out exactly what it is that the funding body is looking for. There is no point in wasting your time, or theirs, by submitting an application that is even slightly off-target. They want to fund what they want to fund. Just because your idea has merit, it is unlikely to interest them if it doesn't address exactly what they want. Even when your idea is a direct fit for them, a conversation with their research manager might help you. You might possibly find out a little extra detail about what they are hoping to fund this year. You might get ahead of the rest by addressing an aspect which you might otherwise have passed over.

Make sure that you are eligible to apply. There may be restrictions with respect to age or number of years post-doctoral; there may be rules regarding citizenship or visa status. It is also vital to ensure that the funding body is acceptable to your university (for example, they might not permit you to accept funding from an organization profiting from the sale of tobacco or alcohol). Check that there are no obligations that you would not be able to fulfill. Last, be alert to requirements regarding ownership of intellectual property or to publishing something that might be incompatible with the requirements of your institution.

Read the Guidelines

Your next step is to carefully read their guidelines looking for number of pages, size of font, CV requirements, and submission dates. The funding body takes the trouble to write these guidelines because the rules matter to them. If you decide that an 11-point font is better than the 12-point font they requested, your application may go straight into the bin. If they offer to pay for equipment but not staff, don't ask for a research assistant. If they say "no medical research" don't bother submitting if your field is cardiology.

If you are applying for a grant from another country, remember that they are likely to award funding in their own currency. The National Institute for Health (NIH) in the United States, for example, requires you to supply the budget request in US dollars. If you are applying from the United Kingdom or New Zealand thinking a dollar is a dollar, these numbers would represent widely different values in your currency. NIH also makes the payments in US dollars, so if you are successful and this is not your currency you might need to protect yourself from currency fluctuation.

Define Your Objectives

Before you write a word, have another think about what it is that you want to achieve with your project.

- What do you actually want to achieve?
- Why does it matter?
- Is this a new area of research or has it already been done? If it has been done before, what will be the benefit of you doing it again?
- Exactly what do you plan to do, and why?
- If it doesn't work, what will you do next?
- If it does work, what will you do next?
- Last, very importantly, how does this fit in with the mission of your institution and how will they support you?

You are going to have to include all the answers to the questions above within your application.

This brings us to what you should actually write. Be specific. They don't need waffle. If your application is to a body funding work into climate change, they do not need to be convinced that climate change is an issue. They want to know about solutions, so leave out the background about why your work is important and concentrate on how you are specifically going to address a known problem.

As Jahren [1] mentions in her blog, she, as a potential funder, wants to be convinced that you have really thought through your project properly and can clearly visualize all your steps and your ultimate success. A plan that is still at the stage of "back-of-the-envelope" thinking will rate poorly next to one that is well prepared, however good the basic idea.

Your application needs to briefly but clearly describe an innovative or novel problem, hypothesis, or challenge; a situation where we need to do better. Jahren goes on to recommend that your application should describe how *you* can provide the ideal team, with the right skills and experience, to carry out this research. Using clear language, which avoids too much technical jargon, you need to convince the people reviewing your application that your approach is plausible and will achieve its objectives. At the same time, you must provide evidence for your claims. The funding body is going to be looking for a high-quality outcome and you want them to pick yours.

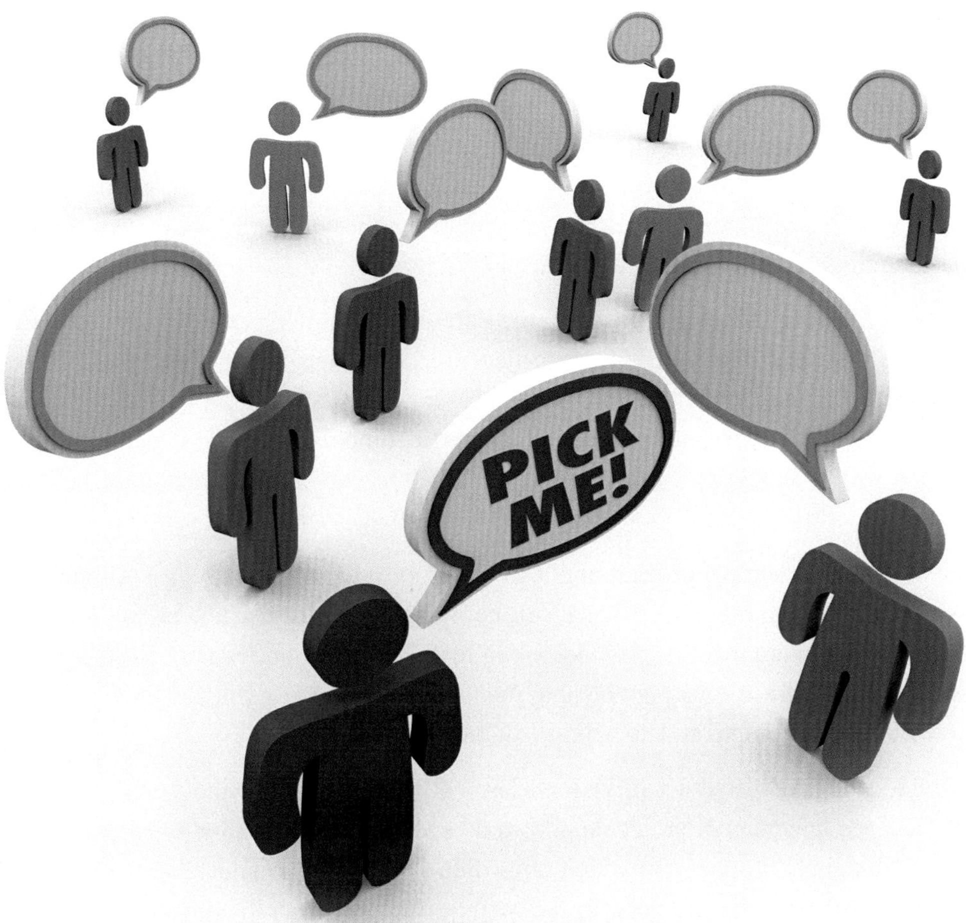

Image Credit: One person says pick me by IQoncept/Shutterstock

When you are considering the actual resources required, don't over-ask and don't under-ask. Put some effort into working out what you truly need. Wanting to do something truly amazing is admirable and understandable but will not look too good if you are then unable to deliver it. Jahren points out that "a lack of realism may create the impression that you have a poor understanding of the problem or poor research methodology." You also must be able to correctly justify each aspect of your proposed budget, making it clear that you have worked out, for example, the level of staff members necessary to support your research and the corresponding cost.

Attack This as a Sales Exercise

Your funding application is a marketing document for your work and your science. You want to it to call out to the reviewers "pick me, pick me". Please remember that the assessors who will be reading your application are people. They probably have to wade through mountains of applications and the ones that are well set out and easy to read will be much more likely to receive a good rating. You don't have to pack the maximum number of words onto every one of those pages. Use figures and tables where you can.

It will help if you use language and formatting to create pointers for overworked reviewers, such as: "The long-term objectives of this project are…"; "The general strategy of the proposed research is to…"; "The specific aims of the present study are to…"; "Three outcomes are planned …"; "In these experiments, molecular genetic, biochemical, and structural approaches will be used to…." When they read indicators like this your reviewers should be alerted to pay attention.

Ask others to read through your draft application and provide comments. It is difficult to proof read your own work. Another set of eyes can be of invaluable assistance in picking up simple errors in spelling and grammar, and omissions of text. By definition, you are close to your topic, but a colleague with fresh eyes may be able to suggest "why don't you put in something about 'this' or 'that'?" which might end up making all the difference.

It is a good idea to take the advice of your research office, even though they aren't subject matter experts. They see hundreds of project applications every year, on all sorts of topics. They know which ones ultimately worked and which ones didn't. They get to understand the needs of the people at the other end, the people with the money. They are also looking with clear eyes, not blinded by their knowledge of the subject matter. They are looking for readability and clarity—and they are there to help you.

The abstract is often, quite understandably, the last thing you will prepare for your grant application, but please don't skimp on effort for it. It is very important and, if it doesn't read well, the reviewer's eyes might glaze over, effectively skipping your application altogether.

The abstract needs to convey the big picture: your general hypothesis and aims, the methodological approach, and the significance of your research. It should also include key words. These really matter as they will be used to direct your application to the correct study section, whether or not you request a particular review group.

In your abstract you should try to avoid technical jargon, instead writing in language suitable for an educated layperson.

What to Do When Your Application Is Unsuccessful?

The sad truth is that, even if it is a good one, it is unlikely that your idea will get funded the first time around. Just as a manuscript rarely gets accepted without changes, it is not uncommon for people to submit an application two or three or even four times before it gets up. Don't be despondent; be realistic. Listen to the reviewers and adjust accordingly. Importantly, note down in your application that you have submitted this grant previously and have responded to review comments by doing x, y, and z. It will stand you in good stead to be seen to be proactive and responsive.

It is vital to conduct a thorough literature search and cite all the relevant literature. Omissions in the literature are often a source of criticism of applications. Your reviewer wants to know you are well informed. Be sure to discuss your work in the context of these published results in your application, and provide your own preliminary data whenever they exist.

The criteria for rating of NIH grant applications are widely applicable for all research applications:

- Significance: Does it address an important problem? Will it advance scientific knowledge? Will it affect concepts or methods in this field?
- Approach: Are the experimental design and methods appropriate to the aims? Does it acknowledge problem areas and consider alternative tactics (in other words, is there a thoughtful backup plan)?
- Innovation: Does it employ novel concepts, approaches, or methods? Does it challenge existing paradigms or develop new methodologies?
- Investigator: Is the investigator appropriately trained to carry out the proposed work? Is the work appropriate to the experience of the principal investigator and collaborators?
- Environment: Does the institutional environment contribute to the probability of success? Is there evidence of institutional support?

Common Reasons for Failure of Applications to the NIH:

- Lack of original ideas
- Absence of an acceptable scientific rationale
- Lack of experience in the essential methodology
- Questionable reasoning in experimental approach
- Diffuse, superficial, or unfocused research plan
- Lack of sufficient experimental detail
- Lack of knowledge of published relevant work
- Unrealistically large amount of work for the given time frame or funding level
- Uncertainty about future directions

Opportunities for Early-Career Investigators

Be aware that there are special grants available specifically for early-career researchers. Take time to find anything that might be applicable to you. Apart from the fact that for these schemes you won't be competing against established scientists, it is likely your application will be acceptable with a lower score and there will be less emphasis on track record than in open schemes.

The NIH is one organization which actively seeks to support early-career investigators. When you apply for your first NIH grant, you may check the box on the application form that indicates to reviewers that you're a new investigator (meaning you haven't been principal investigator on an NIH research grant before). The reviewers are often more forgiving when reviewing applications from novices.

Look for these grants which are available specifically for early-career investigators in the NIH Guide to Grants and Contracts (http://grants.nih.gov/grants/guide/index.html). Each has its own criteria for eligibility and submission of applications. Information on these and other NIH extramural funding opportunities can be found at http://grants.nih.gov/oer.htm.

In addition to NIH, other federal agencies and private sector organizations in the United States and elsewhere solicit and fund research grants, and each has its own application and review system.

You may send the same application to multiple funding sources in the public and private sectors, but to be transparent and to avoid "double dipping" when offers are made you should disclose your multiple applications to each potential funder.

While an individual can muddle through the grant application processes through trial and error, there are major benefits in drawing on existing models and seeking guidance from experienced researchers and the research office. Seek advice from your mentors to help guide you through the process. Later in your career you can make yourself available for peer review panels of grant proposals, another highly valued avenue for learning.

It is also beneficial to have a critical look at the types of projects that have been successful in recent grant rounds. Their outlines might help you rework an unsuccessful grant.

Reference—Applying for Funding

[1] 2014 #HOPEJAHRENSURECANWRITE about things. How to How to Turn a "Good" Proposal into an "Excellent" Proposal in Eight Admittedly Arduous Steps 2014. https://hopejahrensurecanwrite.com/2014/06/02/how-to-turn-a-good-proposal-into-an-excellent-proposal-in-eight-admittedly-arduous-steps/.

Further Reading

Grants.gov lists all current discretionary funding opportunities from 26 agencies of the United States government. https://www.grants.gov/.

The National Institute of Health provides useful information applicable to any grant application.

NIH Central Resource for Grant and Funding Information. https://grants.nih.gov/grants/oer.htm.

Grant application forms and instructions. https://grants.nih.gov/grants/forms.htm.

Examples of Successful Grant Applications. https://www.niaid.nih.gov/grants-contracts/sample-applications.

Every country will have its own sources of funding, but the biggest pool is in the United States. Some of the grants available are open for investigators in other countries.

NIH Guide to Grants and Contracts. https://grants.nih.gov/funding/about-nih-guide-to-grants-and-contracts.htm.

Overview of peer-review process, and within, study section rosters. https://public.csr.nih.gov/StudySections/IntegratedReviewGroups/Pages/default.aspx.

Office of Laboratory Animal Welfare. https://grants.nih.gov/grants/olaw/olaw.htm.

1.6 Preparing the Budget for Your Project

Flossy requested two staff positions and some equipment in her budget. She made two significant errors. The amount she requested for the staff only covered the salary and none of the extras. When thinking she'd asked for £5000, she had actually asked for €5000. Suddenly she hasn't got nearly enough money.

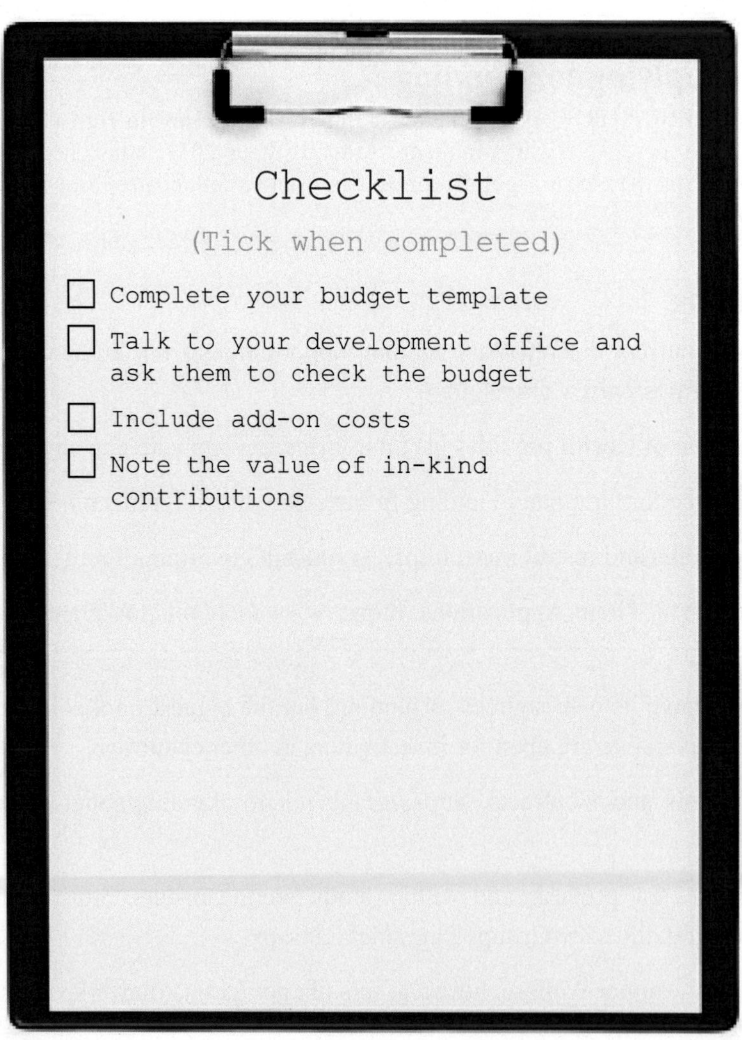

Budgets aren't hard—after all, it is just about numbers. They just take some elementary planning, some background information, and some common sense.

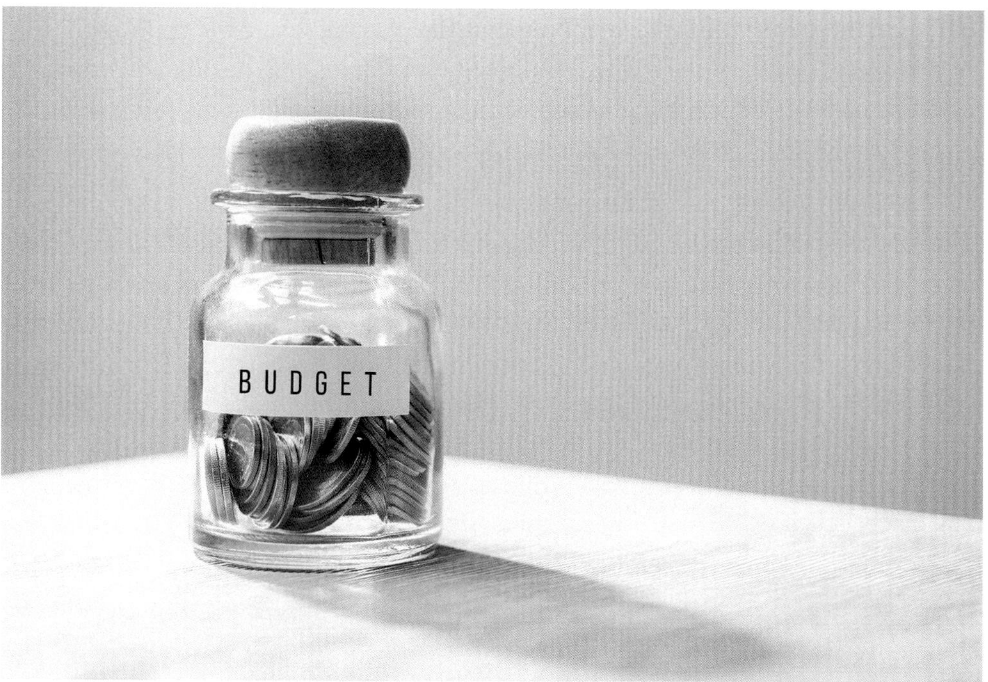

Image Credit: Budget by oatawa/iStock

It is impossible to successfully manage your research if you don't understand how to manage the budget. The step before that is that you can't ask for the correct amount of money in your funding application if you don't understand what the project will cost to run. Forgive me if this sounds obvious, but it is surprising how many people get it wrong.

Your budget should be drafted according to the monies which you know will be available in a given time period. It is advisable to allocate your money to specific project costs, and then spread the expenditure across the time periods for which money is available.

As has been mentioned previously, before you proceed with an application for funding, check the nature of the expenses that the funding agency is prepared to fund. Some will fund people only; some like to fund equipment. Some trusts and foundations have a deliberate exclusion for medical research; others place a ceiling on infrastructure. Don't waste your time and effort on applying to the wrong body. When drafting a budget, it is crucial to know the maximum grant amount awarded by the organization to which you are applying. If you ask for much more, your proposal might be rejected on that basis alone.

I GETTING STARTED

In “The Dream Budget” [1] the author presents information about the budget from the perspective of the funding body. Perfectly reasonably, she emphasizes that you need to explain your requests within your budget justification. As the receiver of the request, she points out that she can’t be expected to understand the hidden detail, providing an example where the applicant was asking for only two months of salary for a twelve-month role because his institution would pay the balance, but without explaining that. She shouldn’t have to guess. Furthermore, she says she will always place the most trust in the applicant who is both transparent and thorough.

The author also recommends that you should visit your development office early in the budgeting process to talk to staff members and learn about their requirements. She has found that most universities and non-government organizations are prepared to reduce their usual overhead requirements to adhere to the guidelines set by foundations. She says she often sees budgets in which the home institution has agreed to provide matching funds to enable its researchers to stay within her foundation’s support guidelines. She recommends that if you are able to access matching funds for, say, salary, fringe benefits, or overhead expenses from your institution, you should show it in your budget in a column labeled “matching funds” or “other sources,” thus indicating that backing.

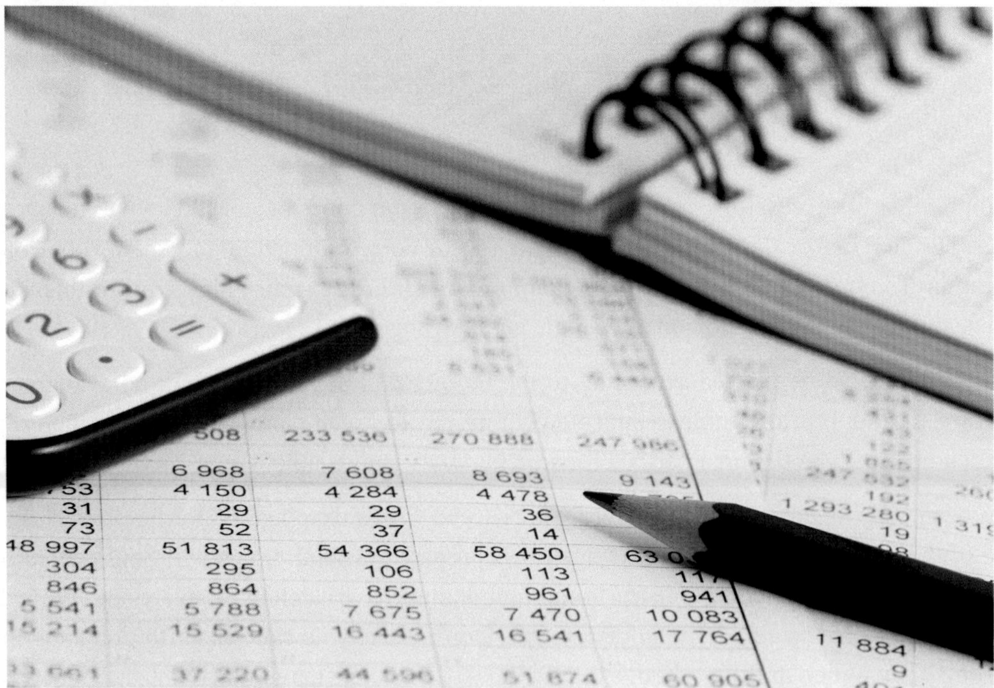

Image Credit: Accounting by Wrangler/Shutterstock

Start With the Basics

You might find it helpful to use 1.6.1 Grant Application Budget Template in Associated Documents at the end of this chapter or a budget template from your institution while working through this section.

When preparing your budget start with the basics. Common project costs are listed in Table 1.6.1.

Something often left out is the costs of communicating with your stakeholders. These costs might include newsletters, special meetings, and travel. Don't stint on them, they are important.

TABLE 1.6.1 Preparing Your Budget

Standard Costs	
Staff costs	Base salaries
	Add-on costs
	Staff training
	Contractors
Laboratory purchases	Consumables
	Samples or cell lines
Data	
Software licenses	
Equipment	Equipment purchase
	Equipment maintenance
Travel	Travel costs
	Conference fees
	Accommodation
Publication fees	
Depending on your institution, you may also need to budget for the following:	
Office costs	Telephone
	Printing
	Stationery
	Computers
Recruitment costs	Advertising

Add-On Costs

"Add-on costs" for staff are the extra costs over and above salary, and they frequently take people by surprise. Unfortunately, they can't be ignored: a staff member costs more than just their salary! When a salary position is supported by a grant, the university might well require the staff member's add-on costs to be paid for out of grant funds.

The size of these costs will depend on your country and your institution, but they could include allowances for pension or superannuation, long-service leave, worker's compensation insurance, and perhaps payroll tax. In some cases, there might be a standard cost per head for desk space or use of a computer, electricity, use of cars or building maintenance. These "extras," which might cost up to almost 30% over and above salary [2], can make a big hole in your budget.

Make sure you find out what add-on costs are required where you work, and add them to the costs of each person.

In-Kind Contributions

An "in-kind" contribution is one where goods or services are supplied without the exchange of money. It could be use of the library, free office space, use of equipment, the gift of consumables, or staff training. It could also be use of a car, provision of a volunteer workforce, or advertising or promotion via an institutional newsletter or website.

For some grant applications, it is necessary to include the in-kind contributions you plan to receive from your institution or some other partner. In-kind contributions are looked on very favorably by funding bodies. Not only do they reduce project costs, but they also add credibility as they confirm the institution or organization's support for your work.

A chief investigator who is not requesting budget for his or her own salary should also note the cost of his salary as an in-kind contribution. This should be an estimate of salary, plus on-costs, based on the proposed proportion of her time to be spent on this project e.g., 40% or 60%.

The Backup Plan

It is not a bad idea, when preparing the budget for your grant application, to have a secret worst-case scenario budget in your back pocket. The budget you present to the funding body is the best possible scenario budget (within funding limits of course). But if you don't get the full amount, there are still things you can do; aren't there? Think of the "bread and butter" budget and then the "icing on the cake" money. This is for the things you'd love to do if you can but which aren't absolutely essential to the success of the project.

The focus of a PhD student's project is sambar deer, which have been introduced to a local forest area. It would be helpful for him to have a really accurate count of the deer and an explanation of their day-to-day behaviors. If he can, he will put electronic trackers on them and that will make his data collection easy. Putting on the trackers, though, will take time and money. To use the trackers, he has first to buy them; then he must track the deer, shoot them with a tranquilizer, catch them, and put on the collar. All this is on the wish list as it would add more solid evidence to his data, but in fact he can still do the core study without this component. An estimation of numbers and generalities about the behaviors will provide adequate information for his needs. The collars are the "icing" part of the budget.

References—Project Budgets

[1] The dream budget. Nature 2015. Available online: http://www.nature.com/naturejobs/science/articles/10.1038/nj7565-379a.
[2] University of Western Sydney on cost for a staff member, 2016–2028%. http://policies.uws.edu.au/download.php?id=251.

Further Reading

University websites often have a comprehensive set of guidelines and a costing template. Check to see if one is available from your research or development office.

Associated Documents—Preparing the Budget for Your Project

1.6.1 Grant Application Budget Template

	Year 1													Year 2	
	Jan	Feb	Mar	Apr	May	Jun	Jul	Aug	Sep	Oct	Nov	Dec	Annual Total	Jan	and onwards
Staff Costs															
Salary Person 1	10,000	10,000	10,000	10,000	10,000	10,000	10,000	10,000	10,000	10,000	10,000	10,000	1,20,000		
Add on costs Person 1	1800	1800	1800	1800	1800	1800	1800	1800	1800	1800	1800	1800	21,600		
Salary Person 2				5000	5000	5000	5000	5000	5000	5000	5000	5000	45,000		
Add on costs Person 2													0		
Training				1000									1,000		
													0		
Conference Fees													0		
Travel and Accommodation													0		
													0		
Consultants Fees									2000				2,000		
													0		
Software purchase													0		
Software licencing or annual support													0		
													0		
Data Fees			1500										1,500		
Data Storage													0		
													0		
Consumables													0		
													0		
Equipment Purchase													0		
Equipment service and maintenance													0		
													0		
Volunteer costs													0		
Volunteer Travel													0		
													0		
Publication Fees													0		
Office Costs													0		
Telephone													0		
Stationery													0		
Printing													0		
Postage, Freight and Courier													0		
Meeting Costs													0		
Total	11800	11800	13300	17800	16800	16800	16800	16800	18800	16800	16800	16800	191100		

1.7 Work With Your Research Office

Investigator A submitted his plan to the research office on the very last day possible (there are so many who do this). As he hadn't bothered to discuss his application with them in the mad scramble to get his information together, he had failed to notice that he needed signatures from the Head of Department and Dean, and signatures of all the co-investigators; that the university was going to charge 20% of his budget to cover overheads and that the document that he had prepared in 10-point type so as to fit as many words as possible had to be written in 12-point type—so now the pages didn't fit. He missed the deadline and has to wait months for the next opportunity. We hope he'll be better organized next time.

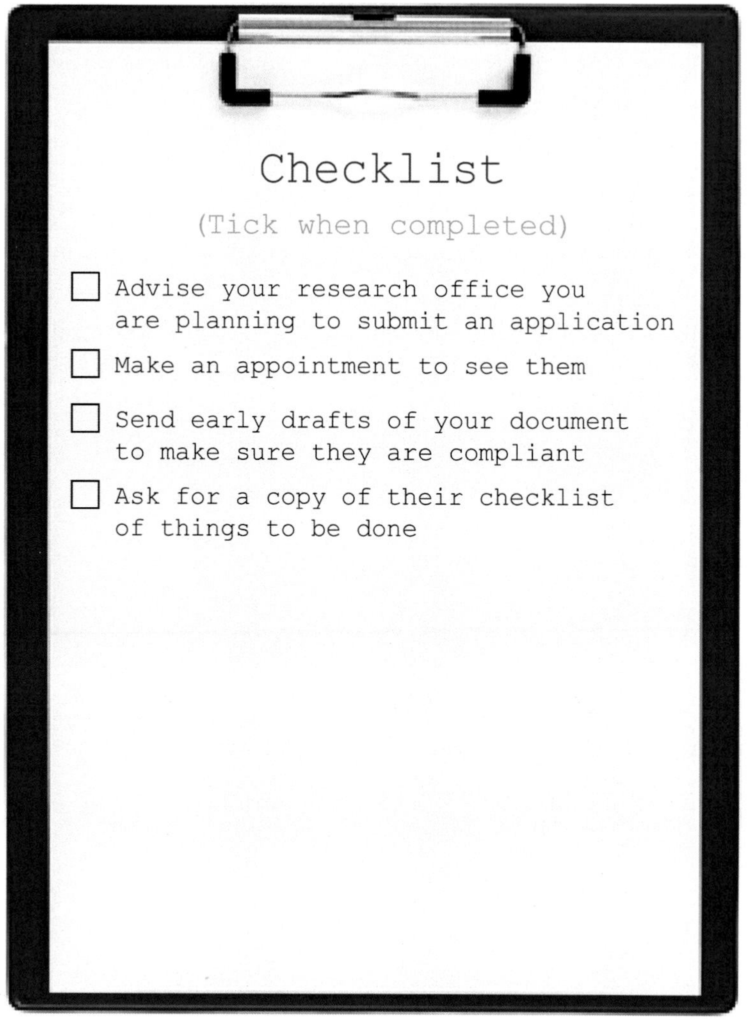

Your research or development office is there to help you.

Yes, they have stringent requirements. Yes, they make you fill in lots of forms which you hate. Yes, they have deadlines you think are unreasonable. Still, they are there to help you. They have, after all, a vested interest in your success. Their aim is to get more grants into the university and that means more successful applicants.

The research office staff will be able to provide advice on the most suitable funding body for your project. They will be able to assist you with your budget, with the proper costs for staff, with reading your application, and making sure you have completed the forms correctly. They may have a writer who can help you put your requests together in a better way.

Remembering that they are only human, and that everyone else in your university is likely to be applying for this range of grants at the same time, it is smart to get ahead of the pack and start early.

The research office is likely to require a draft of your application early on. Don't resent it. Their advice can be very helpful for you, as you might well be on the wrong track.

The research office is likely to require written confirmation from other chief investigators that they agree to be part of your application. This is perfectly reasonable. People do get caught, hoping that Investigator X is going to be part of the team, then suddenly he isn't. Ask for this confirmation and the CVs of the other investigators in plenty of time: not everyone might be as organized as you and might take a while to respond.

1.8 Involving Consumers in Your Research

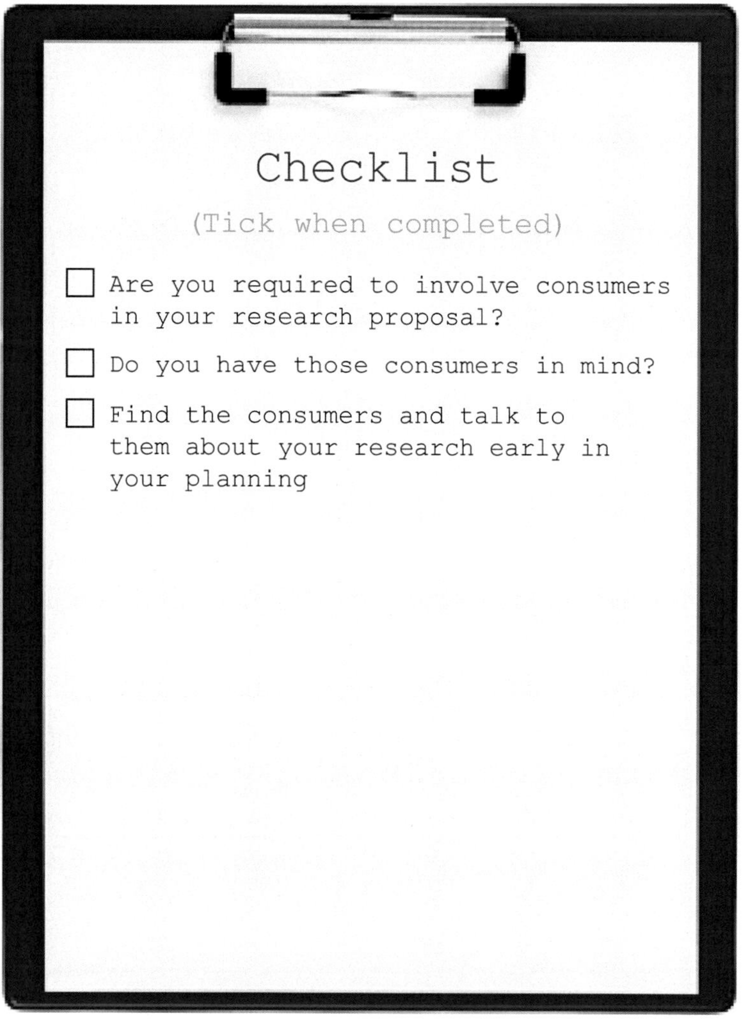

> *The researcher emailed me an overview of his project- the study of the effect (or benefit) of a drug that may ease a specific side effect induced by some chemotherapy drugs. The trial was to be lab based using mice. Although the outline was very technical, I gained a basic understanding of the mechanism of the drug.*
>
> *There were several exchanges of emails. One included an outline of our personal backgrounds. He was amazed by the cancer therapies I had undertaken and the early and late side effects I had experienced from these different treatments. As a lab based researcher I provided a human face to the end result of his work.*
>
> Hunt [1]

A "consumer" in research is a member of the public who is a direct stakeholder, most likely someone who has suffered from, or has been closely connected with, a particular health condition.

> *Before having a consumer representative involved, you think you have a consumer perspective fully in mind. After having a consumer representative involved, you see it is very easy to overlook simple issues that are important to address. With a researcher hat on, it is easy to prioritize what is more easily 'do-able' over what is most relevant to do.*
>
> Crossing [2]

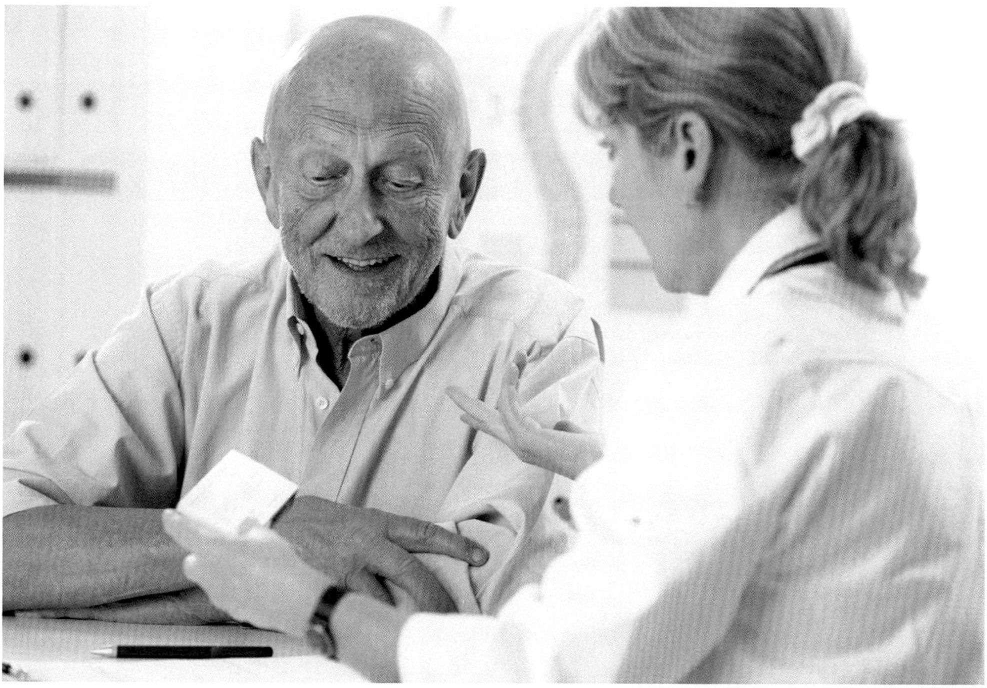

Image Credit: Talking to a senior male patient by Alexander Raths/Shutterstock

There is a growing call for involving "consumers" in research, either as advisors or as part of the assessment process. This is resisted by some researchers as they either see the need for an advisor as a nuisance, or they resent the involvement of the consumers because they might not understand the "basic science" and they feel they should not be able to influence the research direction. In fact, the consumers can add a great deal; it's just that their expertise comes with a different focus.

Think about it logically. If your research is into a human disease or condition, it is only reasonable to assume that the people who suffer from that disease will also have an understanding about it. Indeed, it is very likely that you care about the welfare of people who have that condition. They, or people like them, have probably provided your funding. They, or people like them, have a vested interest in the outcomes. They can provide a very focused view on what matters to them and why. Their perspectives might not be obvious to you without their input.

The moral of the story—be glad to include those “consumers” for a double win.

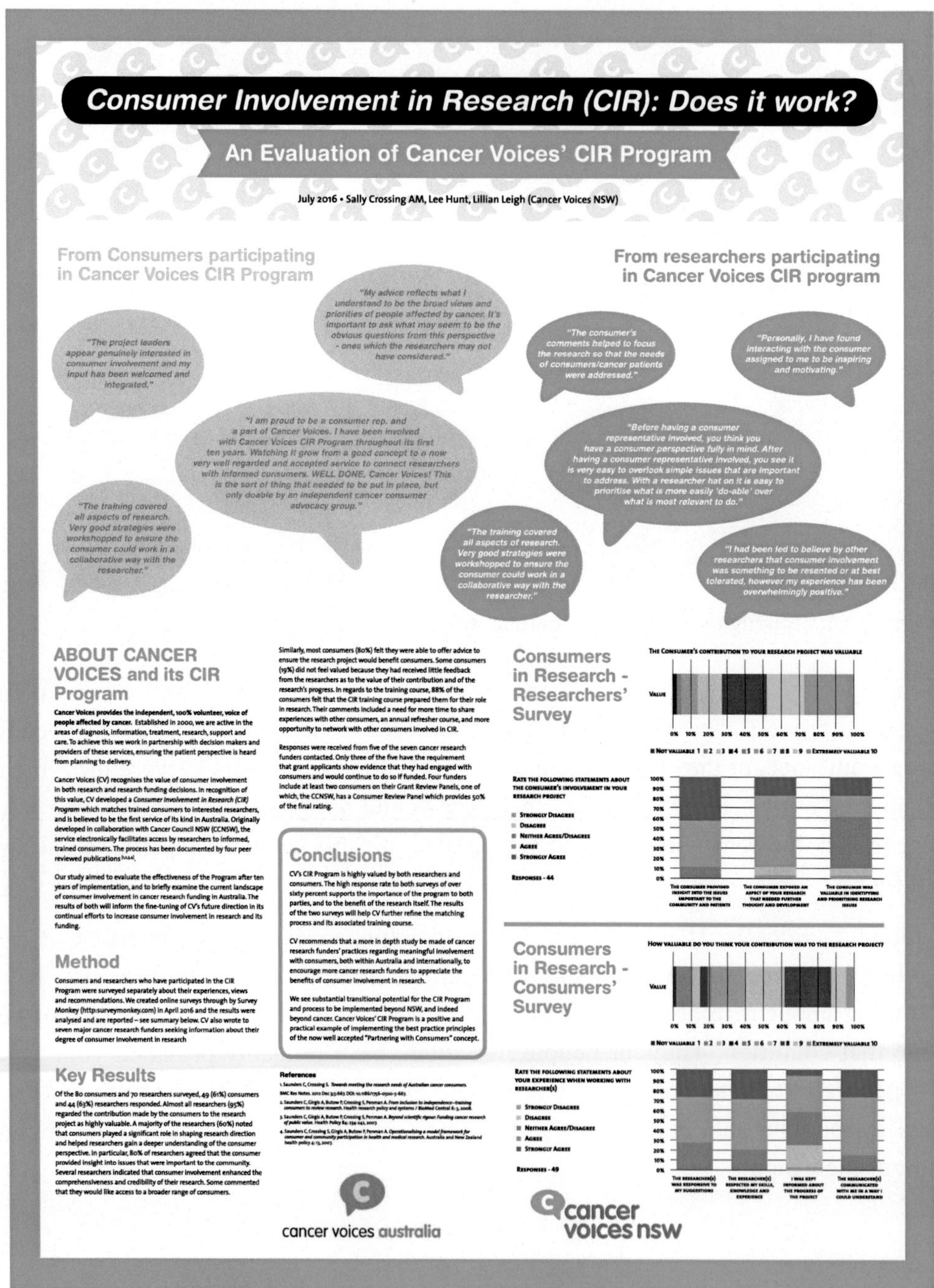

As a researcher, you will win yourself a very powerful ally and extend your network in ways you might not have expected if you are able to do the following:

- Take your consumer seriously
- Speak to your consumer in a language that can be understood
- Keep your consumer informed about your progress

Your consumer will keep you grounded.

Crossing [2] quotes a researcher respondent from a survey: "I had been led to believe by other researchers that consumer involvement was something to be resented or at best tolerated, however my experience has been overwhelmingly positive."

In some countries and for some funding bodies, it is now mandatory to include a consumer(s) in medical research. Where this is the case, it is likely that there will be a community organization focused on ensuring that this consumer involvement is effective and productive. If possible, you should seek out appropriately trained consumers to assist with your research.

Failing that, consider approaching support groups for the disease/condition in question and seek assistance from them. You will be well rewarded for your efforts.

References—Consumer Involvement

[1] Hunt, L., 2017. In: Presentation at Cure Cancer Australia Symposium May 2017.
[2] Crossing, S., Hunt, L., Leigh, L., July 2016. In: (Cancer Voices NSW) Consumer Involvement in Research (CIR): Does It Work? An Evaluation of Cancer Voices' CIR Program.

Valuable information about consumer involvement in research can be found on the Cancer Voices website. www.cancervoices.org.au.

1.9 Enhance Your Reputation

There are so many of them: scientists in the lab, working away quietly in their corner, telling only the people they absolutely have to tell what they are up to. They publish in esoteric journals but it's a bit of a struggle to build their reputation because they're not well connected and they don't have many collaborators. They don't have a lot of contacts within their field, or even their university because they don't get out much. People from outside research who might well be interested in their outcomes never even get to find out about them. They are wasting opportunities!

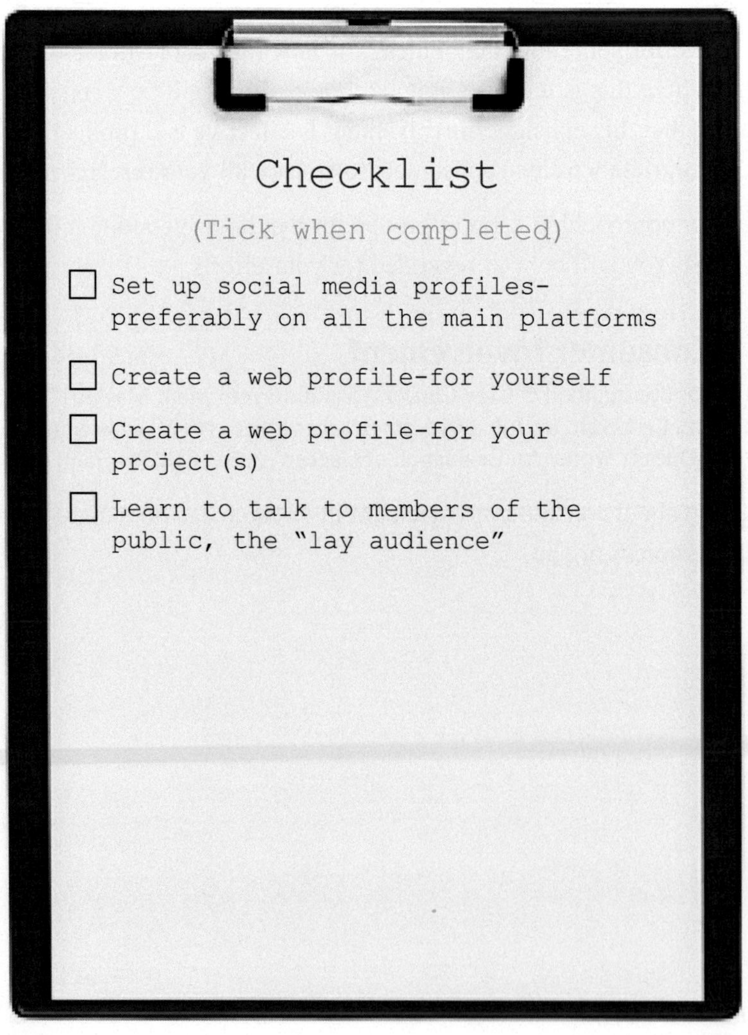

Getting published is not enough to enhance your reputation. You need to do more, and you need to start before publication, right at the beginning. Working on your reputation, your track record and on an explanation of why you are doing what you are doing, and why it matters, should start on day one of your career and should never end.

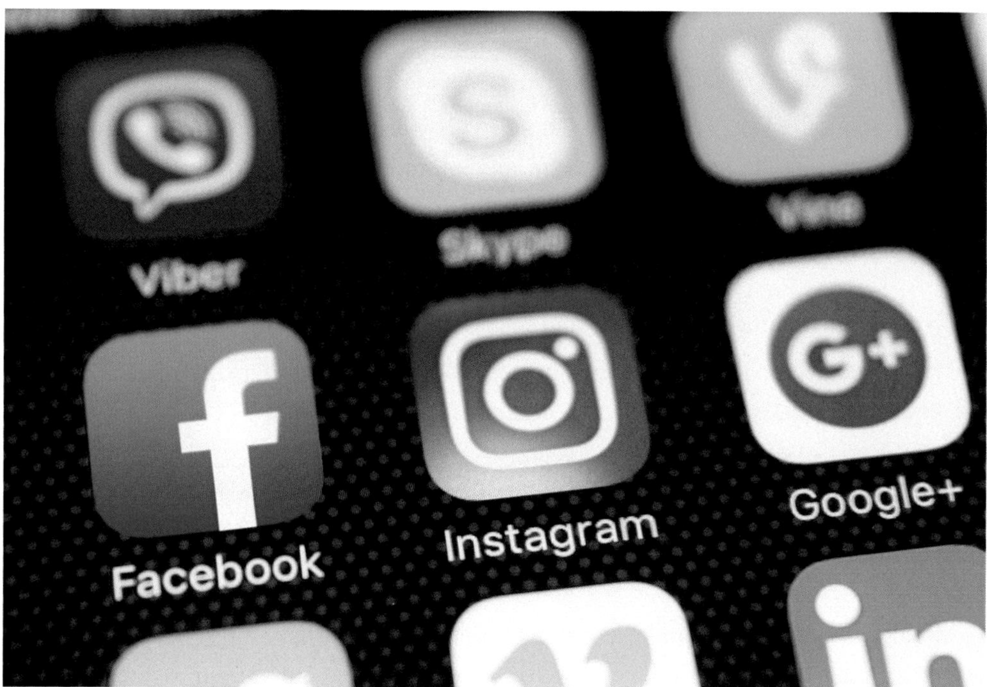

Image Credit: Social media application by alexsl/iStock

Use Social Media

Social media is a great way to enhance your reputation. It costs nothing other than a little time and has the potential for great reach. Social media serves two purposes: providing a way to keep your community informed about your research and means to build your profile.

Twitter and LinkedIn are big social media applications you can use to enhance your reputation. You can also use Facebook, any of the "academic" social platforms, or Instagram, SlideShare—or whatever else is the latest rage. The principle is always the same: it is all about the audience and your ease of access to them.

I GETTING STARTED

Try Twitter

Twitter, the micro-blogging online social networking service, has been in existence since 2006. As you almost certainly know, it allows users to send and read text-based posts of up to 280 characters, known as "tweets." Although the media mainly quote Twitter in the context of celebrity chitchat among the "Twitterati," and/or in the context of political upheavals, it is widely being used as a communication and marketing tool among professional individuals, organizations, and institutions associated with education and research. It can be a great source of up-to-date information.

In their article about the Royal Society of Chemistry's world's first Twitter-only conference, held in 2015, Randviir et al. [1] argue that "social media outlets such as Twitter broaden audiences, speed up communication, and force clearer and more concise descriptions of a researcher's work."

In using Twitter, you can do the following:

- Network with other researchers and interesting individuals by "following" them.
- Keep updated on news and events posted by professional organizations, the government, your institution, and various news channels.
- Discover what's being discussed at conferences, talks, and events by following "hashtags" (#).
- Obtain information or question using "crowd sourcing" techniques (brainstorming online) by using "RT."
- Publicize and share your research findings which you have presented at a conference, written about in a journal or on your blog, or spoken about at your institution.
- Promote yourself—use Twitter to find research posts and projects you can work on, or find collaborators or other like-minded individuals.

There are any number of articles on the Web which can show how tweeting really helps *you*.

LinkedIn

LinkedIn is another useful way to build your profile. LinkedIn is a social networking site that allows you to build a network of business contacts and share content with them. It is a useful tool to expand and improve relationships as well as build trust and credibility among your contacts. Your presence on LinkedIn allows you to post articles, to share links your colleagues might be interested in, and to upload publications. You can boost your audience by joining LinkedIn groups appropriate to your field and by sharing your uploads via your institution's site.

Update Your LinkedIn Profile

Your LinkedIn profile should contain all of the information you want your colleagues, collaborators, or potential funders to know about you. It may seem like simple advice, but you mustn't forget to update your profile. It will have a negative impact on your image if your profile is found to be out-of-date. Just like your Web profile, think of your LinkedIn profile as a shop window or the face of your brand, and ensure you follow these golden rules to make sure your profile is complete.

- Have you completed all sections? An incomplete profile limits your showing up in a search, meaning any potential contacts will not be able to find you.
- You should structure your summary to reflect your research aspirations and focuses. Use it to show off your achievements and passions. Using key words in this section will help your rankings in search results, so make sure you mention those that are pertinent to your research area.
- Make sure your profile image is appropriate and up-to-date. Avoid using holiday and party photos, as this may not reflect the formal image you would like to project. Consider getting a professional photo taken in a formal environment that could also be used on the team page of your project website.
- Include your contact details so that people know how to contact you if they don't want to use the LinkedIn mail service.

Connect

Once you have updated your profile, you might like to connect with other users. You will find that when you are searching for potential contacts to connect with, you will check to see if they have a photo and have updated all the sections in their profile. The people you are interested in might have supplied content-rich and relevant profiles. You can use this information as a "talking point" when they have accepted your connection invitation.

Network Online

To maximize your networking potential on LinkedIn, ensure you remain active on the site so you can stay in the minds of your connections. You wouldn't go to a live networking event and stand silently in the corner, so use your LinkedIn account to your advantage.

Even small actions such as congratulating someone on a new job or "liking" posts can positively affect your reputation, so aim to spend 10–15 minutes per day checking and interacting with the site.

If you wish to project your options and advice, consider updating your status regularly and write blog posts, or comment on articles. Interact with individuals with similar interests, by joining groups and taking part in discussions. These simple interactions will help you seem more personable to contacts. Always remember to remain professional on the site. There are other social media channels for talking about football and your weekend plans; LinkedIn should be for business use only.

"Academic" Social Media Platforms

These academic social media platforms such as Academia.edu, ResearchGate, and Mendeley are gaining importance. While they provide opportunities for collaboration and networking, they are most helpful for promoting publications and increasing citations. See Chapter 7.4 for further detail.

Set Up a Blog

Some academics establish a blog, accessed from their profile page, which allows them to reach a much wider audience than that given by their papers. This provides a platform to mention any subject they are passionate about, to state opinions, essentially unrestricted, and to receive comments—and perhaps start a debate. There are some who might blog every day, but it is more common to post just once a month. When they post on the blog they tend to complement it with Twitter, drawing attention to the blog. They might, for example, write on the blog about a new publication, sharing the link to the abstract; if they do the same on Twitter concurrently, the readership of the paper is expanded significantly.

SlideShare

SlideShare provides an opportunity to upload and share, publicly or privately, your PowerPoint presentations, pdf portfolios, or Word documents. If you can demonstrate aspects of your research visually, make a short video using a smart phone and place it on YouTube and provide a link. Again, link to the video from other social media sites. When you put your presentations on to SlideShare, be sure to put in all the proper key words that will bring you up in a search.

Use Social Media to Raise Community Awareness

Facebook and Twitter are obvious places for raising community awareness. Send out messages with links to your newsletters, or capture text from your stories to stand alone.

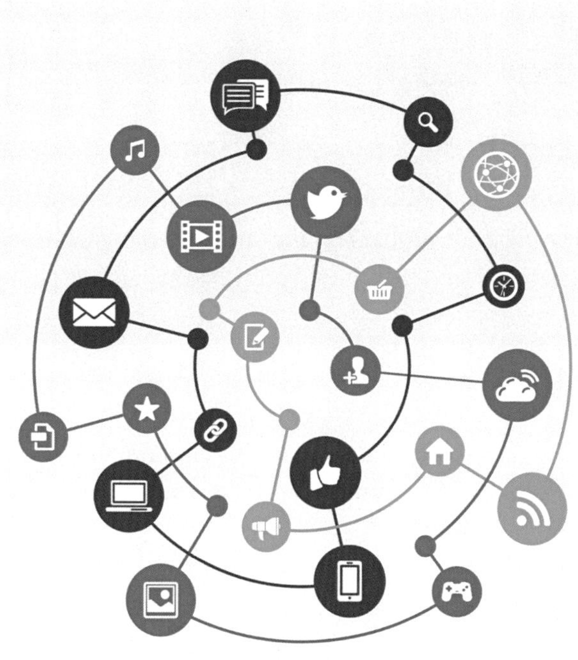

Image Credit: Social media connection concept by Hilch/Shutterstock

You may also like to try Instagram as well as YouTube videos designed for the layman.

If you share your information about your project across these social media sites, suddenly you have the potential to extend your audience a very long way.

Some quick tips:

- Use graphics wherever you can
- Put (limited) text on your visuals
- Include links to the website you want them to visit
- Repeat your posts
- Check to see which times get the best responses

To be sure you get the best benefit from this research dissemination, plan your outputs and create a calendar—and stick to it.

Create Your Web Profile

It is essential that you create a good Web profile for yourself, and remember to keep it updated. You probably look up other people's profiles on the Web as a first step to finding out about them. What you find there makes a difference to how you think about that person, and perhaps about what you do next.

Your Web and research profiles need to be constructed for two audiences: research peers who will be looking to see what you have achieved and how creditable your work is, and others with less knowledge of your field. The latter audience is still important. They might include potential donors, possible research collaborators from other universities, students seeking supervisors, or colleagues within your own university.

You should ensure you have a good personal web page on your institutional website and well constructed profiles through public avenues (e.g., Community of Science database). Include your broad research interests, recent publications, international intersts and whether you are seeking students.

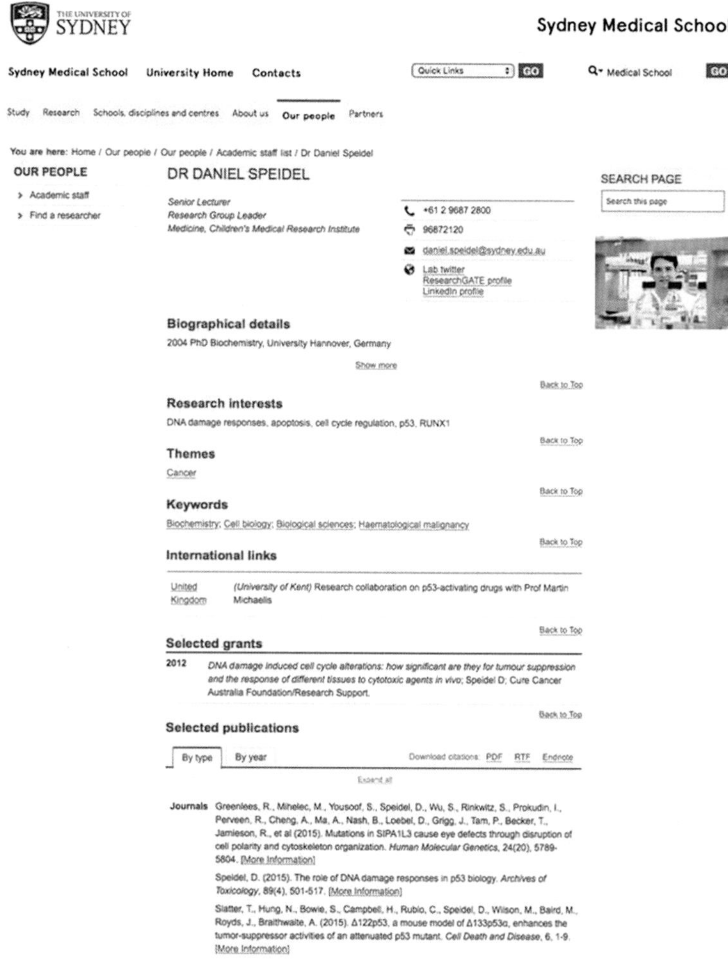

In all cases, it is important to keep your profile current. Set a reminder in your calendar every three months to review your profiles, and keep a list of them to ensure you update them all. This can also be a good time to review your long- and short-term priorities, and whether you are on track. Keeping your profile current is an important professional task. Make sure you keep you list of publications up-to-date.

It can be helpful to have an impartial colleague review your profiles and CV. A mentor can offer very useful insights into how well you are promoting your talents and capabilities. You may also wish to have a non-research acquaintance read your profile. They will give you good feedback on whether it is clear to a layman!

It is a challenge for many researchers to make their profile accessible. As a variation of the "elevator conversation", write a short paragraph on your research focus that would entice others to feel excited about what you do and how it could impact on the community. You might find this hard, don't despair and don't give up! Each time you revisit the statement, you will find it becomes more "people friendly." Think of it as translating from a foreign language. Do it one layer at a time, keeping your audience in mind.

Build a Web Presence for Your Project

You can't get by these days without a good project website. It doesn't have to be complex, but it has to be there. Think about it. When you want to know something, where do you go first? To search on your computer. How often you look up someone else's profile to find out more about them, their work, and their institution?

The same attention that could be directed at you applies to you and your research project. People will search for information about you, your work or for information about the field you are in. If they don't find you, they will find someone else, and you may have lost a potential supporter or investor or collaborator.

The website should reflect your project's general purpose and, where it is appropriate for the information to be in the public domain, its aims and planned outcomes.

The project website should include a little information about the project team and the institutes they represent. It should mention the funding partners and any other important stakeholders. If you wish to profile each team member, include information about their broad responsibilities and their contact email address. If they have their own profile pages on their institution's website, provide a link.

Make sure that the website is correctly branded for all your stakeholders, and include links to their websites.

The project Web pages should include general contact details and, if the detail of the project is not confidential, the latest study updates.

Take care to keep your website up-to-date.

It reflects badly on the whole team if the information is out-of-date or wrong. Add regular checking to your task list, and make it one person's responsibility to diarize a check at least every month. A regular five minute look will ensure your information doesn't become obsolete.

When building your website, consider your objectives and build it around them:

- Is the website only for information?
- Do you want someone to take action?

This website is a marketing tool, so concentrate on the same important things mentioned earlier:

- Why is your work important?
- How are you and your team spending your time and money?
- What difference is your research going to make?

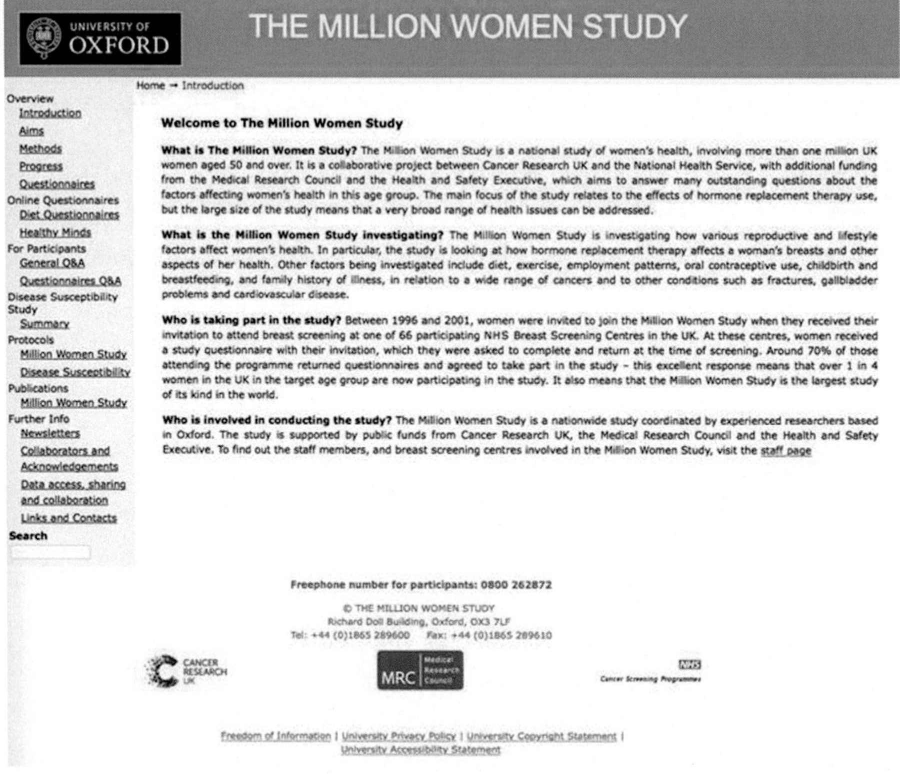

UNIVERSITY OF OXFORD

THE MILLION WOMEN STUDY

Home → Introduction

Overview
Introduction
Aims
Methods
Progress
Questionnaires
Online Questionnaires
Diet Questionnaires
Healthy Minds
For Participants
General Q&A
Questionnaires Q&A
Disease Susceptibility Study
Summary
Protocols
Million Women Study
Disease Susceptibility
Publications
Million Women Study
Further Info
Newsletters
Collaborators and Acknowledgements
Data access, sharing and collaboration
Links and Contacts
Search

Welcome to The Million Women Study

What is The Million Women Study? The Million Women Study is a national study of women's health, involving more than one million UK women aged 50 and over. It is a collaborative project between Cancer Research UK and the National Health Service, with additional funding from the Medical Research Council and the Health and Safety Executive, which aims to answer many outstanding questions about the factors affecting women's health in this age group. The main focus of the study relates to the effects of hormone replacement therapy use, but the large size of the study means that a very broad range of health issues can be addressed.

What is the Million Women Study investigating? The Million Women Study is investigating how various reproductive and lifestyle factors affect women's health. In particular, the study is looking at how hormone replacement therapy affects a woman's breasts and other aspects of her health. Other factors being investigated include diet, exercise, employment patterns, oral contraceptive use, childbirth and breastfeeding, and family history of illness, in relation to a wide range of cancers and to other conditions such as fractures, gallbladder problems and cardiovascular disease.

Who is taking part in the study? Between 1996 and 2001, women were invited to join the Million Women Study when they received their invitation to attend breast screening at one of 66 participating NHS Breast Screening Centres in the UK. At these centres, women received a study questionnaire with their invitation, which they were asked to complete and return at the time of screening. Around 70% of those attending the programme returned questionnaires and agreed to take part in the study - this excellent response means that over 1 in 4 women in the UK in the target age group are now participating in the study. It also means that the Million Women Study is the largest study of its kind in the world.

Who is involved in conducting the study? The Million Women Study is a nationwide study coordinated by experienced researchers based in Oxford. The study is supported by public funds from Cancer Research UK, the Medical Research Council and the Health and Safety Executive. To find out the staff members, and breast screening centres involved in the Million Women Study, visit the staff page

Freephone number for participants: 0800 262872

© THE MILLION WOMEN STUDY
Richard Doll Building, Oxford, OX3 7LF
Tel: +44 (0)1865 289600 Fax: +44 (0)1865 289610

CANCER RESEARCH UK
MRC Medical Research Council
NHS Cancer Screening Programmes

Freedom of Information | University Privacy Policy | University Copyright Statement | University Accessibility Statement

Some extra points:

- Make sure the website is easy to read
- Don't make the text too dense
- Include images
- Link to your publications (e.g., on SlideShare)
- Link to your CVs

As the project develops, include links to publications resulting from the project, as they become available, and include a section for news, and any media releases.

Remember the Lay Audience

Your target audience for your reputation is much bigger than your peers in research. Don't underestimate the importance of being able to explain your research to people outside your immediate group or even right outside research.

Be aware that anyone you meet might just be that person who can open doors for you to the next opportunity. Circumstances might have led them or their friend to have an interest in what you are doing, and you have to be able to talk to them in language they can understand. Similarly, you never know when you may be lucky enough to talk to someone who is interested and has money!

To work out what to say to these potentially important people, envisage yourself with this lay audience in an elevator for 20 floors—and that is the only time you have available to deliver your message. Practice your "elevator conversation" about what you do and why it matters. Your ability to describe what you are doing and why in about two minutes or 100 words, will hold you in good stead for writing lay summaries, for reporting back to funding agencies, for explaining to friends and families what it is you do.

Don't fall into the trap of thinking "they wouldn't be interested" or "they wouldn't understand," "they'll be scared, and they'll think I'm a nerd." They might well be interested (or they wouldn't have asked in the first place), and it is important to be able to make them understand. Just make your elevator conversation *accessible*.

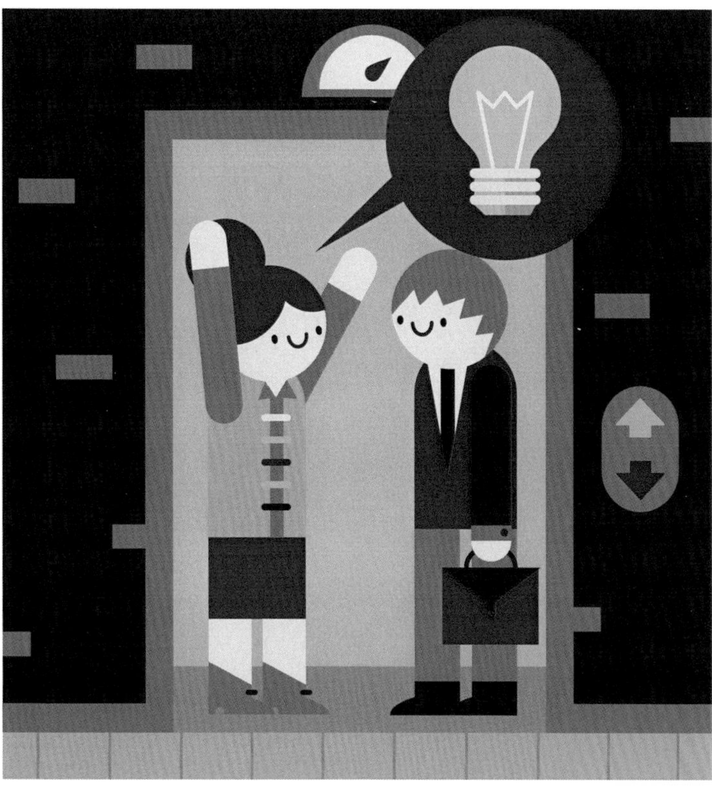

Image Credit: Tell an idea to somebody on an elevator by Team Oktopus/Shutterstock

Practice the five minute version too, the one you might have at a cocktail party. Instead of "I work at a university," a real conversation stopper, make it "I study the lives of some rare beetles which live only in dead trees", and then follow it up with the why "because there is only a very limited population now in Alaska, and we wonder what the birds will eat when they are gone." Not only does this make a more acceptable social banter, but it leads the conversation on to more interesting places.

Test your talk on someone outside your project. Do they understand? The first time round it is very unlikely they will, so go back and have another go.

Don't think of this as dumbing down. Instead regard it as talking to someone who isn't lucky enough know anything about your topic—an entirely different concept. Tell them about what you are doing and why you are doing it. It is the personal touch which makes it interesting, so include some snippets about you and where you came from before you embarked on this project.

You can gain further practice in lay presentation by working on your lay abstracts for your project. Write them out in simple words and explain as best you can what you are planning to do, and for what purpose. Mention the desired outcomes. Read the lay abstract again after a break, and see if it really is lay. Test this out on a friend too or with your consumer. Your lay abstract is important and you want it to be right.

Remember, for all these, practice makes perfect!

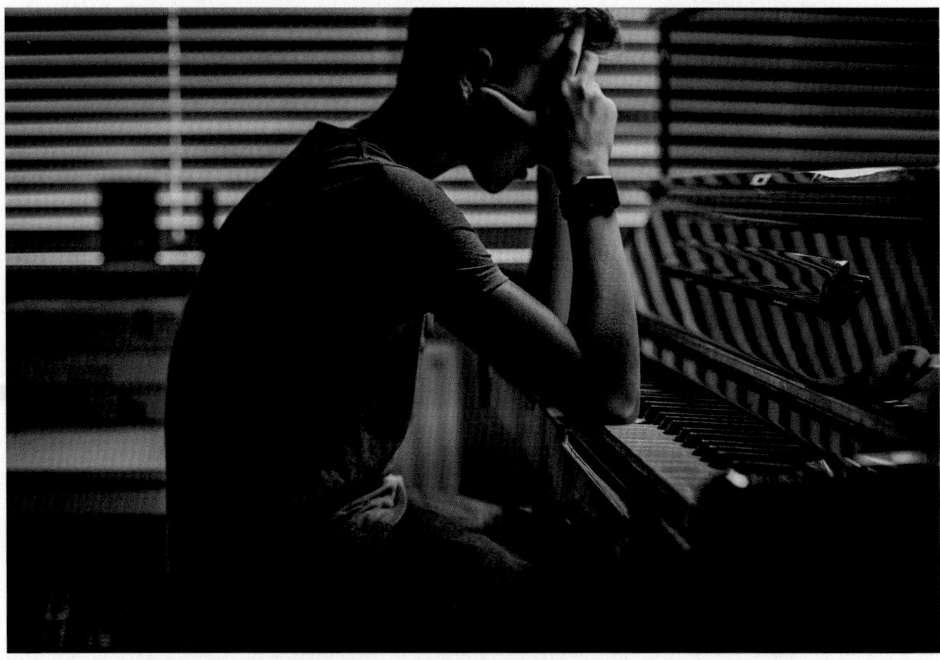

Image Credit: Struggling to learn by DGLimages/iStock

More Interacting With the Community

A very important and often overlooked part of your research communication is interacting with the community. Again, don't dismiss the non-scientist—you'd be surprised how many people in the community are interested to hear about your research. You just need to adjust your pitch to make it understandable to them.

Take the opportunities to attend fund-raising gatherings and information evenings. Instead of treating them as a chore, think of them as a recognition of who you are and what you are doing. You have been invited for a reason, and it's that they actually want to hear from you.

You will probably find that not only can you motivate your listeners, but they will motivate you. You might be surprised at how inspiring it can feel to meet the people who have raised the money to fund your research. In fact, the "conversation" tends to be inspiring on both sides. Every lab tour for prospective donors, or even prospective young scientists, tells the same story: the visitors are impressed and overwhelmed, whether they really understand what they are seeing or not. They love to learn about the research environment you are showing them.

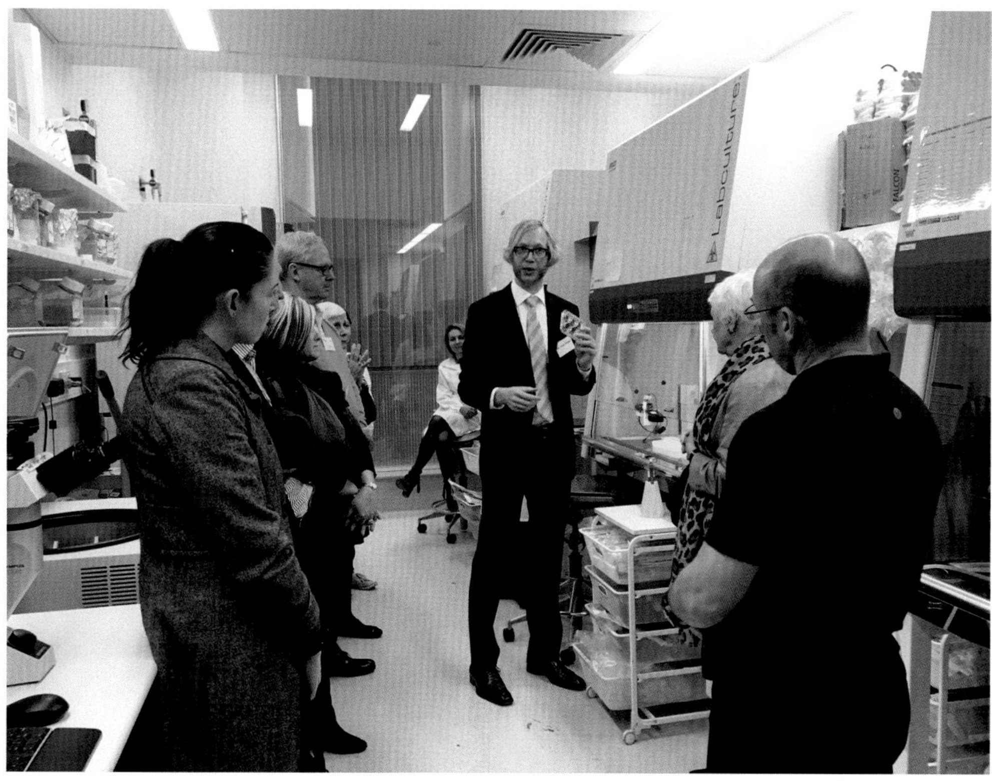

The end result might mean that you have helped generate more funds for your research, or more people who want to become scientists. It is a great way to be able to give back.

Don't forget to record these events to a version of your CV. There are many times when this information about community contribution is considered along with your research work. They matter and need to be recognized.

Reference—Enhance Your Reputation

[1] Randviir, E.P., Illingworth, S.M., Baker, M.J., Cued, M., Banks, C.E., 2015. Twittering about research: a case study of the World's first Twitter poster competition. F1000Research 4 (798). https://doi.org/10.12688/f1000research.6992.3.

Further Reading

Hayes, M. "Postdocexperience", 2013. Become a (social) media butterfly. http://postdocexperience.scienceblog.com/2013/07/29/become-a-social-media-butterfly/.

Total Solution Website Service, 2017. Your LinkedIn profile. https://www.yourfirmonline.co.uk/blog/archive/article/2016/November/using-linkedin-to-improve-your-personal-online-presence.

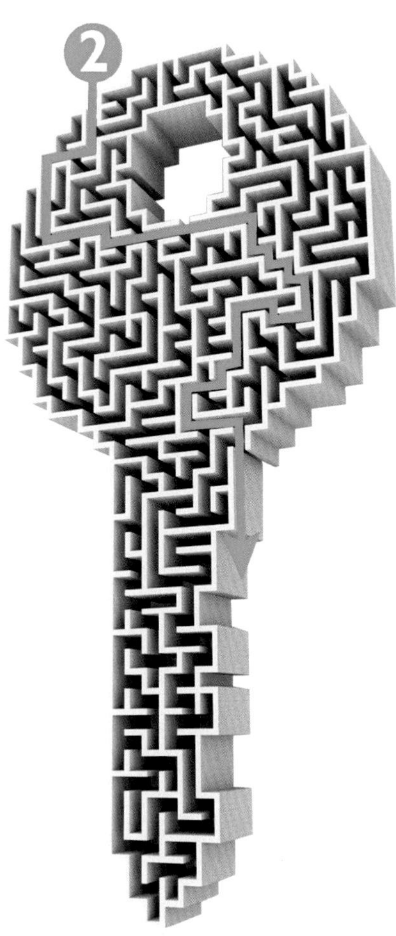
2

2.1 The Recruitment Process—Planning and Advertising

Bill had two research assistants on his project. The first was just great in the lab: quick to understand, clever and inventive, very productive. Until she left. What was in her lab book? Lots of scribble, but nothing that made sense to anyone else. What did she mean when she wrote "again?" What was the time period between one again and another?

Research Assistant 2 was not such a bright spark. She had a little less initiative and took little more telling what to do. The bonus with her was that she kept meticulous records. In the end, her work was much more useful to the study than what was left behind by Research Assistant 1.

Checklist

(Tick when completed)

- ☐ Have you got money for this position in the budget?
- ☐ Find out about human resources requirements
- ☐ Decide what the position looks like
- ☐ Determine essential and desirable skills
- ☐ Write the position description
- ☐ Advertise

Planning a New Position

You find yourself in the fortunate position of having a budget for staff. Now you want to make sure you get the right person or people to fulfill your needs.

This section will deal with selecting your new staff member. Later chapters will cover interviewing, orienting your staff, and then looking after your team, including volunteers and students.

Recruiting the Right Person

As is the case for most management, time spent in planning is well rewarded. Think carefully about the responsibilities of the new position(s) and draft the position description (PD) accordingly.

First, check exactly how much money you have available and over what time period. You might need to consider the benefits of a part-time position versus a full-time position which finishes earlier.

No doubt your institution will have defined processes and requirements for recruitment. You must obviously follow these, so see your Human Resources (HR) department for advice on correct procedures, checking, too, whether there will be any costs associated with the advertising or the actual position. Having done so, the onus will fall to you to take the subsequent steps.

Before you write the PD, think about the nature of the tasks ahead. What do you need done? What sort of skill set will be required for each set of tasks? How do the various tasks fit together to make this job a reasonable one? Think through the amount of time you have allocated for each set of tasks, and, if relevant, the changing nature of this time, as the project progresses.

You should consider whether this position should be short-term or long-term, permanent or casual. If the need really is only short-term, then a short-term appointment is a tempting option, but be aware that your new staff member might not demonstrate the level of commitment you expect if they are only to be there for a couple of months. The other perspective, of course, is that you could end up with someone who doesn't have enough to do, either because the tasks that remain are beyond their capabilities or because they are complete.

Position Description

Whether or not you are to manage the recruitment process yourself, or your HR department does it for you, you will need to consider what should be included in the PD and the detail of the skills required.

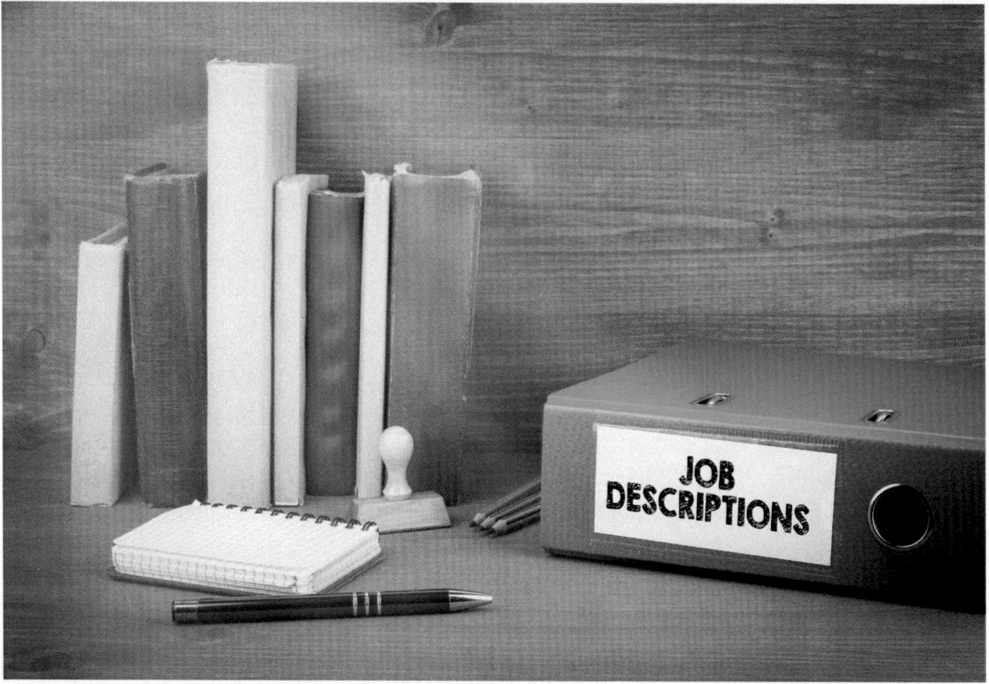

Image Credit: Job Descriptions by tumsasedgars/iStock

The PD typically offers a brief background of the organization, then a broad statement about the role. Following that, it lists the principal tasks for the role and then essential and desirable criteria for the applicant. The latter are very important when you select people for interview—or justify not selecting them—so think them through carefully.

What do you imagine the new staff member's day will look like? Repetitive? Varied? Frantic? People-oriented or a team of one with little interaction with others? There are types of people for all positions. Do your best to match up the characteristics of the person you want with the description you include in the PD.

There will probably be requirements for past training and possibly for the experience they've had. List essential skills and desirable skills. These, along with the defined responsibilities of the position, will give clues to the reader about the nature of the job.

Get your essential skills right. If a candidate meets the requirements for essential skills but is not selected, you could find yourself having to explain why they were not successful and you will need valid reasons.

TABLE 2.1.1 Core Competencies for the Position Description
Leadership
Flexibility
Motivation
Commitment
Initiative
Teamwork
Responsibility
Decision-making
Communication
Trustworthiness
Problem solving
Organization
Resilience

Selection criteria should encompass not only the academic skills and experience required but also any important personal characteristics on which recruitment decisions can be made. You need to choose the right sort of person for the task. You don't want a buzzy extraverted run-about if the role is going to involve a great deal of repetition. For this position you want solid concentration and attention to detail.

Core competencies for the position should be contained within the PD and may include any of the attributes listed in Table 2.1.1.

Some examples of selection criteria, some of which include core competencies, are as follows:

Selection criteria—for qualifications:

- A PhD in bioinformatics
- A background in respiratory medicine or astronomy

Selection criteria—e.g., for experience:

- A history of safe laboratory practice, preferably in the context of virology
- Experience with mass spectrometry
- Well-developed track record in field of public health
- Active in, and with a long-term commitment to, fieldwork

Selection criteria—e.g., for personal characteristics:

- Excellent written and oral communication skills
- Demonstrated ability to work under pressure
- Proven ability to work as a member of a team
- Ability to communicate with staff at all levels of the organization
- Capacity to interact with technical staff
- Good time management and organizational skills and willingness to take responsibility

The HR Council of Canada provides a PD template within its HR Toolkit [1], a comprehensive online resource designed to help managers, employees, and board members better understand, address and manage issues relating to HR in nonprofits.

Advertising the Position

While it is sometimes possible to appoint someone to a position without first advertising it, it is usual to have to advertise first. This obviously gives you a chance to recruit the best available person at the time and widens the field beyond people you already know. It also avoids accusations of nepotism or lack of transparency.

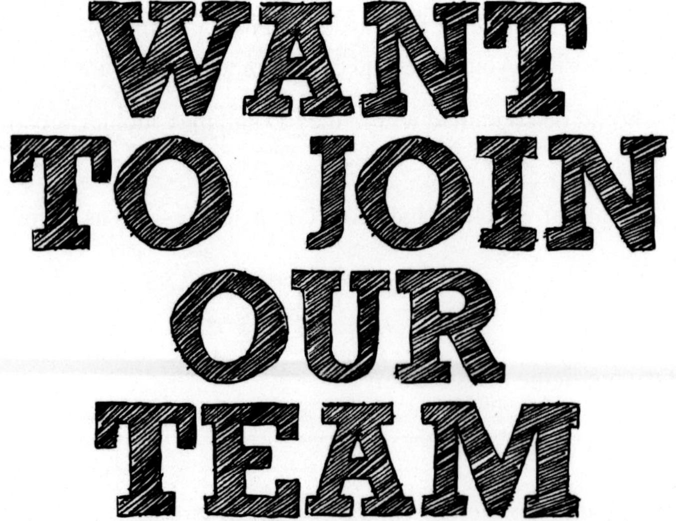

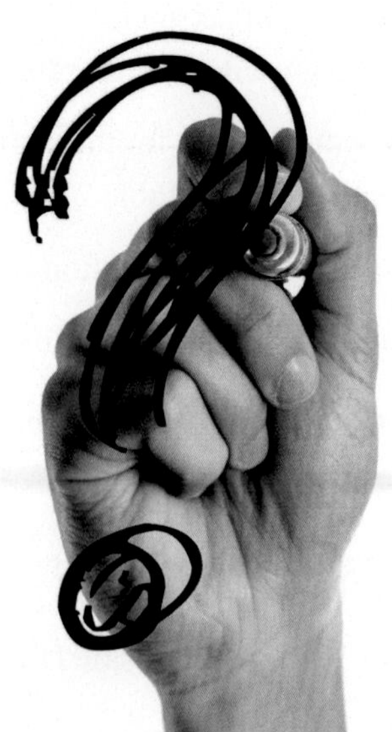

Image Credit: Want to join our team by gustavofrazao/iStock

There are times when a direct appointment could be valid. Sometimes, you might want to appoint someone already in your team, perhaps someone with a contract coming to the end. Alternatively, you may wish to appoint an individual who has been named in a successful grant application document, or employ someone to meet pressing short-term needs with a casual appointment. Employment by invitation, say short-term employment of a person on loan from a collaborator, would also be an exception.

For any of these situations, check with your HR department to see if you may go straight on to offer your desired candidate the position.

Your position will be advertised via the institution's usual networks. This might include the institute's website, online recruitment sites, a university bulletin or even notice boards. Advertisements in the newspaper are used less frequently these days except for very senior positions. You can increase distribution of your ad by including it, and its corresponding documentation, on your LinkedIn profile or by emailing your network and asking your contacts to send it onto potential interested parties. Remember to include the advertisement on your project website (and take it down when the position is filled!).

References—Planning and Advertising

[1] The HR Council of Canada. http://hrcouncil.ca/hr-toolkit/home.cfm.

Associated Documents—The Recruitment Process—Planning and Advertising

A PD template can be found at http://hrcouncil.ca/docs/Template_JD.doc.

The following documents sourced from Business Victoria can be found at http://www.business.vic.gov.au/#1007711.

2.1.1 Job Description Template

Job title: (insert job title here)

Reporting to: (insert supervisor's title here)

Salary: (insert salary per hour/annum or total package including base salary, superannuation, commissions or benefits here)

Hours: (insert average number of hours per week or type of employment such as casual, full-time here)

Location: (insert location of the position and any travel required)

Purpose of the position (insert short paragraph which describes the overall purpose of this position and how it contributes to the goals or function of the business, include the authority level (e.g. manager or support staff) here)

Key responsibilities & duties

(insert the main responsibilities and duties of the position here. Then list the skills or competencies which the candidate will need in order to complete those duties. It's also worth thinking about how important each duty/competency is e.g. how much of the job will be spent on each duty and is it a must have competency or can you train someone to do it?)

Duties of the role	Time spent	Competencies sought	Must have or optional (can be trained)
e.g. Respond to enquiries – over the phone and face-to-face from the staff and public	70%	Communication skills including conflict resolution and friendly manner	Must have

Duties of the role	Time spent	Competencies sought	Must have or optional (can be trained)
e.g. Miscellaneous admin duties and support business team	20%	Good organisational skills and attention to detail Team orientated approach	Must have
e.g. Data entry	10%	Excel database skills	Optional

Academic or trade qualifications

(insert list of desired academic and trades qualifications here, e.g. Certificate in Office Administration. If none are necessary state this as it could increase the number of applicants for the job.)

Work experience and skills

(insert list of work experience and skills needed to perform the job here, e.g. general administration/ reception experience)

Manager Signature:

Date:

2.1.2 Detailed Job Description

Job title: (insert job title)

Reporting to: (insert supervisor's title)

Salary: (insert salary per hour, per annum or total package including base salary, superannuation, commissions or benefits)

Hours: (insert average number of hours per week or type of employment such as casual, full-time)

Location: (insert the location of the position and any travel required)

Purpose of the position

(Insert a short paragraph which describes the overall purpose of this position and how it contributes to the goals or function of the business. Include the authority level, for example, "manager" or "support staff")

Responsibilities & duties

Responsibility 1 – (insert responsibility or duty of the position including frequency or duration of work, effort and skill required, complexity of tasks and equipment required)

Work standard: (insert what aspect of the responsibility will be reviewed to determine if the job is being done correctly, for example, time frame, or number of completed tasks per week)

Responsibility 2 – for example, "to manage the daily operations of the office including organising mail, couriers, catering and travel. Staff need to be able to use MS EXCEL confidently, to arrange global travel and to work on their own."

Work standard – for example, "at the end of each working week, all catering events for the following week must be finalised."

Responsibility 3 – (insert additional items as needed)

Work standard – (insert additional items as needed)

Academic & trades qualifications

Essential qualifications

- (insert list of essential qualifications, for example, Certificate in Office Administration)

Desirable qualifications

- (insert list of desirable (but not essential) qualifications, for example, Advanced Excel course)

Work experience & skills

Essential experience

- (insert list of essential experience, for example, Minimum two years general administration/ reception experience)

Desirable qualifications

- (insert list of desirable (but not essential) experience, for example, Experience working within a manufacturing environment)

Personal qualities & behavioural traits

Essential qualities or behaviours

- (insert list of essential qualities or behaviours, for example, Written and verbal communication skills)

Desirable qualities or behaviours

- (insert list of desirable (but not essential) qualities or behaviours, for example, Attention to detail)

2.1.2 Detailed Job Description

Relationships

Details of relationships relevant to this role

- (insert position name and details about the supervision given and received, for example, "This position will trained by the General Manager with ongoing support and supervision")
- (insert details of the relationships involved both internally and externally. An example of external relationships would be "customer relations")

Employee signature:

Manager's signature:

Performance review period: (insert review period, for example, "every three months")

Next review date:

2.2 The Recruitment Process—Interviewing and Selecting

A reputable university employed a scientist from another university. He had a great CV; all were sure he was going to be really helpful to the team. But he wasn't. He was useless and had no idea how to do the things he was employed for. He had committed academic fraud. The papers listed on his CV weren't true, the work supposedly behind them wasn't true. Money was wasted; the project was delayed; and the institution's reputation was damaged. It wouldn't have been hard to check up on him in the beginning.

Checklist

(Tick when completed)

- ☐ Shortlist your applicants against the selection criteria
- ☐ Appoint a selection committee
- ☐ Make the interview times, preferably all on the same day
- ☐ Draft the interview questions
- ☐ Select your candidate, again against the selection criteria
- ☐ Check the references of your preferred candidate
- ☐ Make your offer
- ☐ Advise the unsuccessful candidates
- ☐ Diarize a time to evaluate the candidate before the end of the probation period

Shortlisting

Sometimes you hear of people being swamped with applications for a position. It does happen and can be enough to make you resist even advertising the job. Sorting through literally hundreds of applications is exhausting, but you have to start somewhere. Be ruthless.

Apply your selection criteria to all applications, especially the essential skills, right from the beginning. If they haven't followed your guidelines, don't give them the benefit of the doubt. Cut them out immediately. If "excellent written and oral communication skills" is one of your criteria, reject an application with spelling mistakes. The same applies if you asked for "careful attention to detail." If you asked for the application to be a response to the selection criteria and they only sent a CV, don't give them a thought. They haven't followed instruction, so you don't want them. (Note that there is always a corollary. If attention to detail is not a key criterion, you might judge someone who has made a minor mistake a little less harshly).

A good rule of thumb is to invite the best three for interview. Save the next ten, just in case these three are not suitable.

The Selection Committee

Invite some of your colleagues to join you on the selection committee. Three people is a good number. Try to have a gender balance. One of the others on the committee should be part of your project team or work closely with you. Do not include anyone who has a lesser position on the institutional hierarchy than the new position.

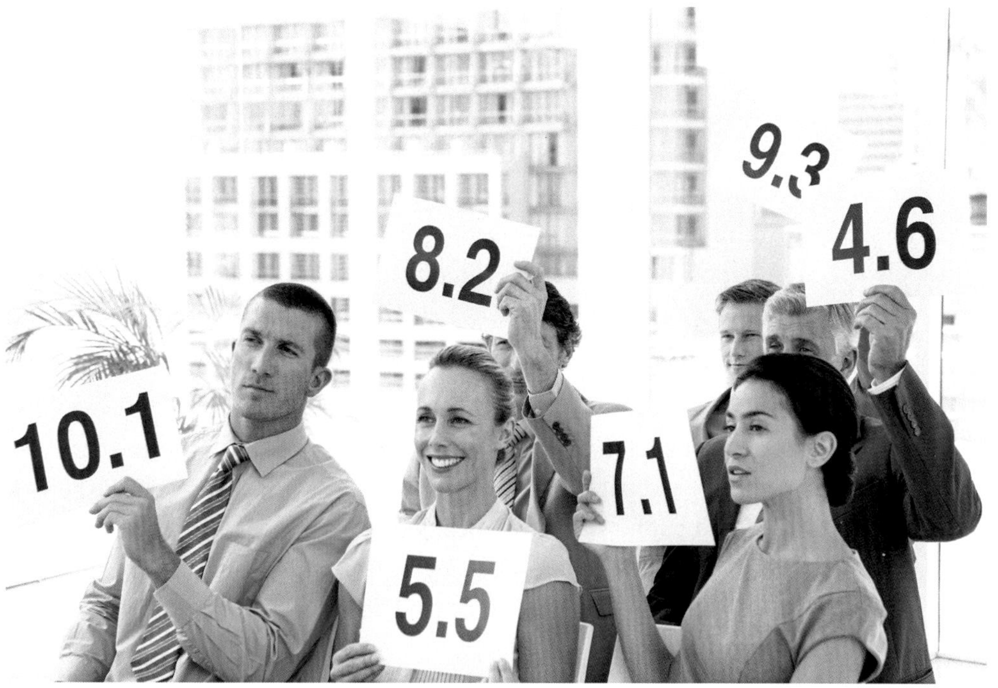

Image Credit: People holding grades by wavebreakmedia/iStock

Check the availability of your team, and try to have your interviews on the same day, or as close as possible to one another. Wherever possible, the interview panel should be the same for all applicants. These practices allow you to be fair to the candidates.

Circulate the PD and the applications, and the proposed interview timetable, to the other committee members in plenty of time. At the same time, write out the set interview questions, allocate them to each committee member and share them in advance.

The Interview

The interview provides the opportunity for the selection committee to appraise the value of the leading candidates selected for interview. You will aim to judge the fit of the person to the position based on their personal characteristics, their previous experience and their education. By the end of the interview, the interviewers should have learned more about the applicant's background and experience and how effectively they would integrate into your working environment.

There is much to recommend the set "situational" or "behavioral" question method of interviewing, rather than the alternative of just telling about the position and asking if the person thinks they would like it. They wouldn't be there at the interview if they didn't want the job. The question is whether *you* want *them*, and you will learn this from the behavioral method of questioning.

Behavioral interview questions provide an opportunity for you to assess the applicant's current skills and knowledge with respect to the core competencies of the position because when you place the applicants in a hypothetical or remembered "situation," their answers give you good guidance to their understanding and experience. The situational questions don't help them learn about the role, but they have had the first clues from your well-written PD, and, after all, you can deal with their questions at the end—if you think they are worth telling.

Give careful thought to the set of questions. If the job is going to involve a great deal of action and possible stress, include questions about a time they had to deal with such stress. If the tasks are going to be very repetitive, find out how they will deal with the repetition and keeping their mind on the job. If they have sensible answers, it is probably because they have done this sort of work before and know they can manage what others would find boring.

Make sure that your questions require an open response, not a yes/no answer.

There are probably interview guidelines set down by your university. Make sure you read and understand these so that you can be certain you are following best practice and are meeting all your legislative requirements.

Harvard Law School has published a list of sample behavioral interview questions complied by the Office of Public Interest, shown in Table 2.2.1. There are further questions in Associated Documents, at the end of this chapter.

Selecting Your Candidate

As you interview each candidate you should record comments about their responses, their attributes and their apparent strengths or weaknesses. It is useful to use a selection criteria form such as Form 2.2.1 in Associated Documents at the end of this chapter.

TABLE 2.2.1 Sample Behavioral Questions

Tell me about a time you had to make a quick decision.
Tell me about a difficult experience you had in a clinic or internship and how you overcame it.
Tell me about a time you had too many things to do and had to prioritize.
What did you do the last time things didn't go according to plan?
Tell me about a situation where you failed. Why did you fail and what did you learn from it?
Tell me about a time you had to work with someone who did things very differently from you.
Tell me about a time when you had to deal with a difficult client or coworker.
Describe a situation in which a detail you thought to be unimportant turned out to be very important.
Tell me about a time you had to persuade a colleague to accept your point of view.
Tell me about a time you went above and beyond the call of duty.
Describe a situation where your efforts had a direct impact on the outcome.
Tell me about an ethical work situation you had to deal with. How did it turn out?
Tell me about a time when you had to act in a leadership capacity.
What have you done in the workforce that shows initiative and creativity?
How would you handle a situation where you and your supervisor disagreed about an issue or course of action?

Checking References

It sounds obvious, but when you ask for references from your prospective staff member, you should undertake your due diligence and check them properly. Make sure your selected applicant was employed where they said they were employed. Even more important in an academic environment, check to see if they have published what they said they have published. If you don't, you might be sorry. See Reference Check Form 2.2.2 in Associated Documents at the end of this chapter.

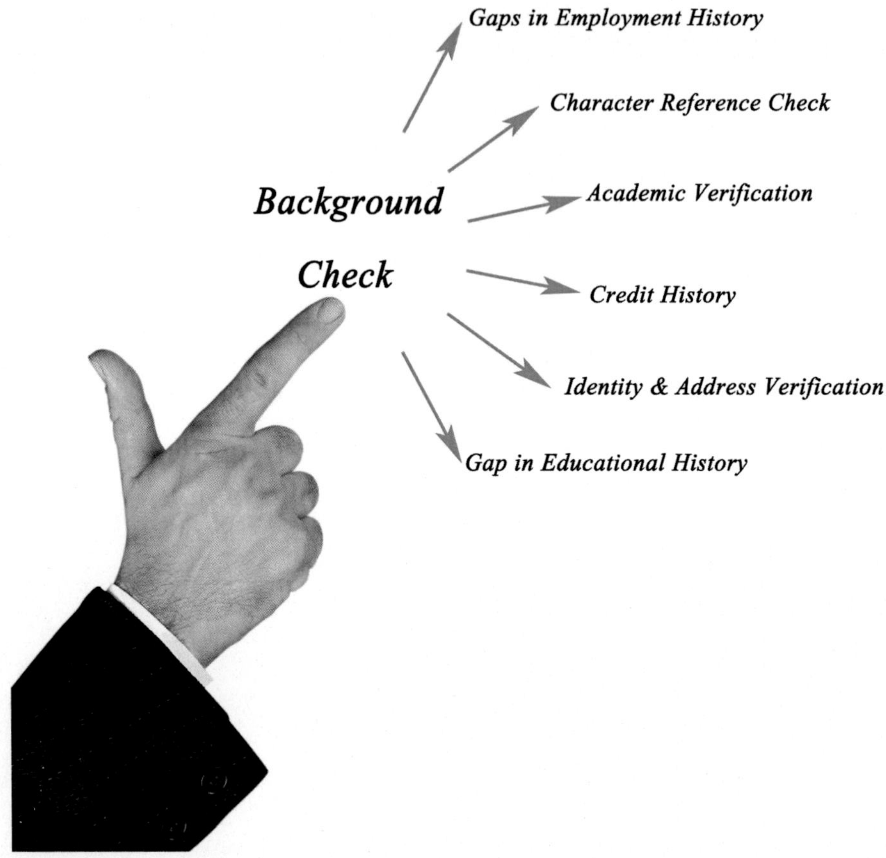

Image Credit: Diagram of background check by Arka8/Shutterstock

Make Your Offer

It is an exciting time when you find the candidate who has the right fit for your position. What a relief! Be careful now to follow the correct steps so you don't mess things up.

It is probably wise to check in now with your HR team to check on steps they need to have followed. You will need to discuss salary, start date, and terms and conditions of employment. Remember that your applicant will probably have to give notice at their current place of work, and you must allow for that in your plans. In some countries a notice period of up to three months can be the norm.

Advise the Unsuccessful Applicants

A very important step, sadly often neglected, is to advise the unsuccessful candidates that the position has been filled. Everyone who applied for the position should be thanked for their application and told they have been unsuccessful.

Extra courtesy is due to those who came for interview, and best practice is to phone them to let them know they have been unsuccessful, and another candidate has been selected. Try to avoid detailed discussion about why the candidate did not get the job, especially avoiding criticism of their application or interview. Useful expressions include "there were a number of very high quality candidates," or "the person we selected appears to have the best fit for the selection criteria." You might be unfortunate enough to lose your first pick, for any number of reasons, so be careful not to "burn your bridges" with near-miss candidates. It is wise to keep the top applications on file for a few months just in case.

Probation

In most countries, a new employee is offered employment on the understanding that there is to be a probation period, and they will be offered a permanent position or contract after that period (perhaps six weeks or three months), provided they have met expectations. The probation period is for the benefit of the employer. Make use of it if your new employee does not fulfill your needs. It is very difficult to dismiss a staff member after probation is finished, so take the time to evaluate the situation, and take action in time. It is a good idea to diarize a reminder about the end of the probation period so you don't miss it, and to hold a meeting with your new employee to discuss progress. You can use Form 2.2.4 in Associated Documents at the end of this chapter to help you with the conversation.

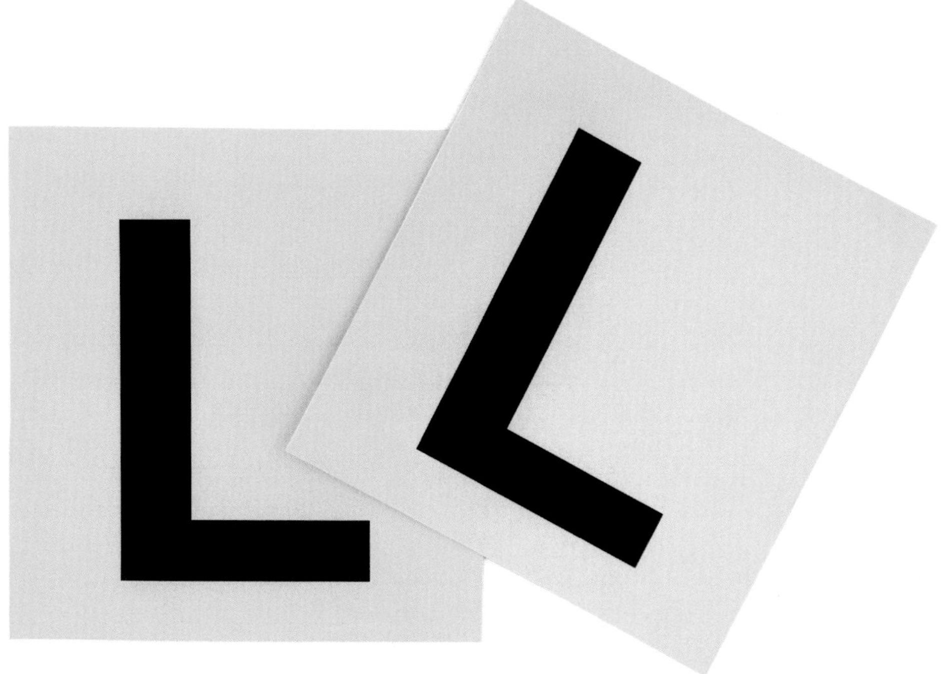

Image Credit: L plate by Jamesbowyer/iStock

Associated Documents—Interviewing and Selecting

The following documents sourced from Business Victoria can be found at http://www.business.vic.gov.au/#1007711.

Form 2.2.1 Selection Criteria Template

(Insert Position title here)

(Insert Organisation name here)

- Use your job description as a basis for your candidate selection.
- Make sure your selection factors are based on the competencies you need e.g. communication skills (and the questions you are asking will test how the candidates have demonstrated this in the past).
- You can identify as many selection factors as you like but we suggest no more than 10.
- Keep in mind how important each selection factor is e.g. is it must have or optional, will half the job require this skill or will it only be needed occasionally?
- Once you've held the interview, rate each candidate on each selection factor. The easiest way to do this is to score based on doesn't have the competency (1), partially has the competency (2) or has the competency (3).
- The highest score should be the preferred candidate. It might also be worth considering whether the other candidates would be suitable for the job if the preferred candidate doesn't accept the job.
- Your worksheet should look like this:

Selection factors	(Insert Candidate Name here)	(Insert Candidate Name here)	(Insert Candidate Name here)	(Insert Candidate Name here)
1. *e.g. Communication skills. (Mandatory)*				
2				
3				
4.				
5.				
6.				
7.				
8.				
9.				

Form 2.2.2 Reference Check Template

Date: (Insert date here)

Reference Check for: (Insert Candidate's name here)

Position Applied for: (Insert position title here)

Referee's Name: (Insert referee's name here)

Title & Company: (Insert Referee's position title and company here)

Phone: (Insert Contact number here)

Candidate's role at this company: (Insert role candidate held here)

Dates candidate was employed: (Insert date of employment here)

Questions for Referee

Effectiveness in role

- "How effective was (insert the candidate name here) in the performance of their role?
- "Why do you say that?"
- "How was their performance measured?"

Strengths

- "What do you think (insert the candidate name here) strengths are?
- "Why do you say that?"

Technical Competence

- "How would you describe (Insert the candidate name here)'s level of technical skills and knowledge?
- Ask any questions that you have specific to the position

Deals with pressure

- "How well do you think (insert the candidate name here) deals with pressure?
- "Can you give me some examples of times when (insert the candidate name here) was under a lot of pressure?"

Supervisory skill and style

- "Did (insert the candidate name here) supervise anyone in their position?"
- If yes, "Can you tell me about (insert the candidate name here)'s supervisory skills and style?

Areas of improvement needed

- "Based on your experience of (insert the candidate name here) what areas did you note as needing further development?

Interaction with all levels of management and staff

- "How does (insert the candidate name here) interact with different levels of management and other employees in the company?"

Reason for leaving

- "Why did (insert the candidate name here) leave your company?"

Honesty and integrity

- "Are company values important to (insert the candidate name here)?"

Management Style

- "What is the best way to manage (insert the candidate name here)?"
  i.e. Micro-managed, given clear objectives, given some autonomy etc.

Rehire

- "Would you rehire (insert the candidate name here)?

Other

- "Are there any other comments you would like to add?"

Points to Follow Up in Next Reference

Points to follow up with candidate

Selection factors	(Insert Candidate Name here)	(Insert Candidate Name here)	(Insert Candidate Name here)	(Insert Candidate Name here)
10.				
TOTAL				
ASSESSMENT				

***Rating:** 1 = Does not Satisfy 2 = Partially Satisfies 3 = Fully Satisfies

Assessment P = Preferred S = Suitable U = Unsuitable

Form 2.2.3 More Sample Interview Questions

Questions about experience at work

- Give an example of when you worked in a team and what you found the most rewarding thing was in doing that.
- Can you tell me about a job you have done in which you worked with private and confidential information? How did you protect the privacy of whose records you were working with?
- This job is very multi-faceted. Give me an example of a time when you had to deal with conflicting / competing priorities. What did you do? What was the effect of your actions?
- You will be largely unsupervised on a day to day basis. What would you describe as the most important job you have done that was largely unsupervised?
    - What was the level of input from your ultimate manager?
    - What did you do to ensure that that supervisor was informed about what you were doing?
    - What steps did you take when you were unsure about how to proceed?
- This position needs you to maintain effective working relationships with your staff. Tell us about a difficulty with other people in the workplace or other people with whom you have interacted in your job and what you did about it.
- Tell me about your most recent publication and the processes you went through to do the research and bring that paper to fruition.

Questions to ascertain interest in, and suitability for, the job:

- What is it about this organization which appeals to you?

- Why did you apply for this particular position?
- In what sort of environment do you like to work?
- What do you hope to be doing in 5 years time?
- Why should you be the successful candidate?

Questions to ascertain personal skills/attributes:

- Tell us about yourself. How do you believe others see you?
- What do you believe are your greatest strengths? In what areas could you do better?
- Tell us about an achievement of which you are particularly proud.
- Give an example of how you have recently used your initiative.

Form 2.2.4 Three Months Probationary Period Review

Objective

The purpose of this meeting is for the employee and the Manager to discuss the past three months and highlight any areas that may need to be addressed as we move forward to ongoing employment.

Typical examples are:

- Planning – or lack of
- Communication
- Work load
- Expectations and deliverables
- Training
- Retention
- Presentation
- Follow through

Attention to detail

- Adherence to deadlines

Initiative

The team member will have an opportunity to communicate how they feel they are performing within the guidelines given for the role. We will discuss what areas are enjoyed, what areas if any, are proving difficult, expectations and accountability.

Three Month Review – Expectations

Within the initial three months, the basics of the role should be under control; a good grasp of the broad business offering, strong ownership of the role, competence across the business administration and relationships developed with key clients and stakeholders.

Format

Recap on outcome of previous Reviews, Invite employee to talk about the past three months in total, talk about issues and improvements that they have made.

(Document issues or concerns raised and come back to them at the close.)

Manager gives feedback on performance over the past three months.

(Highlight any relevant issues with examples if possible here)

Discuss issues raised

(Insert document specific action or outcome here)

Set expectations for the next 3 or 6 months which will be reviewed at the next performance review.

Discuss appropriate training, retraining, refocus and appropriate time lines. The Team member will receive a copy of documented Action Plan.

End positively.

2.3 The Recruitment Process—Orienting Your Staff

Three months after she started work, Sally was still struggling to get the rhythm of the place. She didn't understand where they all disappeared to at 3 o'clock on Wednesday afternoon, and now she felt it was too late to ask. They didn't mean to leave her out, but it would have helped if someone had explained in her first week that Wednesday was the day they all went next door to afternoon tea, and she should come too.

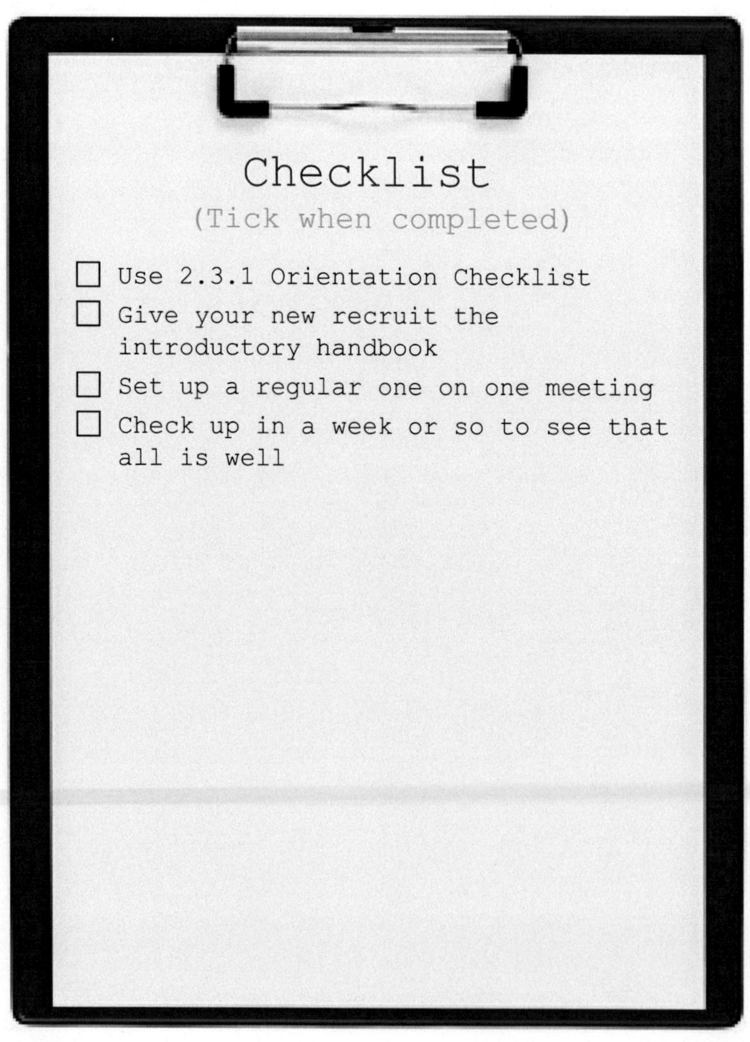

Remember to take the time to properly orientate your new team members when they arrive. Allowing them to "suck it and see" is not good management. You will get them up and running and productive quickly if you spend the first day with them, explaining their new environment, and your expectations.

As a first step, there are practical matters to attend to which will allow them to settle into their new environment. They need to meet the other team members, find their way around the building and know where to have lunch. See Orientation Checklist for a full list of things to cover on day one.

You may need to allocate your whole day to your new staff member, but it will be a worthwhile investment of your time. If there are other people from your group available, they could take the tours, or act as mentor for the new recruit for the first couple of weeks.

Take care with work, health, and safety. Show your new person the fire exits and describe procedures if you need to evacuate. If you work in a lab with hazardous products or equipment, remember to brief them on safety procedures. Check that their desk and chair suit them and if they have any special needs.

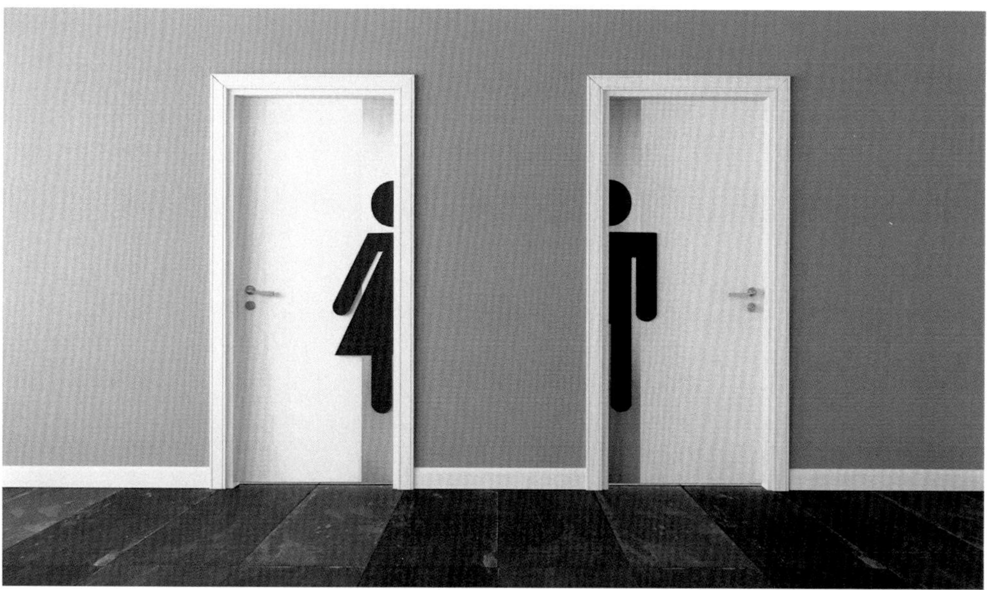

Image Credit: White doors by tomap49/iStock

You should take the time, as soon as possible, to fully explain your project and its purpose, and give them background material to read. You will be much more likely to get full engagement of any of your staff when they understand the big picture and how their own part fits in.

Discuss with them the terms of probation and plans for performance review. Later, you will need to have discussions with your new starter(s) about their career path and opportunities for professional development and training. You should also plan regular sessions where you can discuss performance and provide constructive feedback.

If you are employing a post-doc or taking on a PhD student, don't forget that they will have special additional requirements. Students receiving a stipend from a research grant will have to comply with university procedures relating to admission, candidature, enrollment, and thesis preparation and submission, and you will need to also provide appropriate supervisors for them.

See the sections on Managing your Team and Managing Students for further detail.

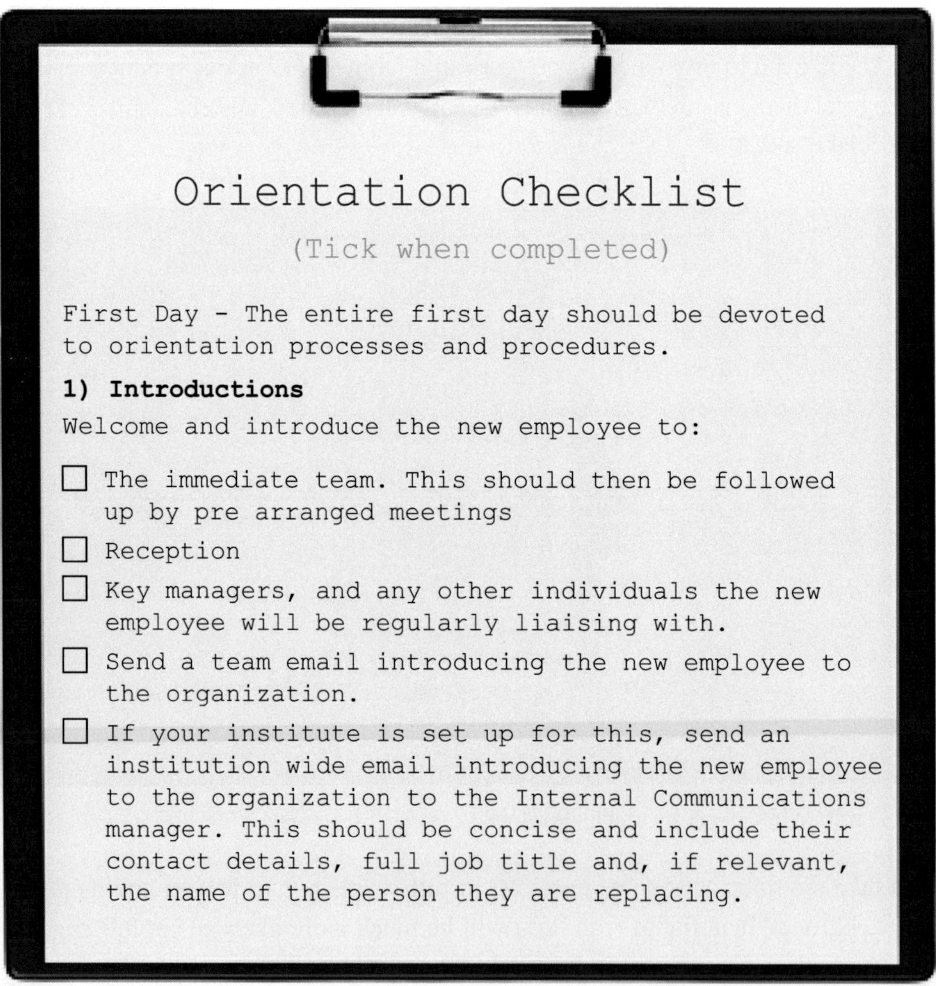

Orientation Checklist

(Tick when completed)

First Day - The entire first day should be devoted to orientation processes and procedures.

1) Introductions

Welcome and introduce the new employee to:

- ☐ The immediate team. This should then be followed up by pre arranged meetings
- ☐ Reception
- ☐ Key managers, and any other individuals the new employee will be regularly liaising with.
- ☐ Send a team email introducing the new employee to the organization.
- ☐ If your institute is set up for this, send an institution wide email introducing the new employee to the organization to the Internal Communications manager. This should be concise and include their contact details, full job title and, if relevant, the name of the person they are replacing.

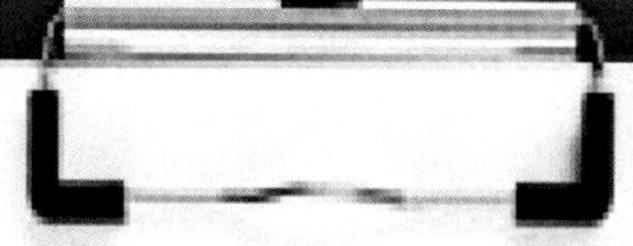

Checklist

(Tick when completed)

2) Office Tour

- ☐ Discuss building access and give the new employee their access card Show the new employee -
- ☐ Out of hours entry and exit (if applicable)
- ☐ Kitchen facilities
- ☐ Toilets
- ☐ Utility room
- ☐ Fire exits and fire equipment. Explain the emergency procedures
- ☐ First aid kit and room
- ☐ Relevant notice boards including the Occupational Health and Safety notice board
- ☐ Library
- ☐ Where to eat lunch

3) Everyday Office Procedures and Information

- ☐ Advise best place to put personal belongings
- ☐ Explain how the telephone operates
- ☐ Explain key computer software and systems they need to access
- ☐ Provide an overview of the intranet; how to navigate the various sections
- ☐ Conduct a basic ergonomic checklist
- ☐ How and when to use Voicemail and Out of Office Assistant

In a separate step, give your new staff member a booklet which summarizes all this information, together with key phone numbers, room/lab numbers, email addresses and, if you have one, a map.

2.4 Involving Volunteers

Beryl and Marjory were faithful volunteers who came every week and would turn a hand to anything they were asked to do. They treated their volunteering like a job and would be there on the dot on the appointed day. Woe betide you if there was nothing for them to do. They had to be treated with respect. If there was actually nothing to do, they were given the day off!

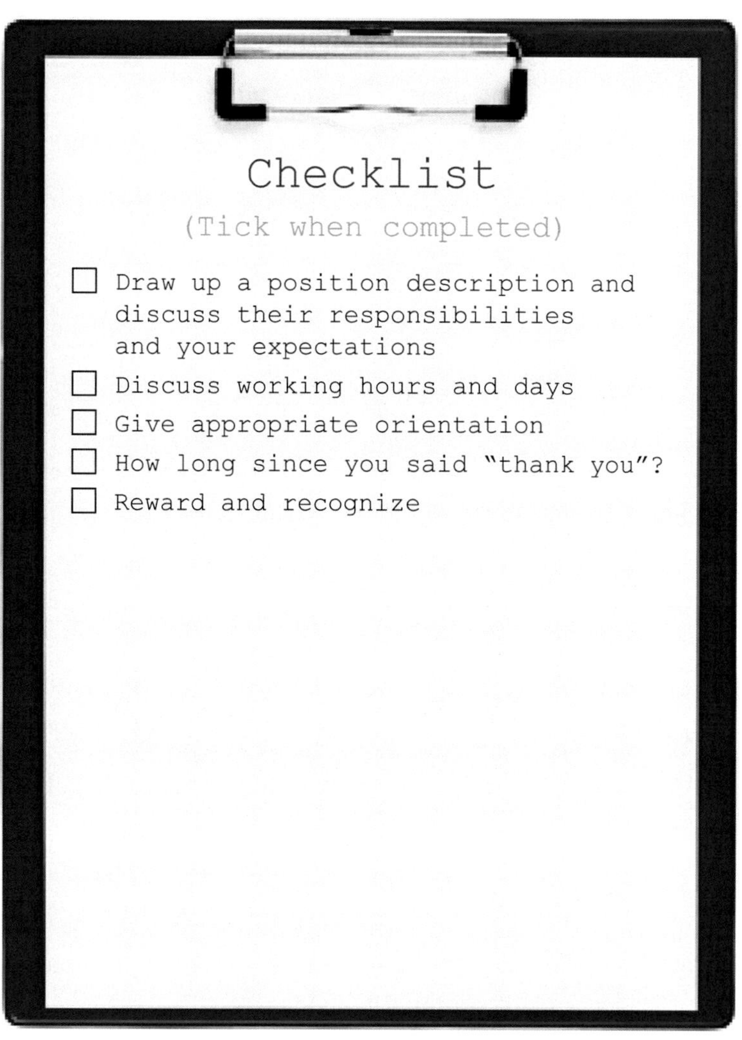

② BUILDING YOUR TEAM

Involving volunteers is a great way to increase the size of your project team at a minimal cost. Volunteers, however, are not staff members and must not be treated in the same way as staff members.

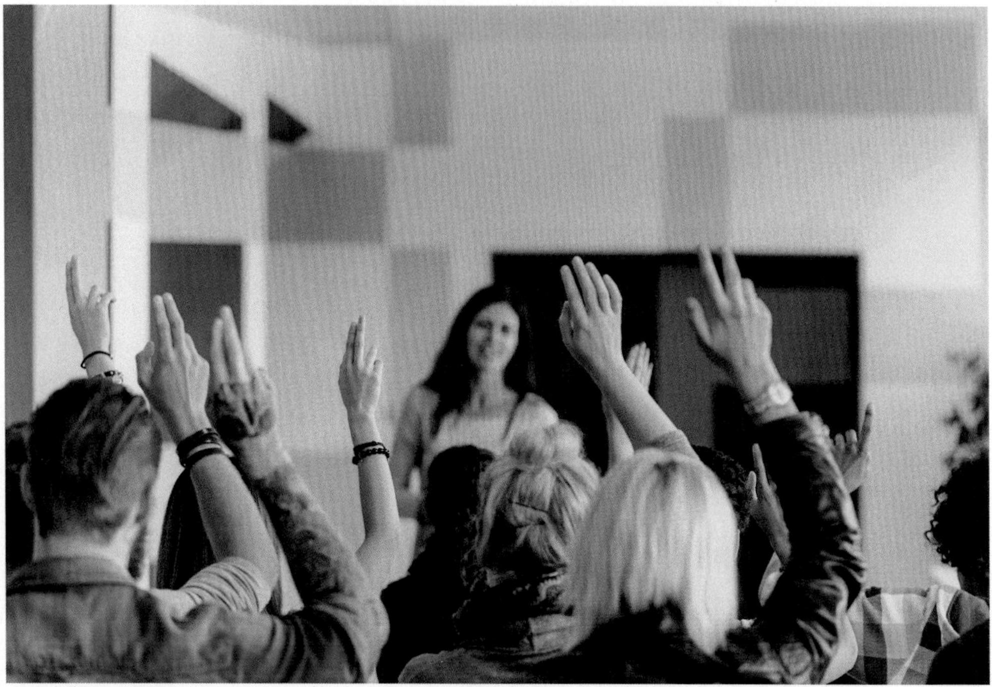

Image Credit: Voting on seminar by izusek/iStock

In best practice your volunteers must

- not take a staff position
- not work full-time
- be treated with respect
- be afforded the same work health and safety conditions as staff, and
- be offered appropriate opportunities for personal development.

In short, you must look after them and not take unfair advantage of them.

Volunteers can provide a fantastic resource. If you are lucky enough to attract skilled volunteers they might be happy to come to your workplace once or twice a week and perform a range of regular tasks, thus contributing enormously to the productivity of your project. Other volunteers might be able to assist with less frequent routine tasks or help with one-off unskilled jobs.

The key is giving the volunteers defined tasks and precise expectations to encourage them to treat their work for you as seriously as they would a paid job. It is best practice to interview people for your "permanent" volunteer positions, provide a job description, explain your expectations, and have an annual review. You should offer appropriate training, while also explaining that with this training comes an expectation that they will stay with you for a period. In short, you should treat them with the same overall processes and courtesies as you would a person in a paid position.

> Any organization which uses the services of volunteers must ensure that those volunteers are managed within a well-defined system and by capable staff who have the authority and resources to look after them appropriately. [1].

Typical volunteer tasks can include the following:

- Data entry
- Literature searches
- Writing routine letters
- Routine management of study participants
- Preparing routine mailings

Remember that if aspects of your project or the work your volunteers will be involved with are confidential, ask them to sign a confidentiality form.

Ways to Attract Pro Bono Help

You will find the best volunteers when you search for people in situations where both parties are advantaged. This might include the following:

- Employees of big companies where they need to fulfill corporate social responsibility needs, where the company wishes to be seen to be doing good for the world at large. These companies often offer their staff the opportunity to perform volunteer work in a field of interest to them during paid work time.
- Expert volunteers who have recently retired from the workforce and who would like to offer the benefit of their years of experience.

- Final year university students seeking unpaid intern positions or students who have formed groups wanting to provide free "management consultant" advice to broaden their experience before they reach the workforce.
- Students considering a career in research.

Offer to provide a reference for anyone who may be using this experience with you to assist them to get a paid position in the workforce.

You must remember, of course, that volunteering is voluntary and experience will demonstrate that you often can't rely on a volunteer quite as much as on a person with a paid position. You can expect that other calls on their time such as family needs might, quite reasonably, take priority.

Look after your volunteers well, and you will be amazed how advantageous the relationship is to both sides.

References—Volunteers

[1] Volunteering Australia National Standards for involving-volunteers in not-for-profit organizations. https://volunteeringaustralia.org/wp-content/uploads/VA-National-Standards-for-involving-volunteers-in-not-for-profit-organisations.pdf.

Further Reading

501 Commons Volunteer Management Guide. https://www.501commons.org/resources/tools-and-best-practices/volunteer-management.

Volunteer Now Ireland. http://www.volunteernow.co.uk/.

2.5 Managing Students

Students are part of the fabric of the research environment. You were one once, after all. Part of your career progress will involve supervising students, being a good mentor and, with luck, you will mutually benefit from the outcomes. Remember that your student's success or failure will reflect on your institution as well as you.

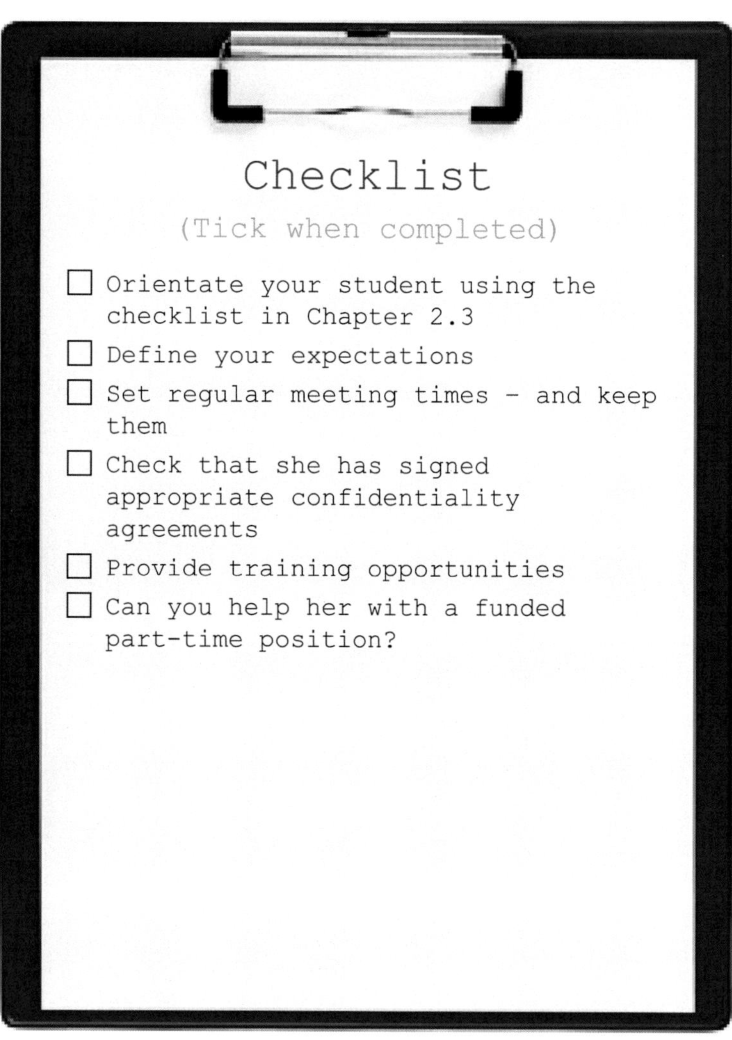

Day to Day Student Management

Taking on students is a serious responsibility. There are considerable supervisory obligations. You must treat them as you would a member of staff—seriously. It is up to you to see your student through to the end.

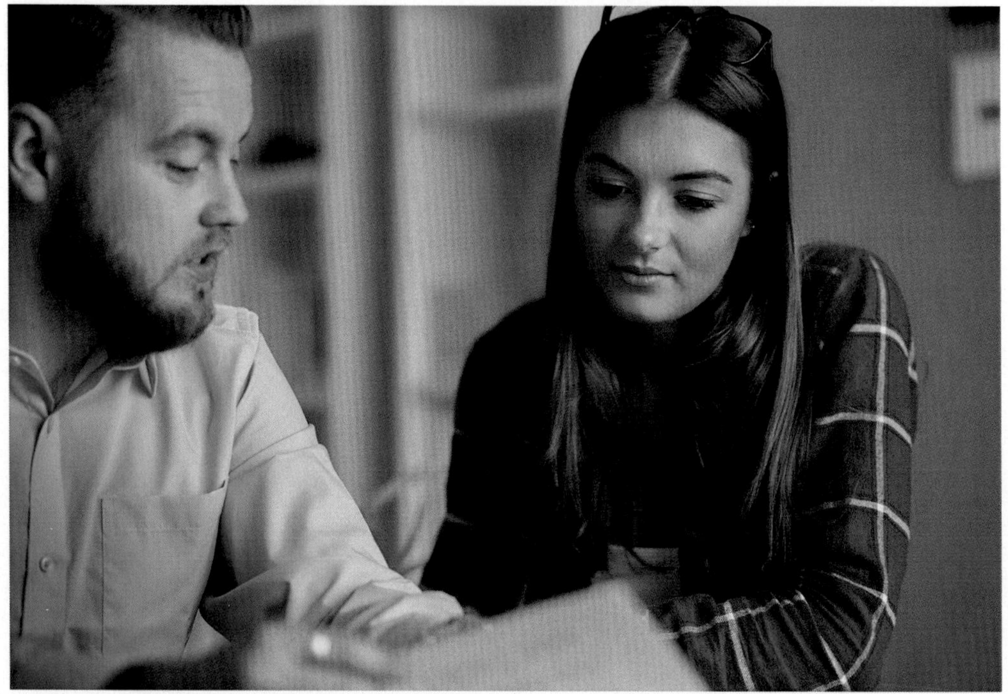

Image Credit: Teacher and student by sturti/iStock

Take time to explain your expectations and learn about those of the student just as you would for a staff member.

Set your ground rules early. Make regular appointments to catch up, and keep them.

Ensure that your students are keeping appropriate records so that their research can be validated and intellectual property (IP) can be claimed. Check these records regularly.

You must all understand your rights and responsibilities from the start. This will include you teaching your students good governance in research. Your students will need to be aware of the relevant codes of conduct, as well as how to comply with the institution's requirements for legal and safety compliance. Right at the beginning, you must discuss any need for approvals relating to human or animal ethics; formal safety training or training for use of equipment.

The Future Leaders Research Program [1] lists the following items, many of which are matters may need to be considered for the typical research project:

- Human ethics approval
- Animal ethics approval
- Gene technology approval
- Biosafety approval
- Import approval for material
- Licenses to access certain areas
- Licenses to use certain materials
- Permissions from government agencies or communities

A student's research may also involve the following:

- Native flora and fauna
- Historical or cultural artifacts
- Travel permits
- Access to premises or regions
- Scheduled poisons
- Scheduled carcinogens
- Radiation sources

You should assume your students may not think about any of these matters without prompting from you. Whether or not they do, as their supervisor, it is *you* who is responsible for getting the permissions right.

You must remember that your students are not employees of your institution or university and are therefore not bound by the same agreements for either privacy and confidentiality or IP as your staff. Before they start with you, you must check that the students have signed the appropriate privacy and confidentiality agreement to protect both your project data and their IP. This sort of agreement might form part of the university's usual procedures, or you may need to contact your legal or HR office for the correct form. See the section in Chapter 4.6 on IP as it relates to students.

2 BUILDING YOUR TEAM

During her first days, orientate your student to your team and your institution. You are likely to be working together for at least three years so it is in your interests to make the time as productive as possible. The time taken to mentor your students will be well rewarded.

Later, introduce your student to your colleagues in your network. Just as with your staff, you should provide opportunities for her to attend meetings where she can start to form her own network as well as learning new information about your field.

Your management plan should include regular progress meetings with your student who should always be treated as part of the team and have the same involvement in team meetings as employed staff.

Watch out for signs of stress or struggle in your students. It is not uncommon for a student to be way overcommitted, trying to balance the need to complete her research with earning some money, and maybe even having fun. They are usually young, after all. As well as striking troubles with their research, students often struggle with sleep deprivation, financial worries, and associated personal difficulties. If you think you see signs of trouble, take the time to quietly and confidentially make inquiries. If it is something you can help with, start sooner rather than later. If not, direct your student to the right place.

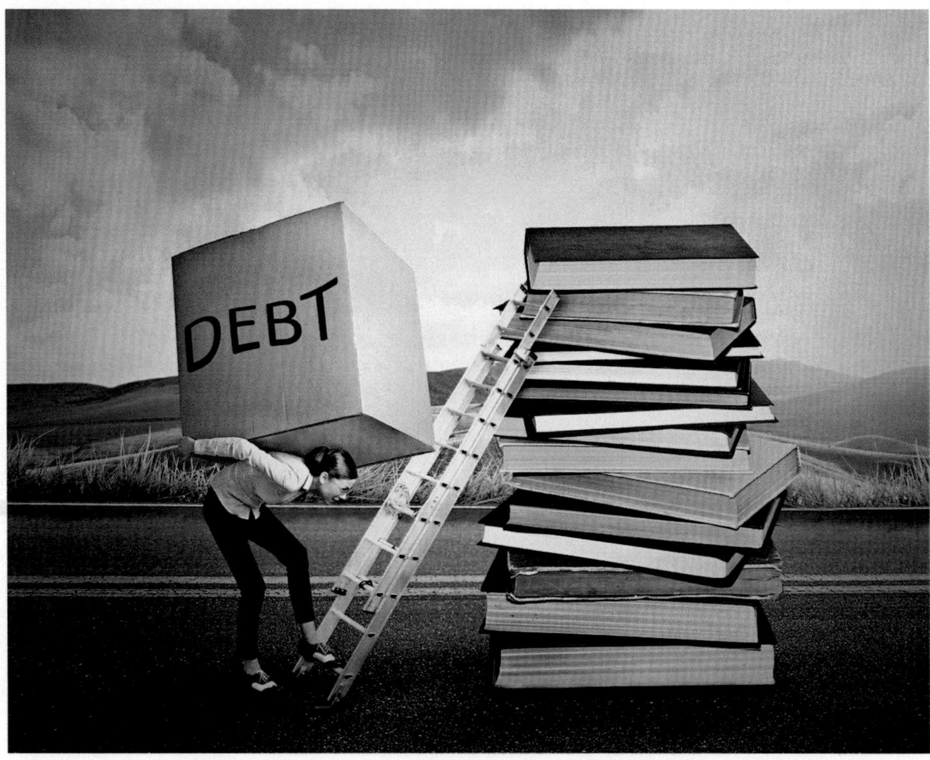

Image Credit: Student loan debt concept by Siphotography/iStock

Note that students on PhD or Masters scholarships who are working as part of your research project will have specific reporting requirements—to the university, and sometimes to an external funding agency, if the scholarship is externally funded. Help make sure these requirements are met.

Provide Training Opportunities

Your students are *not* research slaves to do your bidding. While your PhD students can and will generate data that will be used in your publications, the students are there to learn and to contribute knowledge to your mutual field. Your students are research trainees, and you must see that they are trained. Allow your students to take the opportunities offered by the university and encourage attendance at personal and career development courses. Make them read this book!

Provide Funding for Your Students

You may wish to plan your grant applications to include funding for Honors or PhD students. This provides a win-win situation. The scope of the project can be extended at minimal cost (but with the cost of your supervisory time). Your student gets to be part of a larger project which is good for building a track record. At the same time her work can contribute to the project's publications. Take care if there are special confidentiality or IP obligations to the funding body. You must ensure that the student is able to have her thesis marked and her research published. Note that in many countries students automatically own their IP unless it is formally assigned to the institution. Seek advice from your legal office concerning student IP issues if this could cause difficulties.

If you have included students in your grant proposal, you will have identified the training that is to be provided to the students involved in the project and may have nominated the supervisors. It is important that suitably qualified supervisors are available to guide and advise the students for the duration of the grant/degree. If the original supervisors are no longer available, you must find appropriate replacements.

Note that payment of a student's stipend may not be able to commence until all agreements or contracts are fully executed, and sometimes this involves a considerable delay. If you have a particular student in your sights, make sure you keep her up-to-date about any delays and her likely start dates. If there is other funding available, it might be possible to start the student before the grant documents are signed; however, if you do that it is possible that you will be unable to use the grant funding to reimburse the payments made from elsewhere.

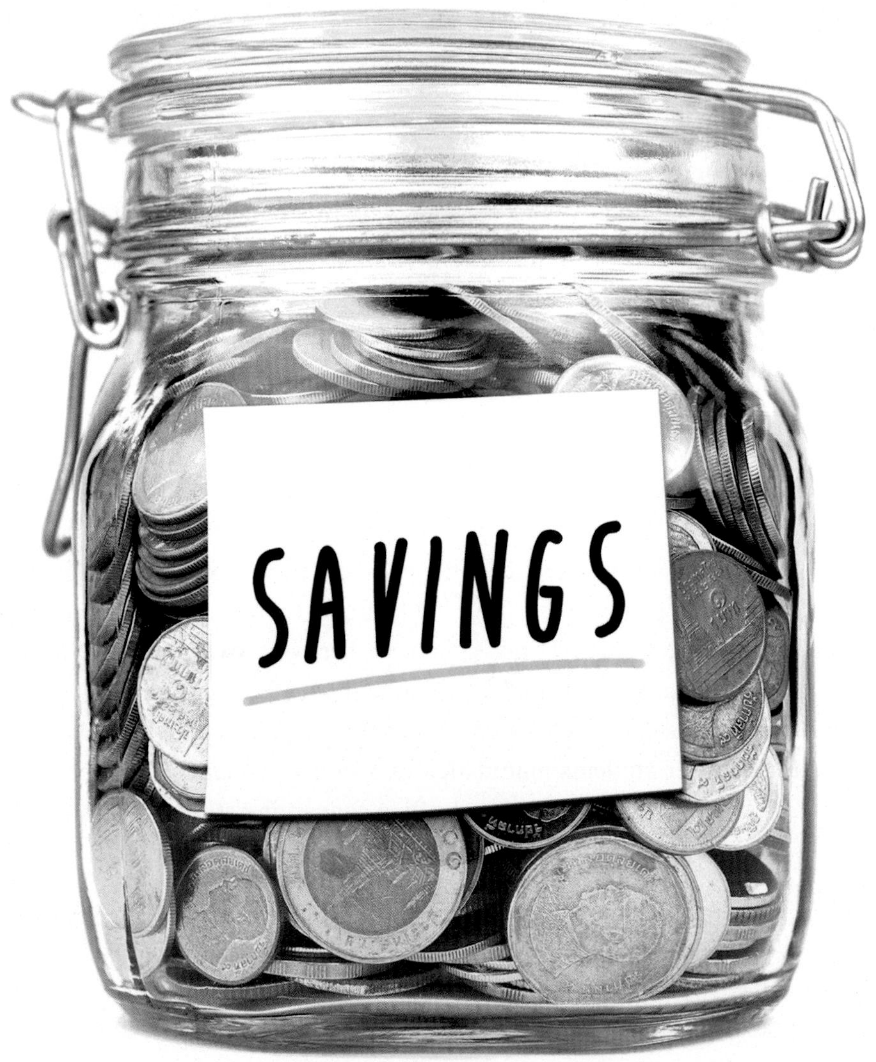

Image Credit: Stack of coins in money box by Component/Shutterstock

Alternative Ways to Provide Student Funding

If you do not have grant funding for a PhD student's stipend, you might be fortunate to be able to attract a self-funded student or someone with a scholarship to join your project because they are interested in your research. Be sure to promote possible topics or research areas of interest for higher degree students on your project's web page. Include your research areas of interest on your own profile page, and indicate you are willing to consider student supervision. Some universities have special websites which act as a dating agency to match students and supervisors, such as University of Sydney's Research Supervisor Connect [2].

It is sometimes possible to provide a student's stipend by means of a scholarship funded by a specific philanthropic donation. This scholarship for this position must be a true scholarship, awarded competitively. The donation will need to be channeled through the university's scholarship office with an undertaking to fund the whole term of the scholarship, although funding is usually only required one year at a time.

In many countries there are student fees for a PhD; in some there is no charge. Whichever the case, be aware that the student still needs money to live. It is usually better for the students to receive a tax-free PhD stipend than to receive a salary. If they have a strong enough track record, they might be able to attract a university or publicly funded scholarship, but sometimes it might take a couple of years of higher degree research before they are successful in obtaining this funding.

Manage Your Student's Needs and Expectations

Higher Degree Research students are usually working on a project to generate research results which will be useful for their thesis. Inevitably they have a schedule to meet, and the university has obligations to provide them with appropriate supervision. Your role as supervisor includes ensuring they receive support and that your project plan's timing takes their needs into account. It is also important they get the opportunity to gain proper recognition of their efforts through the publication of papers, since this is the key to developing their track record.

Make sure you provide your students with enough challenges by setting them open-ended tasks where they can choose a direction rather than just giving them predictable and repetitious chores.

Do remember that many students need to balance their studies with paid work to support them financially. This may put a constraint on their flexibility, and the conflicting demands of the project and their outside employer may cause stress. If paid work is available within your institution, it can greatly help reduce the pressure. An even better scenario can be providing some paid work within your project.

References—Managing Students

[1] Future Leaders Research Program. http://www.frlp.edu.au/.
[2] Research Supervisor Connect. http://sydney.edu.au/research-opportunities.shtml.

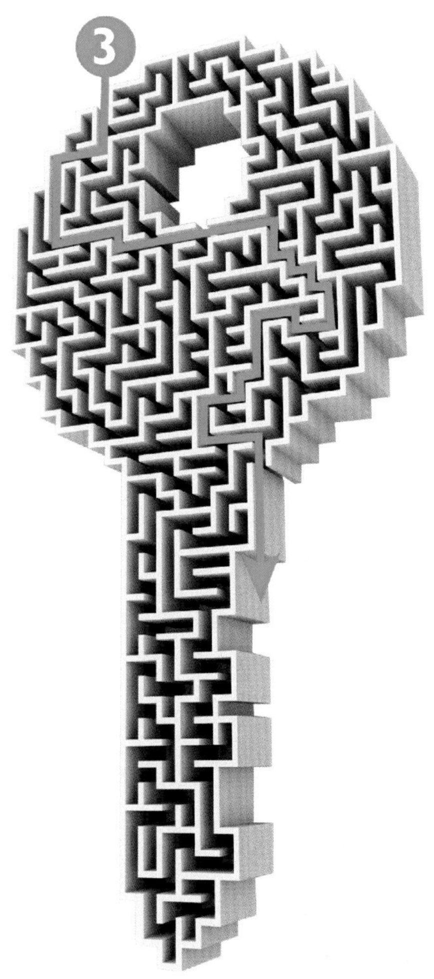

Collaboration drives innovation. It matters. Successful collaborations will underpin your career.

3.1 Finding the Right Collaborators

Post-doc Jessie was proud to be able to tell people she had established a collaboration with Professor BigWig. Sadly, it wasn't all plain sailing. She wondered if Professor BigWig had only agreed to be part of the team so his post-doc could use her institution's equipment. Milestones were being missed and he wasn't answering her phone calls or emails. People told her this was how he always behaved. She didn't know what to do…. If only she had done some more research about him before she asked him to work with her.

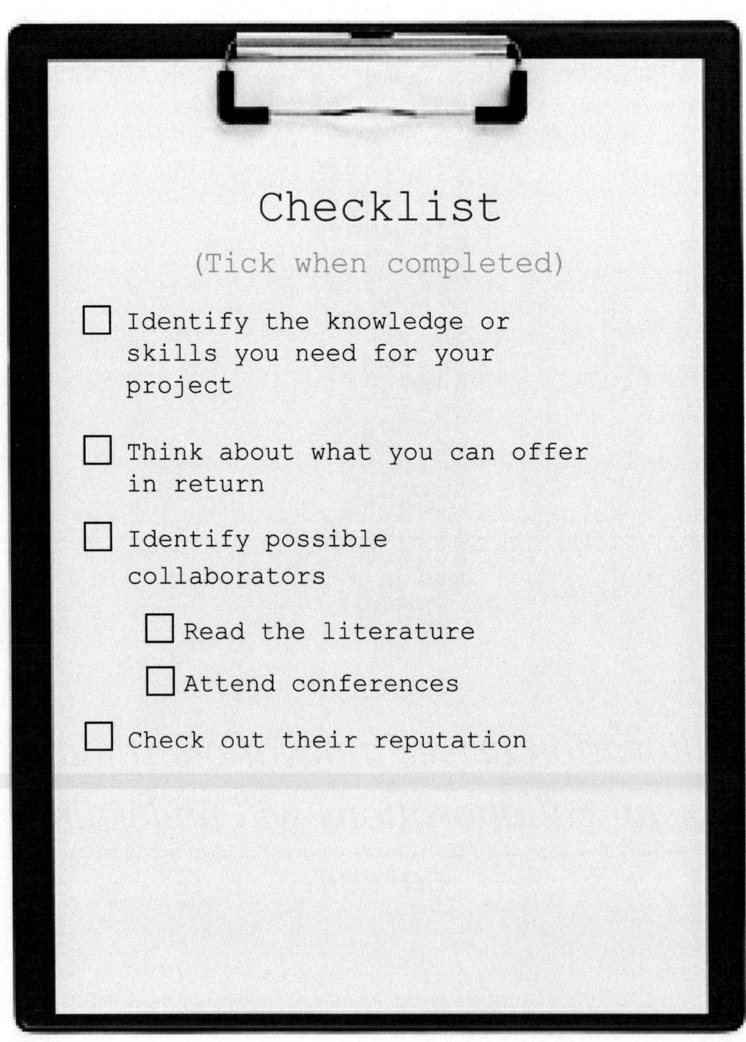

There has been enormous progress in collaborative research in the past couple of decades. This has been facilitated first by the fax machine, then cheap long-distance phone calls, followed by the ubiquitous and accessible internet and email and open document sharing. It is now entirely possible to collaborate effectively with someone on the other side of the world.

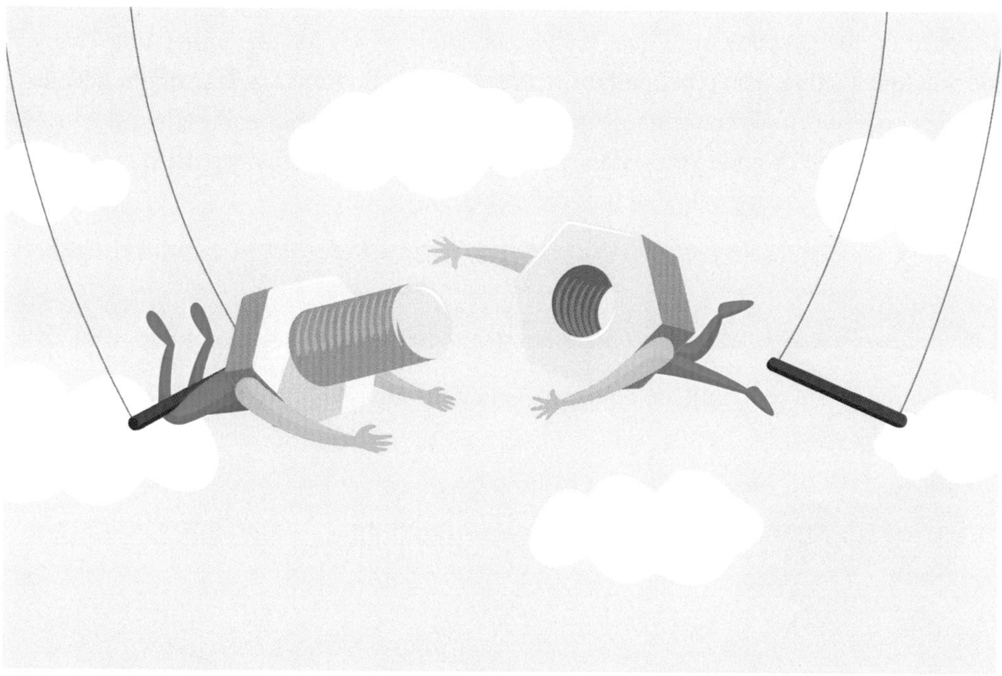

Image Credit: Nut and screw jumping on flying trapeze by CurvaBezier/iStock

There are two very valuable things to understand about collaborations:

- They must provide a two-way partnership. The value might not be equal, particularly when there is a very senior collaborator involved, but it must be a win-win situation for all parties or it is simply not reasonable.
- Communication is key. In each collaboration it must be clear to all partners who is doing what and why.

Some people like to work with a wide network of collaborators. Others stick with a favorite few. There are no hard and fast rules. You should aim to build collaborations with people who help you fill a gap in your knowledge or in your team. These people may be from within your usual or local network, but you might choose to look more widely. There can be great benefit in looking outside your network for your collaborators as they might bring an entirely new approach.

3 COLLABORATIONS

The process of finding collaborators is similar to that of finding mentors. Keep your eyes open, ask questions, read the literature to see who is doing what in your field, and quietly identify people who would be suitable.

Endeavor to form your partnerships with people or organizations which will be better off with you than without you. It sounds obvious, but you'd be surprised how many people try to partner with people based on their reputation alone. If there is nothing in it for the "other side," they won't provide you much value. You must partner with someone who thinks he/she might become more successful as a result of an enterprise with you. When pursuing a collaboration, try to look for collaborators who can provide you with something of value—such as expertise or equipment—and to whom your research group can provide something in return.

> Things always work best when they are for mutual benefit.

At the beginning of the courtship, be ready to explain the advantages to them. Also, be ready with answers about the risks.

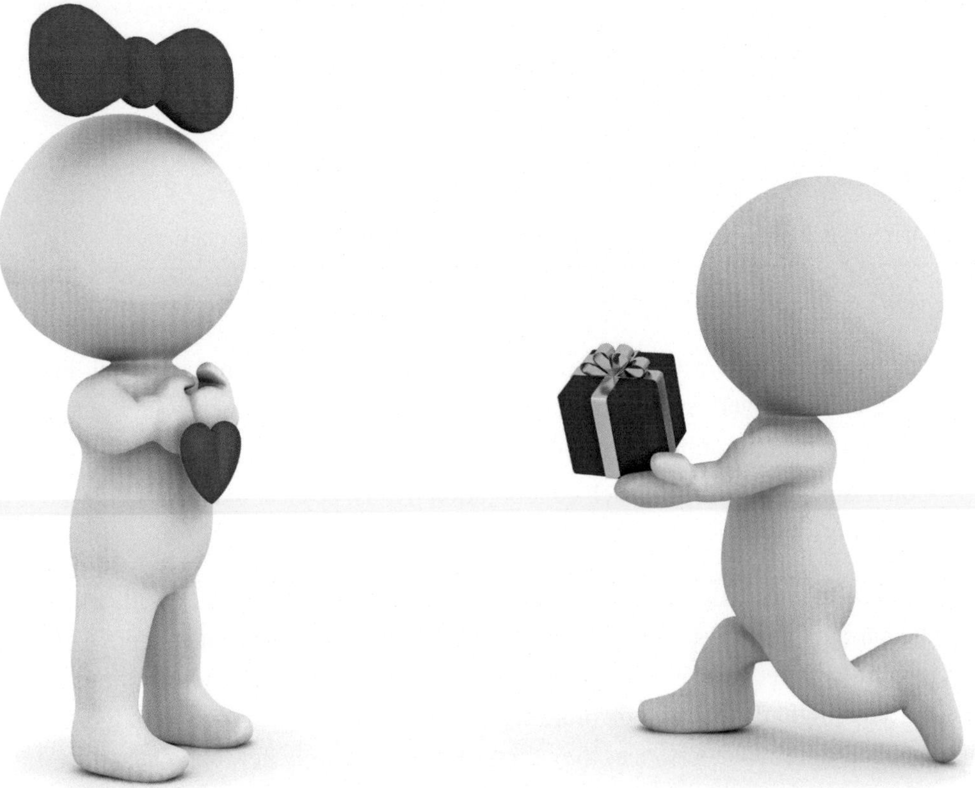

Image Credit: Offering a gift box by Lucian3D/iStock

Early in your career, you can aim to form collaborations with others in the same position. They, too, will be looking to grow their networks and enhance their research through collaboration. Your new collaboration stands every chance of becoming very productive and will help you all build your networks inside and outside your institution. Take every opportunity to meet other early-career researchers and chat to them about your mutual interests. You will be surprised how many doors will open.

Who Can I Trust?

It is a great shame, but out there in the wide world you will find that not *everyone* is necessarily on your team. This is a dog-eat-dog world, and realistically, others will mostly be putting their own interests first. Be aware. Forewarned is forearmed.

As mentioned earlier, the best thing to do is to create situations where your success is of mutual benefit to those you are working with. Include members of your team in your ideas; be open with your collaborators; share the successes. This should create an environment where others will want to share back.

So where to begin? Think where you might find appropriate collaborators from within your university. Which faculties does your faculty have synergies with? Where do you know people already? Perhaps you should invite key people to chat over coffee about common research interests.

If you are looking externally, think about which other organizations are interested in your area of research. Check the literature. They all don't have to be your competitors. You might be able to join forces with them and build on work together. Think, too, about who might have funds!

It is always a good idea to chat to your colleagues about where they have found collaborators and listen to any tales of disastrous collaborations. Not only can you avoid these people, but you can also learn from your colleagues about how things went wrong.

A good way of finding contacts in your field is to involve yourself by volunteering to serve on a committee organizing a meeting, or serving a specific research interest group. Volunteer contributions are nearly always welcomed, and this can provide a great way to extend your network.

There is one downside to extending your network of collaborators to be aware of. Once you publish with someone, that person will be unable to review your work for five years.

More Ways to Build Your Network

Do your very best to get out of your "silo," your own work area, and explore research environments outside. This might mean attending events or seminars, not only outside your discipline but also outside your faculty!

Take the opportunities to interact with people from other disciplines. There is great advantage in understanding how other research environments work, and how others conduct their research. At enlightened universities, attendance at cross-disciplinary seminars is encouraged and resulting conversations can be fantastic. Research is a state of mind, not just a job, and there is much to be learned from the ways other people approach their work. Read the UC Davis article [1] which describes how "UC Davis scientists ride the Colorado River to break down jargon and overcome silos" on their now annual trip that brings together "fish people" and "rock people" with huge success.

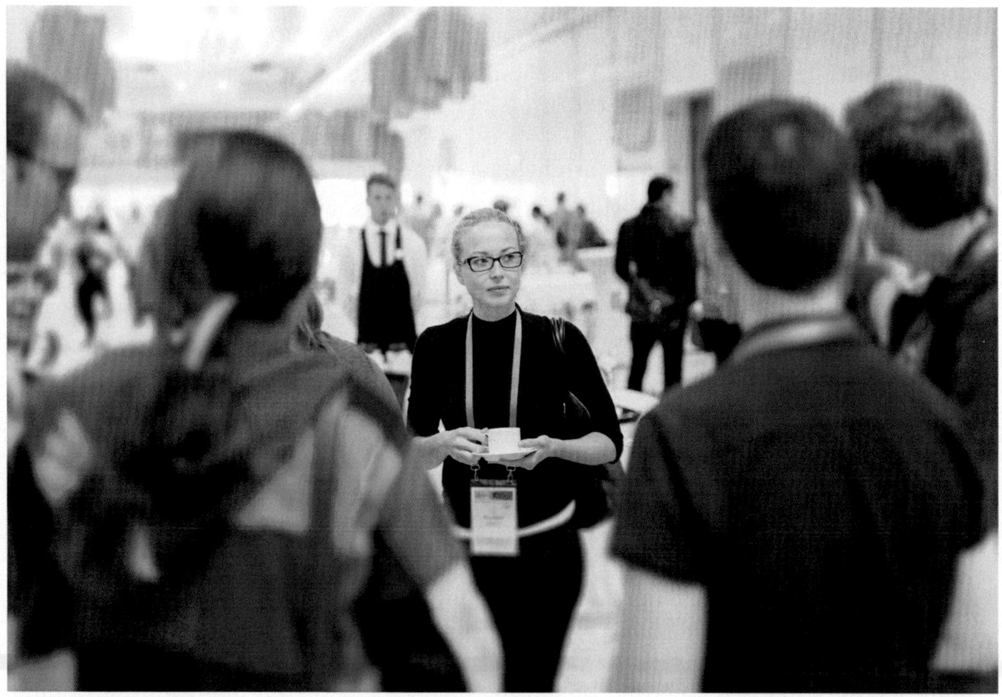

Image Credit: People interacting during coffee break by Matej Kastelic/Shutterstock

Another great way to grow your network is by attending conferences. Hayes [2] recognizes that this can be scary, but it can also be very rewarding. She recommends that while you are at the conference, you take your courage in both hands and attend networking functions. At each one, aim to meet at least two new people.

If there is an opportunity to do so, book in for, and participate at, conference workshops. These smaller and less threatening environments can provide a perfect way to meet people with like interests.

Always take, or create, the opportunity to report on what you have learned when you get home. Preparation of your presentation for your colleagues will help you consolidate your thoughts about what you have learned. You might also pick up a potential collaboration on your home turf.

Collaborations Outside Academia

It is worth noting that there can be useful collaborations between a researcher at a university and a government body or commercial organization. Of necessity, these relationships will be different from a collaboration between researchers at universities.

Collaborations with government may require a great deal of red tape, and the wheels are likely to move very slowly. The government priority will always have to be consideration for the tax payers' money. The plus side, though, is that government can be a very good source of funds and may be looking for a research expert to lead a project. This can lead to a highly successful collaboration for mutual benefit. Opportunities that could open to you might include a consultancy, a placement within government to access equipment or technology, or joint initiatives.

Keep your eyes open for opportunities to collaborate with a commercial organization. Although there is often reluctance for people from an academic or not-for-profit environment to go "to the dark side," your research might well benefit the prospective corporate collaborator, and equally their money, equipment, or technology might benefit you. The fact that the company's first responsibility is to its shareholders doesn't mean that they will not want to conduct research to your mutual benefit. Opportunities might include short-term placement within a company, joint funding bids or joint commercialization of your research.

References—Finding the Right Collaborators

[1] How rafting in the Grand Canyon is creating better scientists. http://www.chronicle.com/paid-article/How-Rafting-in-the-Grand/12.

[2] M. Hayes, An introvert's guide to conference networking. http://postdocexperience.scienceblog.com/2013/08/01/an-introverts-guide-to-conference-networking/.

3.2 Establishing Your Collaborations

A PhD student and his supervisor were burned by his supervisor's new collaborator who provided samples which they analyzed (genotyping many DNA markers) and interpreted. They were dumbfounded when the new collaborator demanded first authorship on the resulting paper, which was based about 90% on their work. This was almost certainly not intentionally malicious; it's just that there was no discussion at the beginning of the relationship.

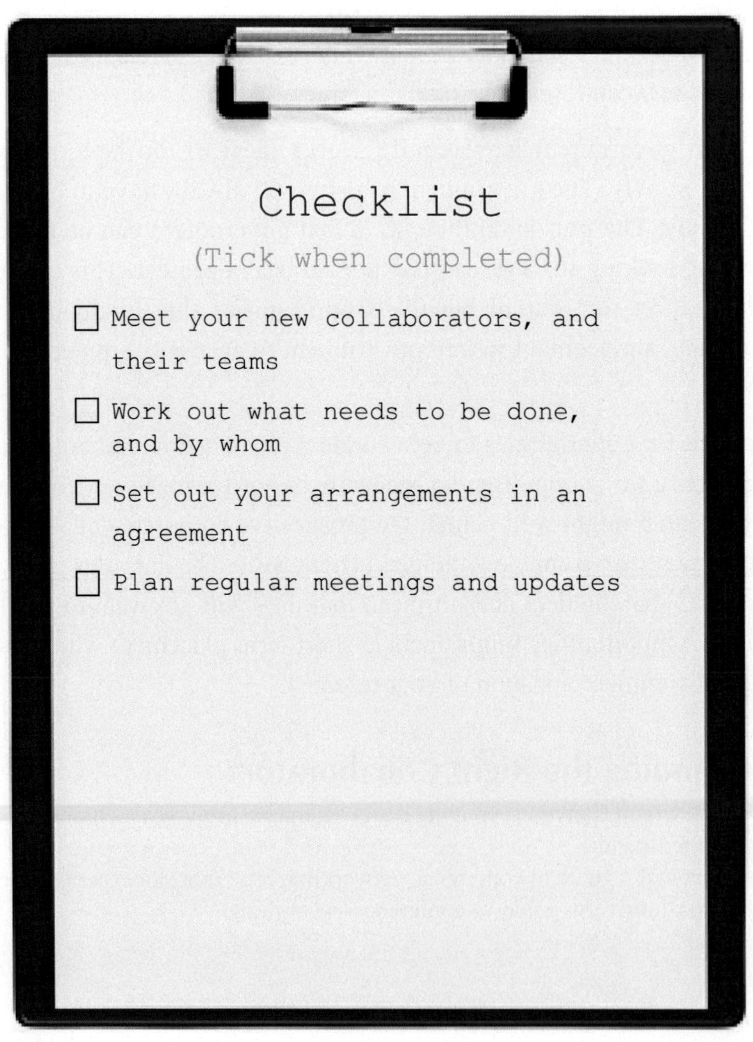

Once you have identified your new or potential collaborator(s), do your best to get to know them and let them understand you.

- Search the collaborator's work
- Exchange CVs
- Find out what they are hoping to achieve from the collaboration

If possible, you should meet face to face. Arrange for them to visit your institute and to meet your team, preferably having them spend some time with you. You want them to be able to understand the nature of your team and the facilities you have (or do not have). You also want your team members to meet the collaborator so they have an understanding of whom they are working with. This all builds trust and understanding and will make it easier to pursue your common goals. Use this time to get to know one another. It is particularly important to work on understanding one another when the two sides come from different backgrounds, say from different countries, or if your partnership is from different worlds, as for a university partnering with a commercial organization.

If you can't meet face to face, have teleconferences. Take your time and involve the team wherever possible.

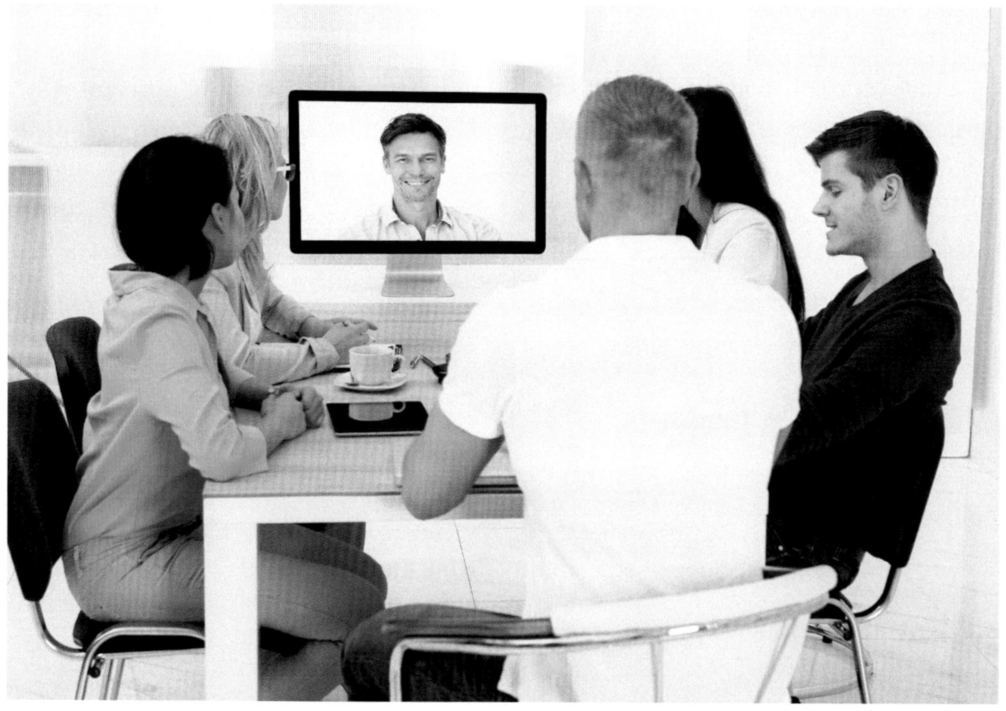

Image Credit: Business team attending video conference by Andrey Popov/Shutterstock

3 COLLABORATIONS

After your preliminary meeting and after every stakeholder meeting, gather your team and discuss the key outcomes. The team members are all part of the collaboration too, and they will contribute valuable perspectives if they have had a chance to really engage with your collaborators.

Above all, allow plenty of time to build your new collaboration. This is particularly important when preparing for a grant application. Many a budding collaboration has been brought into early stress over the documentation required for each investigator. *Do not leave the collection of important information to the last minute.*

As you develop your project's team, have conversations with each collaborator about his/her desired outcomes. Do they need PhD students, equipment, and/or access to data? If the collaborator is from another institution they might be able to offer quite different development opportunities. They might also have quite different needs from you. Make sure your conversations include discussion about the time they will have available to give to your project.

While you are having these conversations, remember to consider and discuss up-front ownership of intellectual property (IP), plans for publication, presentations, authorship, any payments and, where appropriate, material transfer agreements. You all need to be clear about expectations from the beginning. Once it is all worked out, record your decisions in a collaborator agreement (see Chapter 4.3).

Be aware that your collaborator(s) might be used to working in an entirely different way from you, particularly if they are from another country. This difference doesn't matter, as long as you understand one another. The most important characteristic of a successful collaboration is that you work well together. For that to happen, you must share the dream, be aiming for the same goals, and be helpful to one another.

In the long term, collaborations can be further enriched by the exchange of staff, or short-term placements in one another's institutions.

Collaborating for a Project

Application for a joint grant will cement a collaboration and commit the relationship to the research target.

If you are to work on a project together, carefully define the project goals:

- Write the goals down
- Attribute tasks to each team member

- Assign due dates
- Discuss the points above
- Draw up a collaborator agreement (see Chapter 4.3 agreements)

Remember that while the goals of the project team will overlap at times, they will not necessarily be the same for all. Similarly, you will need to be aware that the various stakeholders may value all outputs differently.

Communication in Collaboration

Once the project is underway, you should hold regular meetings and keep minutes.

The world is littered with "broken promises" which were, in fact, merely misunderstandings. Just because *you* know what you mean doesn't mean that the other side understands.

Above all, communicate with your collaborators about your progress. They need to know about your successes and your failures, your time delays and your problems. Remember these are relevant to the other side too.

Marketing and Branding Your Project

You should remember to discuss the marketing of your research and the branding you will use for the project. If this is a multi-institutional collaboration, each of your institutions will probably require its logo to be displayed on presentation materials or media releases. Define a template for your slides and a letterhead or document template for your mutual use. Agree on the wording you will use for acknowledgments. These small steps of recognition can prevent much unnecessary heartache.

Information Exchange

In your planning stages you should discuss *how* information will be exchanged between you and *when*. Identify your processes for collection, storage, and dissemination of information.

Talk about any ethical requirements for the project, remembering that the requirements might be different in different locations or countries. You need to make sure the ethics requirements are adhered to in all locations in a way that will be compliant in the place where the requirements are most stringent.

Intellectual Property in Collaborations

It is most important to have a clear understanding of how the collaboration's IP will be managed and the ways in which ownership and responsibility will be assigned. Your partnership relies on a strong basis of trust and respect for the other individuals as people and as reputable researchers.

3 COLLABORATIONS

Your need to share ideas and contribute to a collective research strategy also requires you all to be willing to operate flexibly and constructively.

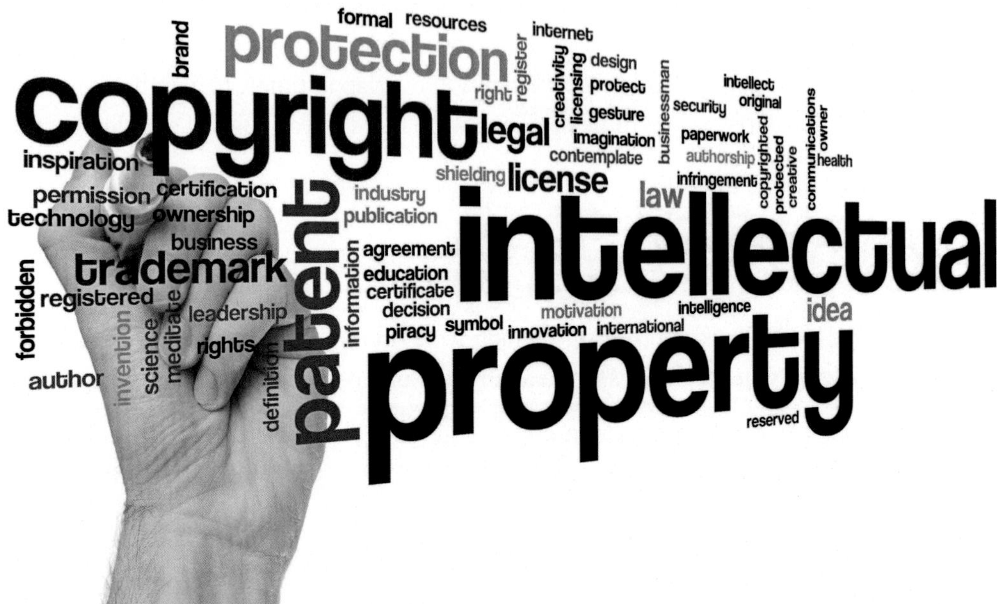

Image Credit: Intellectual property word cloud by ibreakstock/Shutterstock

At the beginning, it is important to consider whether there will be "background intellectual property" (background IP) brought into this collaboration, and whether this is to be recognized as such. In research, background IP would be existing IP, tangible expertise, methodology or data, already developed and owned by one of the collaborators, to be used as a platform for the new project. You must negotiate appropriate guidelines for the use of the background IP as well as for the IP which you will create together in your project.

While it is usual for partners to agree that IP created during a project will be owned and shared equally, someone who is engaged (and paid) as a consultant will not usually be able to claim ownership of the IP they have generated unless this has specifically been included in their consultancy agreement.

It is important to establish the ownership, or otherwise, of the IP generated by any student involved in the project. In many countries the IP generated by a student is owned by the student. In others, it belongs to the university. You must be careful not to permit any restrictions requested by the partners in a collaboration which could make it impossible for a student to publish her thesis (just as you must consider any implications your agreements for publishing your own work).

3.3 Collaborations Over Distance

Project Dynamo was led by Investigator Apple from New York with Investigator Orange in Dublin, Silk in Shanghai, and Devi in Delhi. Project meetings were held by phone, but Apple inevitably set them to suit him. He was Principal Investigator, after all. Too bad that it was always the middle of the night in India. He also failed to notice, or care, that things happened differently in China and India. Nor did he understand how very difficult it was for his international colleagues to get that extra $100,000 in funding he so lightly asked them to source.

Checklist

(Tick when completed)

- [ ] Plan regular meetings by phone and in person
- [ ] Be fair with your meeting times
- [ ] Try to understand cultural differences
- [ ] Check the laws as they apply in each country and make sure you're compliant

3 COLLABORATIONS

One of the biggest changes in research in recent years has been the development of technology which makes it easy to collaborate from afar. Nowadays, instead of relying on the mail, research collaborators who are separated by time and distance rely on many different forms of electronic communications: teleconferencing, electronic brainstorming, group display screens, discussion threads, and internet meetings. "Virtual teams" are a common component of modern research.

In 1994, when virtual teams were really new, Jarvenpaa [1] described a virtual team as one where members (1) physically remain on different continents and in different countries, (2) interact primarily through the use of computer-mediated communication technologies (electronic mail, videoconferencing etc.) and rarely see each other in person. She pointed out then that trust is pivotal in preventing geographical distance from leading to psychological distance in a global team. This remains just as true today.

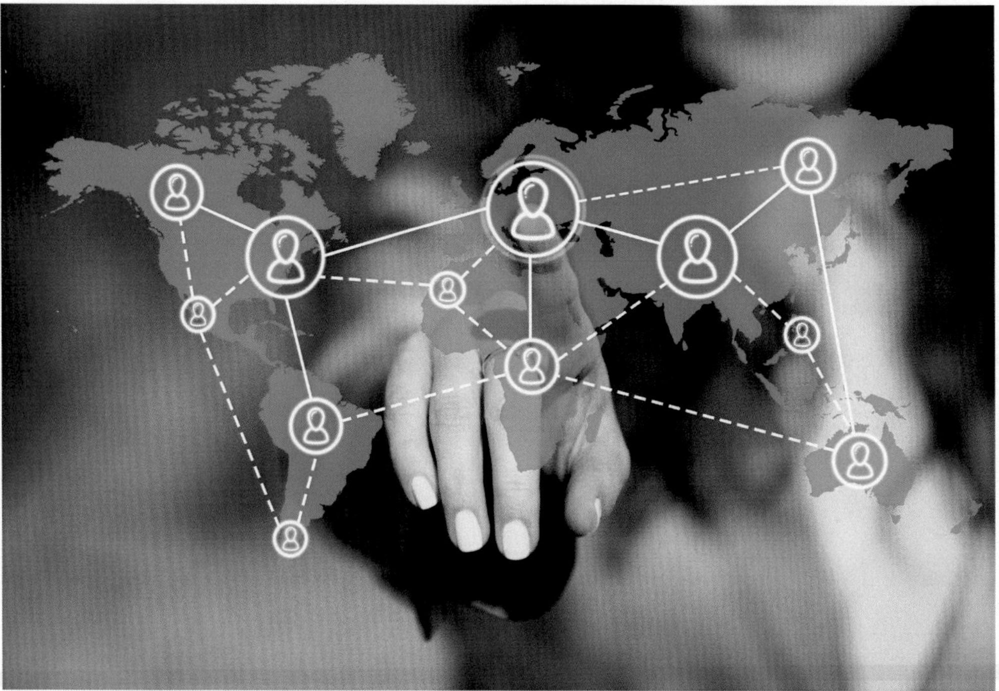

Image Credit: Worldwide team building by FotoCuisinette/iStock

Virtual research teams should maintain regular communication just like any "normal" team. You should set up scheduled meetings to ensure both accountability and the maintenance of group cohesion. Your team members will rely on these meetings to share issues, discuss decisions and their implications, and explore new ideas.

Trust in each other is always necessary for successful collaboration and can be especially difficult to build when people are elsewhere. You should understand that it is all too easy to misconstrue one another's intentions and actions when you are not meeting face to face.

Although essentially aiming his article at virtual teams in a corporate scenario, Reiche [2] provides ten tips on managing virtual teams which are just as applicable for a research collaboration. Those that particularly relate to research, and have not been covered already include the following:

- Be available—something easily overlooked when you are across the world
- Encourage informal conversations
- Where practical, organize visits for team members to the other locations
- Treat time zones fairly; don't expect the people in the "other" time zone to take the night call every time

Strong leadership is always needed to maintain virtual team cohesion. Virtual research teams require particularly strong and involved leadership to ensure their connectedness across the electronic divide. Team members need to develop a proper sense of themselves as part of this scattered team and must come to know the other members as individual people. Sharing regular project updates and regularly reviewing your agreed commitments in your team meetings will remind everyone where their piece fits in the puzzle.

From the beginning, try to set up protocols for your meetings (especially when your meetings are by phone, not videoconferences). Set an agenda, just as you would do for a face-to-face meeting, and appoint a chair. Establish practices that make life easy for everyone, such as asking people to state their names when they start to speak. It can be helpful, too, to ask people to clarify their understanding of points made.

You can set protocols, too, for "discussion" via written communication, (usually email), such as determining the time by which a response should be expected.

In all cases, keep in mind that words, whether written or spoken, often have different nuances in different cultures.

Last, you should aim to recognize and reward performance just as you would in a locally based team.

Issues and Concerns in International Research Collaborations

International research collaborations can be as rewarding as any other collaboration, but they can come with some special difficulties in addition to those caused by the tyranny of distance. The European Association of Research Managers and Administrators [3] has identified the following issues and concerns in international research collaborations which you should be aware of.

Cultural Differences

As mentioned above, differences in culture can cause unintentional but significant challenges for international research collaborations. These differences may include "normal" acceptable behaviors or differences in ethical standards.

Differences in Ethical Standards

Differences in ethical standards may be a result of either cultural or economic differences. What you see as "standards" for the protection of research participants, for example, or the "proper care and use" of animals may be completely different, or indeed not even thought about, in another country. You must balance the requirements for complying with internationally accepted ethical concerns along with an understanding of local customs.

Responsible Conduct of Research

It is essential to maintain public confidence in academic research, wherever it is carried out. Public confidence in research can be diminished when people think that it might be biased or influenced by financial, political, or other pressures. You need to lead by example and also train your colleagues in the accepted practices of responsible research to the highest international standards.

Intellectual Property

There is no common international approach to the protection of IP, despite efforts to develop one. Be aware that there are some countries where IP protection is either questioned or simply ignored.

Liability and Insurance

You would already be aware that the different laws between states or provinces *within* a country can provide challenges for legal matters or insurance. The difficulties can be much worse across borders.

Research Integrity

As discussed in Chapter 8.1, there are many challenges in setting rules for defining, investigating, or prosecuting cases of scientific misconduct. There can also be similar difficulties in dealing with instances of questionable practices of data manipulation or fabrication.

Safety and Security

You need to think about your team's personal safety and security if you are conducting research in locations where there is social or political instability or where there could be the possibility of natural disasters. Don't leave them to work it out for themselves. This is your responsibility too!

Currency and Other Financial Issues

Currency differences and other financial issues can impact international research projects all too readily. Early in your project you should specify which currency will be the basis for payments, so you can try to manage the impact of changes in the exchange rate.

Export Controls

Many countries are sensitive about the transfer of knowledge and technology. Needless to say, this issue has implications for international research.

Contract Law

You should make sure that you and all your collaborators understand which laws apply to your contracts and agreements, and how they should be interpreted. Similarly, make sure you are aware which country's laws apply in the event of any difficulties.

References—Collaborations Over Distance

[1] Jarvenpaa, S.L., Leidner, D.E., 1998. Communication and trust in global virtual teams. Journal of Computer-Mediated Communication 3, 0. https://doi.org/10.1111/j.1083-6101.1998.tb00080.x.

[2] Prof. Sebastian Reiche, Professor of Managing People in Organizations at IESE Business School, Forbes. https://www.forbes.com/sites/iese/2013/06/20/managing-virtual-teams-ten-tips/#1923d3d4198b.

[3] European Association of Research Managers and Administrators. www.earma.org/.

Further Information

Further information about international collaborative research is available from the European University Association (developed to deal with collaborations between European industry and European publicly funded research institutes), including general information that can be applied to all collaborative research projects.

Responsible Partnering. Joining Forces in a World of Open Innovation: for Collaborative Research and Knowledge Transfer between Science and Industry http://www.eua.be/Libraries/Publications_homepage_list/Responsible_Partnering_Guidelines_09.sflb.ashx.

Further Reading Could Include:

Barnes, T.A., Pashby, I.R., and Gibbons, A.M. Managing collaborative R&D projects: development of a practical management tool. International Journal of Project Management 24 (2006) 395–404. http://www.sciencedirect.com/science/article/pii/S0263786306000482.

Background to Intellectual Property, including global IP rights on the IP Australia website https://www.ipaustralia.gov.au/understanding-ip.

The GUIRR International Research Collaborations Project: towards a greater understanding of international collaboration http://www.udayton.edu/law/_resources/documents/law_review/the_guirr_international_research_collaborations_project.pdf.

Online Ethics Centre Collaborative Research between Scientists and Industry/University Collaborators Bibliography http://www.onlineethics.org/Resources/Bibliographies/CollaborativeResearchBib.aspx.

4 RUNNING THE STUDIES

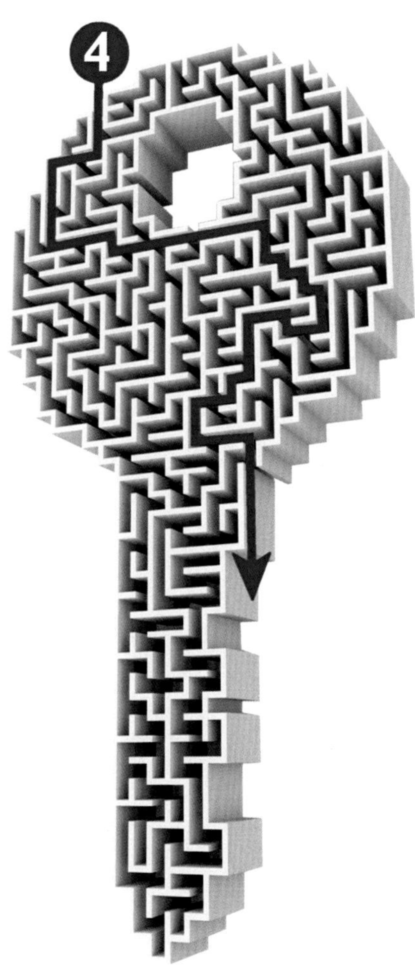

4 RUNNING THE STUDIES

4.1 Elements of Project Planning

Mike the inventor had a dream to develop a cattle handling system that made use of electronic ear tags, telemetry, and solar power. Great idea. Great idea, too, to incorporate weighing, yarding the cattle based on that weight, tracking the water the animals drank when they came into the yards—and much, much more.

The trouble was that Mike couldn't get one idea finished before he went on to the next. Instead of demonstrating one idea to his stakeholders, and keeping the clever extension ideas for later, he tried a bit of this and a bit of that and never got anything quite to the end. The ideas were still good, but he had nothing absolutely perfect to demonstrate and nothing either to show for the many thousands of dollars that had been invested in his ideas.

The design developments were perfectly reasonable changes, but they all led to delays and then the grant ran out.

To make matters worse, Mike only kept the very sketchiest records.

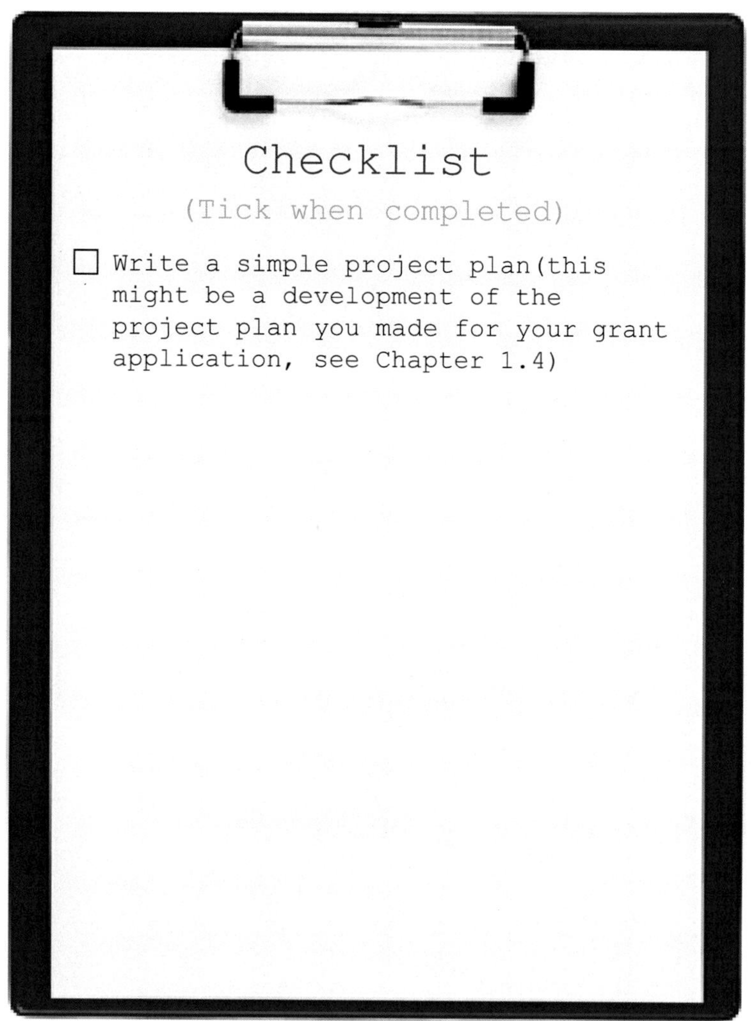
Checklist
(Tick when completed)
☐ Write a simple project plan(this might be a development of the project plan you made for your grant application, see Chapter 1.4)

❹ RUNNING THE STUDIES

You have your funding and you have at least the promise of project staff. Now you need to work out *what* is going to happen, *how* it is going to happen, and *when* it is going to happen during the life of your project.

You will reap the rewards of good project planning just as you will have benefitted from planning well for your grant application. This good planning takes time but will save a lot of heartache on the way.

Project planning is simple, really. Start with your goal, consider the steps you need to take to reach it, and work out how much time you need for each step. Some steps can be done in parallel and some need to precede others.

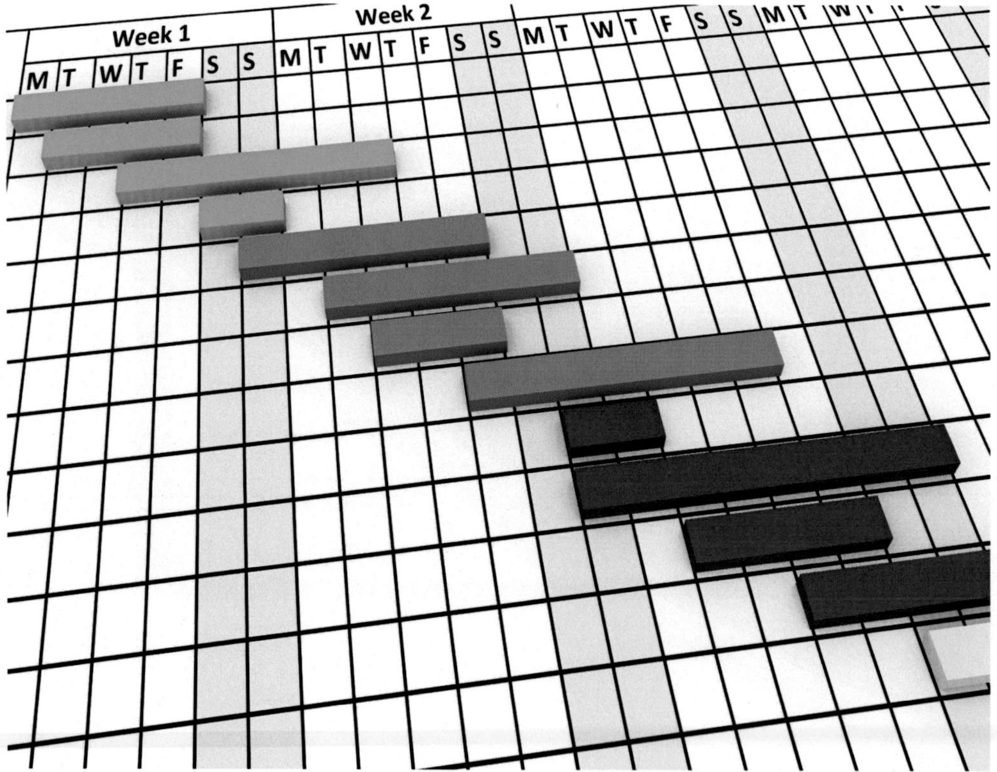

Image Credit: Closeup of gantt progress chart of project by nasirkhan/Shutterstock

First Steps for Project Planning

- Break the project into definable and logical phases or streams
- Break the phases into identifiable tasks
- Understand the order in which the tasks need to occur, including the following:
    - Predecessors, the task that the successor is dependent on
    - Successors, the task whose start or finish depends on another task
    - Time lags between tasks
- Work out how long each of the tasks will take, calculating a start date, end date, and duration
- Identify your milestones, i.e., key events in the project
- Work out who is doing each task (and their cost, if applicable)

Your first plan should focus on the tasks and timeframes, rather than on your deadline. If you see that you aren't going to make the deadline, you will need to go back to the tasks to make adjustments to the steps leading up to it.

You can see that during your planning phase, you must think about the timing and management of a very big list of tasks, while mapping out who will have responsibility for doing what and when. The list of actions in Table 4.1.1 covers some of the many, many *initial* steps, roughly in chronological order, which need to be considered and built into your project plan. They all take time and all that time needs to be factored into the project's time period. All this must be managed inside the available funding.

This phase of the planning might identify the need for a pilot study for proof of concept. A pilot study can rapidly identify weaknesses in your plan, and ultimately save a lot of time and money.

Before you embark on the detailed project planning, you should consider the roles you have available and the responsibilities that go with them. Now is the time to plan to plug any gaps.

When you are fine-tuning your project plan, focus on doing everything you can to achieve early results. You will be amazed how quickly a typical three-year project grant flies by. If you can manage to carry out your research in the first year, then you will have the subsequent years to write up and fine-tune. You can also use these early results as the justification for further grant applications.

TABLE 4.1.1 List for Project Planning
Development of any agreements between stakeholders
Development of study protocols
Refinement of objectives
Staff recruitment
Managing the budget
Obtaining suitable infrastructure for the staff—desks, computers, and laboratory space
Student recruitment and funding
Ethics applications
Requirements for compliance—for the funding body or the university
Requirements for compliance—for example, for using dangerous chemicals or approval to use animals in research
Completion of legal documentation, including approval of agreements
Establishment of a steering committee, if required, and nomination of a chair
Appointment of consumer advisers, if required
Staff training
Consumables procurement
Equipment procurement
Identification of external service providers
Management of team meetings and other collaborator management
Risk management
Reporting
Stakeholder communication planning
Setting up a website
Conference attendance and other networking opportunities
Publication planning
Commercialization opportunities (if relevant)
Applications for further funding—and so the cycle goes on

It takes roughly a year to submit a grant application and receive an answer. If you can submit an application for further funding, which includes your results at the beginning of the third year, you may be fortunate to receive a grant to allow the project to flow on smoothly from the beginning of the fourth year, thus keeping up your momentum and maybe even keeping your team together.

Aim to get your papers published within the three-year period. This takes enormous energy and discipline but is the key to success, particularly early in your career. You will be judged by your track record, and this is the way to build it.

Experienced researchers warn that where research is concerned, it's always later than you think!

More About Project Management

The PMBOK model (Project Management Body of Knowledge) [1] represents best practice for project management. PMBOK recommends use of a basic framework made up of four distinct development phases—design, planning, implementation, and closeout—and nine knowledge areas that require planning and control across those four phases.

The nine PMBOK knowledge areas to consider when mapping out your project, plus two extras for research (research management and stakeholder management) are as follows:

- Scope management
- Time management
- Cost management
- Stakeholder management
- Research management
- Quality management
- Risk management
- Human resources management
- Communication management
- Procurement management
- Integration management

References—Project Management

[1] PMI, 2008. A Guide to the Project Management Body of Knowledge, fifth ed. Project Management Institute. http://www.pmi.org/pmbok-guide-standards/foundational/pmbok.

4.2 Detailed Project Planning

Joe ordered a new instrument that was critical for the project and arranged for it to be shipped from Europe. It was heavy, so it had to come by sea. He didn't think to ask how long that would take. He employed a technician to run it, sent him for training, and then they waited, and waited.

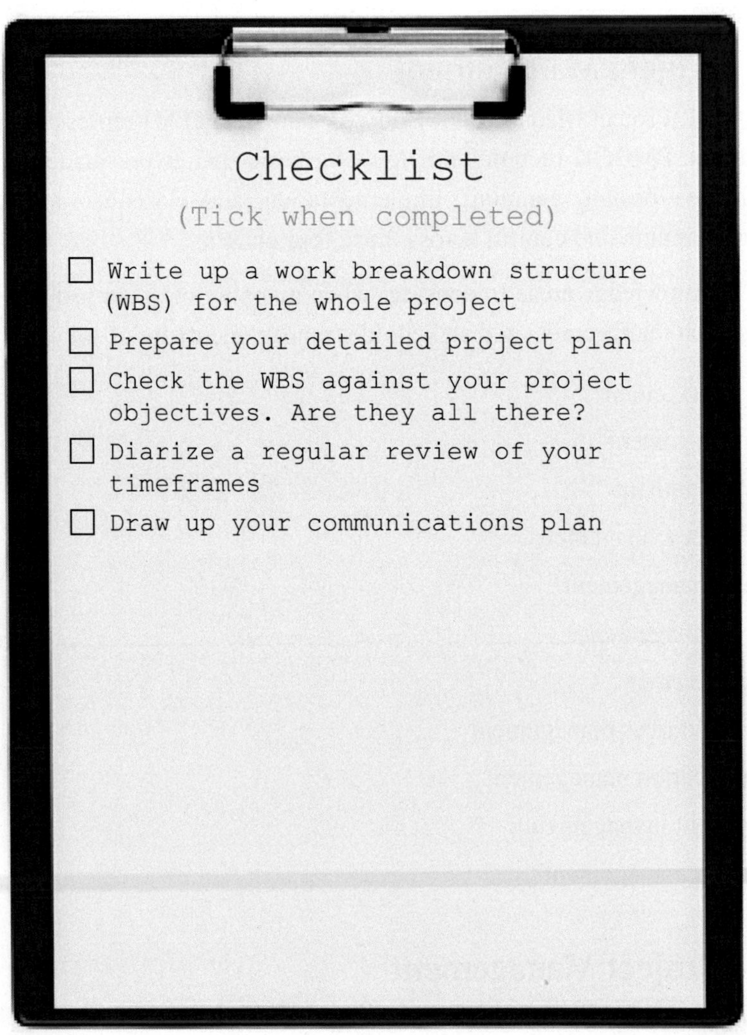

Understanding the Work Breakdown Structure

Those tasks listed in Chapter 4.1 can now be planned in greater detail by use of a "work breakdown structure" (WBS). Your WBS is a valuable tool for working out how the parts of the project fit together, especially for working out estimates for time, resources, and costs. It will help you identify the various tasks that need to be undertaken, when they need doing, and by whom. It also shows the inter-dependencies of the elements of the project, making it clear which steps have to come before, or after, others.

This detailed planning will allow you to make sure you have understood the likely timing for each section of your project and the corresponding personnel requirements. It helps you understand the consequences of delays to your projects. You don't want to have study staff standing around with nothing to do for three months while they wait for the next stage. When you get your timings right, you can be ready to make use of a piece of equipment as soon as it has arrived, and your staff have been trained, or issue your already approved study consent and recruitment forms. The WBS should also help you plan your expenditure in balance with the arrival of your expected income.

If you plan your WBS as a project team, you can allocate responsibilities together, which should help you avoid overloading a particular individual with many tasks that have to be carried out at the same time.

The top of the WBS hierarchy, the big picture, gives a broad description of the activities. Further down, each activity is broken down into defined tasks with people attributed to them and firm timeframes. The inter-dependencies with other tasks is noted. At the next level come the many detailed tasks that contribute to actually *doing* the project.

You can use the list of management tasks in Table 4.2.1 as a prompt to map out the tasks for your project. You may find it helpful to use the Project Management Template 4.2.1 at the end of this chapter. There is also a separate Project Communications Plan Template 4.2.2.

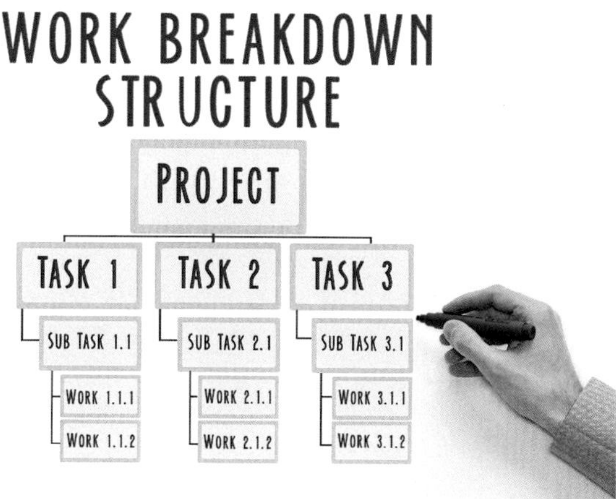

Image Credit: Work breakdown structure by astephan/Shutterstock

TABLE 4.2.1 List of Management Tasks

Meet university requirements	Contact with your research services to discuss the project and its management. Check what processes need to be completed or approvals sought.
Legal matters	Liaise with your legal services to ensure all necessary contracts and grant documents are signed off.
Project budget	Set up the project fund account and identify the budget to be committed to each element. Prepare your budget according to your planned activities and the timing of grant monies. Establish protocols for expenditure, with one or two people maintaining oversight of the budget. Plan for regular reports on expenditure and regular reviews of project costs for particular components.
Ethics approval	Do you need to seek ethics approval? Get started as soon as possible to ensure compliance. Obtain all ethical clearances for the conduct of your research from the Research Integrity Office
Project staff	Plan for recruitment of staff based on human resources policies and protocols. Plan induction of all team members.
Higher Degree Research students	If you plan to include Higher Degree Research students in your project, liaise with the graduate research and scholarships office to identify requirements or issues to be addressed.
Establish your study processes and systems	Establish some procedures and templates for recording the results and observations so that you have a consistent approach and documentation. Set up templates for reports, progress logs, and other processes.
Agreements	Establish agreements with staff and collaborators for confidentiality, intellectual property, and dissemination of research findings
Setting up your research space	Can the research be accommodated in existing facilities? What equipment do you need? What is already available in your faculty/university?
Equipment and consumables	If you plan to share available equipment, how will that be managed? Is it better to buy in bulk for the whole project? When?
Meetings	Set up your regular meeting schedules for staff, collaborators, and stakeholders
Training	What training will your team require and when?
Pilot study	Do you need to undertake a pilot project for proof of concept? If yes, it will need its own complete set of milestones. Then they will be replicated for the "real" project
Plan for communications management	How often do you plan to meet with your research team, partners, and stakeholders? Develop a communication protocol to explain who will be responsible for which elements.
Work health and safety management	Is your research using dangerous processes or chemicals? Is fieldwork involved? Contact your safety and health office if there are issues that need to be managed.
Risk management	Establish a risk log and encourage all members to identify potential risks that require consideration.
Check grant conditions	Review the conditions of the grant and ensure any reporting or deliverables are included in your project planning.
Establish project website	Set up your website for the project, including staff profiles, an overview of the project, and contact details.
Advisory group	Should you establish an advisory group to oversee the research? When? Who should you invite? Determine terms of reference and the role and responsibilities of members.

How to Draw Up a Work Breakdown Structure

At the simplest level, you can use a whiteboard or a very big sheet of paper to map out the individual objectives of your project, their timings, and their co-dependencies. Pads of Post-it notes in assorted colors make very effective planning tools, particularly when mapping out allocation of resources as you can move the notes about.

If your project is very complex, it might be worthwhile using project management software such as Microsoft Project, but it is usually good to try the whiteboard method before committing your thoughts to the software. Involve several members of your team in this process. Remember that the end result needs to be clear for all, including people with limited experience.

Start by marking out your time line across the board. Add Post-its with the high-level task descriptions above the time line, then fill in your detail with more Post-its below in the appropriate time columns. It can be helpful to note the planned duration of each task on the Post-it. You can add the initials or position name of the people or person to do the task, or perhaps use a different color Post-it for each position and attach them to the task. It is then easy to spot if one person is doing too many jobs in the same time period.

Once you have finished, check with your list of project deliverables. Have you managed to include the whole list?

Remember to add routine tasks, including regular team meetings, standard operating procedure (SOP) reviews, and audits. You need to keep on top of your income and expenditure, so set aside a time every month to review your costs against budget and make adjustments where necessary.

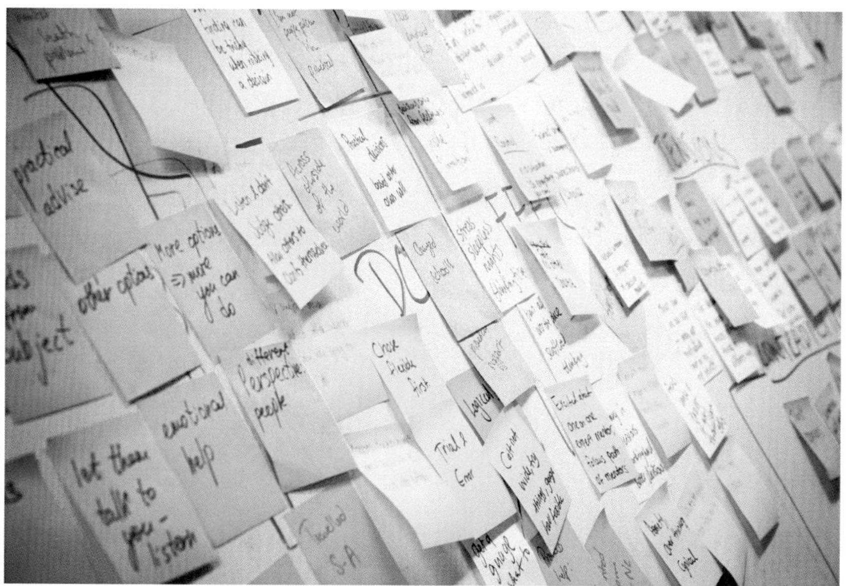

Image Credit: Whiteboard post-it colored notes by SkyLynx/Shutterstock

You can now capture all this information in a document using a table, spreadsheet, or a Gantt chart. It is useful to allocate a hierarchical number to each task, as below:

1. Purchase equipment
   - 1.1. Research suppliers
   - 1.2. Arrange suppliers to come for site visits
     - 1.2.1. Site visits freezer
     - 1.2.2. Site visits centrifuge
   - 1.3. Purchase a liquid nitrogen freezer
     - 1.3.1. Seek approvals for nitrogen connection
     - 1.3.2. Arrange nitrogen connection
     - 1.3.3. Freezer delivery
     - 1.3.4. Team training
   - 1.4. Purchase centrifuge
     - 1.4.1. Centrifuge delivery

In separate columns note the time and person/position allocated to each task.

Review Your Timeframe Regularly

At the beginning of your project set yourself a timetable of tasks to be done in a particular timeframe. Inevitably there will be slippage. During the life of your project you must review your planned work schedule with respect to time and expected milestones and make the necessary adjustments.

You might need to rearrange the order of some tasks to keep staff fully occupied—or to avoid them having to do three months of work in one fortnight. It is good to review the tasks against time in your regular team meetings.

Other Tools for Project Planning

For a big project, it may be worthwhile using a Gantt chart or Microsoft Project as your tool. It's an easy way to provide a snapshot where you can see all the above project elements and identify the critical path.

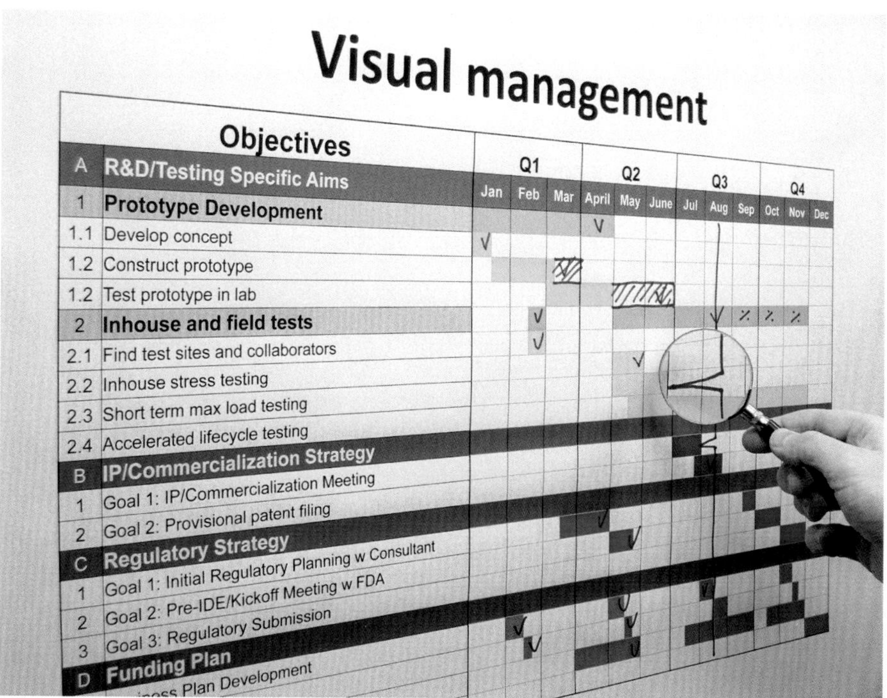

Image Credit: Project plan using visual management by jazz42/iStock

Associated Documents—Detailed Project Planning

4.2.1 Project Management Template

1. Name of Research Project
2. Lead Institution and Other Partners
3. Sponsor's Name, if applicable
4. Research Leader's Name
5. Stakeholders (i.e. those who may need to have their issues addressed or who are otherwise involved in the research project background or outcomes)
6. Location of Research Project, if focused on a geographic place(s)
7. Project Lay Summary (100 words or less)
8. Research Scope
9. Research Aims
10. Objectives of the Research
11. Potential Benefits of the Research
12. Deliverables
13. Context of the Research Project and any Relevant Background (including related research projects)
14. Research Constraints
15. Potential Research Topics which are Beyond Scope
16. Work Breakdown Structure
17. Projected Timeline, Milestones and Activity Schedule
18. Projected Cost and Breakdown into Key Expenditure Areas
19. Roles and Responsibilities
20. Risks and Contingency Planning
21. Quality Assurance Mechanisms
22. Communication Strategy
23. Procurement Plans

4.2.2 Project Communications Plan Template

Stakeholder for Communication	**Objective**	**Type of Communication**	**Frequency**	**Level of Communication**	**Individual(s) Responsible**
Funding Agencies	Demonstrate project progress for continued funding	Progress Report	Annually	Scheme/Project Manager	Research Leader
Research Managers/Administrators					
Ministerial Assessors and Reviewers					
Auditors					
Collaborators – Industry (business development, legal, academic)					
Collaborators – Academic (inside institution, outside of institution)					
Internal Administration – host institution and other institution – Executive					
Internal Administration – host institution and other institution – Administration					
Internal Administration – host institution and other institution – Legal Office					
Internal Administration – host institution and other institution – HR					
Internal Administration – host institution and other institution – Finance					
Internal Administration – host institution and other institution – Marketing					
Project Staff and Students					

4.3 Understanding Agreements

I didn't know that they expected me to do that.

He said he would do x by y, and now I can't make him.

That part of the data was mine, I brought it into the project, what makes him think it's his now?

Does this sound familiar? Did you get it in writing? If no, you might well have some sorting out to do.

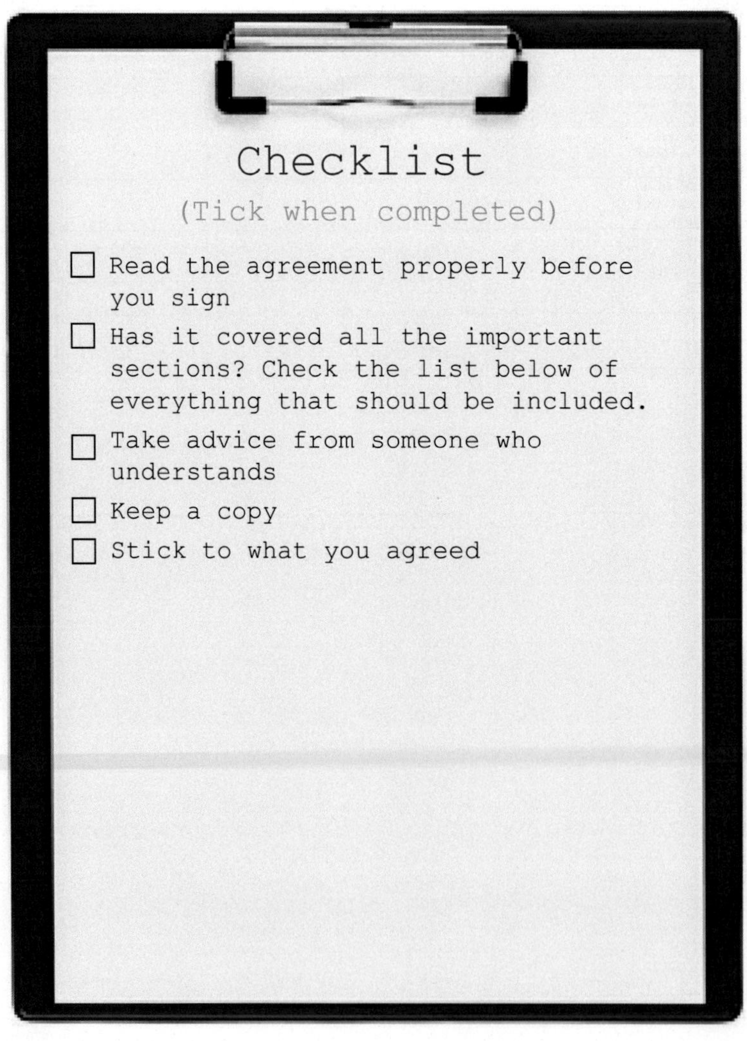

Yes, agreements are a nuisance. Yes, you mightn't understand the legal language. Too bad. In this chapter we discuss setting up formal agreements with institutions, collaborators, publishers, and/or suppliers because they are a necessary part of research life. It is very important to have agreements in place to cover all your arrangements, and you must be able to understand their meanings. Your agreements will take you some time and trouble, but they'll save a great deal more in the long run.

An agreement should be seen as a confirmation of understanding. It provides certainty and transparency. Don't be frightened of agreements—use them to your benefit. Remember the following essential rules which appear in the earlier checklist and which apply to *every* agreement:

- Read before you sign
- Take advice from someone who understands
- Keep a copy
- Stick to what you agreed to

Some of the material to follow might seem complicated. Please read it and try to understand the nature of the types of agreements you can expect to encounter or need.

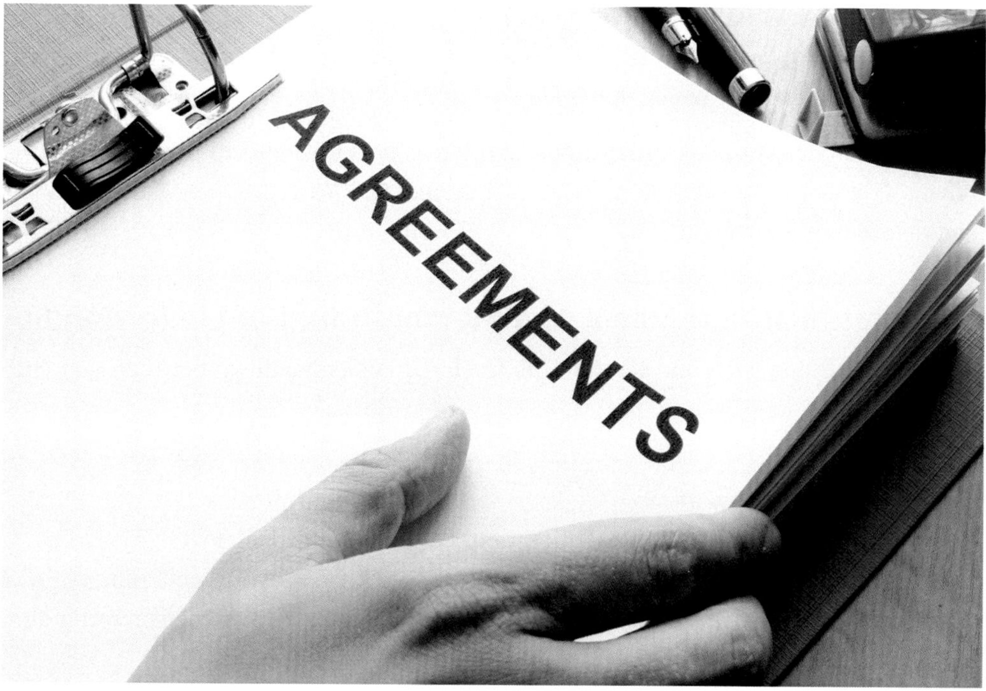

Image Credit: Agreements on a table by Designer491/Shutterstock

The main types of agreements you will encounter include the following:

- Funding agreement
- Multi-institutional agreement (MIA)
- Memorandum of understanding (MoU)
- Non-disclosure or confidentiality agreement (NDA)
- Data use agreement (DUA)
- Material transfer agreement (MTA)
- Publication agreement
- Consultancy agreement

Your research or legal offices will be able to help you with agreements, but the information that follows will give you a basic understanding of the most usual types of agreements you might need to use.

Funding Agreement

The funding agreement will usually be handled by the funding body and the institution.

Make sure you read it. It will include promises on your behalf. Note that it will almost always state that the intellectual property (IP) created by your research will become the property of the institution, or perhaps, in rare cases, the funder.

The agreement might also place restrictions that make it apply only to your current place of employment. If you are considering moving institutions, take care that you understand whether your funding can move with you.

Multi-Institutional Agreement and Memorandum of Understanding

The purpose of both the MIA and the MoU is to clarify understandings between you and your fellow investigators for a particular project or series of projects.

Multi-Institutional Agreement

An MIA will set out the terms of collaboration on an institutional level. Typically, it will provide terms of agreement for all legal matters such as IP, publication and authorship rights, and confidentiality, and might also deal with allocation of funds between investigators and institutions.

A standard MIA (or where there is no MIA, a standard MoU) for a research project might be made up of a long list of sections, including any (or many) of the items on the list in Table 4.3.1.

It might also contain sections listed in Table 4.3.2.

It is likely that your institution will have a template that you will be required to use; however, templates can readily be found online, including the current version of the excellent MIA developed for the Australian Group of Eight (Go8) universities [1].

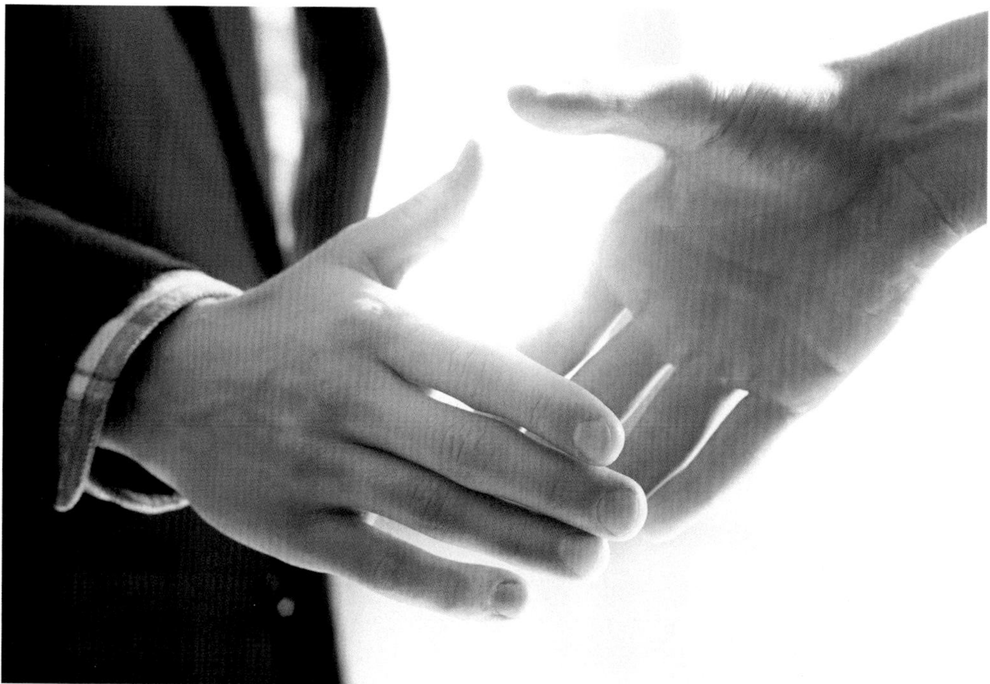

Image Credit: Handshake by pikcha/Shutterstock

TABLE 4.3.1 Standard Sections for an Agreement
• Background
• Details of parties
• Term
• Milestones
• Intellectual Property
• Confidentiality
• Budget or funding
• Allocation of tasks and responsibilities
• Sharing of infrastructure in cross-institutional projects
• Planned meetings
• Publications and authorship
• Signature and date
• Addendum or schedule
• Research protocol
• Grant application

TABLE 4.3.2 Additional Sections for an Agreement
• Definitions
• Privacy and confidentiality
• Ownership of and access to research data
• Storage and transfer of data
• Need for changes in the research design
• Ethical requirements
• Payments between institutions or to suppliers
• Responsibility for reporting
• Conflict resolution
• Termination
• Notices
• Liability and indemnity
• Responsibility for public representation on behalf of the collaboration
• Exchange of staff
• Placement of students
• Exchange of data

Memorandum of Understanding

An MoU will provide the grounds of understanding between you and your individual collaborators on a project or a more general collaboration. The MoU doesn't need to be complicated. It should spell out who has agreed to do what, and when, who is in charge, and the consequences in the case of non-delivery.

The aim of an MoU is to facilitate productive research collaborations that, with any luck, will result in high-impact research and research outputs. It may be legally non-binding.

This MoU does *not* replace or take precedence over the funding agreement for a project or the successful grant application that forms the background to that funding agreement. That grant application will have specified work to be undertaken by different investigators and institutions. The MoU is drafted to clarify the actual delivery of the undertakings you made together in the grant application.

Similarly, the MoU does not replace or take precedence over any formal MIA in place which will take precedence over all other agreements.

Where there is an existing over-arching agreement such as an MIA, an MoU might simply outline agreement between collaborators about, for example, division of specific duties and responsibilities, their timeframes, and plans for collaborator meetings. Use the list of possible sections for an MIA to prompt you to make sure you have suitable agreements in place with your collaborators for all facets relevant for your project. If there is a disagreement later, on any of these topics, your MoU should help prevent conflict in the collaboration.

Material Transfer Agreement

An MTA is a contract that formalizes the arrangements for the transfer of research materials (for example, cell lines or tissue samples) between two organizations. It defines the rights of both the person who supplies the material and of the person who receives them, as well as the terms of acceptance. This might include the conditions of use of the materials and/or anything that is created from it. An MTA will typically also outline the conditions for dispatch and delivery and might include reference to payment and to return or a prohibition of sharing.

An MTA should be exchanged whenever institutions are buying or selling research specimens. There should also be an MTA even if you are simply sharing and there is no money to be exchanged. The MTA benefits both parties as it makes sure that the terms of the exchange are perfectly clear to both sides of the transaction.

A good MTA template is provided by the Medical Research Council, UK [2].

Data Use Agreement

A DUA is an agreement that defines terms and conditions related to the transfer of data. Those data are usually not public or are otherwise subject to some usage restrictions.

As with the MTA mentioned earlier, a data transfer agreement is there to protect the supplier as much as the person who receives it. In these days where data are very portable, it is vital to place protective conditions around their transfer.

A DUA defines the data that are to be shared, and the terms under which they may be used. It will define ownership of the data, ownership of the data once they have been manipulated, and any restrictions regarding their sharing.

Non-Disclosure Agreement

An NDA is a legal contract between two or more parties which gives permission to discuss another person or organization's business *with appropriate privacy and discretion*. The NDA protects non-public business information.

An NDA is more than a token piece of paper. If you are required to sign an NDA, take it seriously. It does not give you permission to discuss confidential matters with the person at the next desk.

An NDA might also be known as a *confidentiality agreement* (CA), *confidential disclosure agreement* (CDA), *proprietary information agreement* (PIA), or *secrecy agreement* (SA). In all cases its purpose is the same.

Remember that if there is a possibility you might want to lodge a patent application for your research outcomes, you must not disclose your invention publicly before lodging the application. Public demonstration, sale, or public discussion of the invention may well invalidate the patent application. Any discussions with your colleagues or partners must always be on a confidential basis, and they should complete an NDA early in the life of the project.

Publication Agreement

It is usual practice for journal publishers to ask authors to assign copyright to them, although many now allow self-archiving of the final accepted manuscript version in an institutional repository. Since the requirement to make your papers publicly available has become commonplace, it has become important to make sure that your publication agreements allow you to meet your requirements.

Macquarie University [3] provides excellent online advice for the many variations of publishing agreements and how to manage them. This is a rapidly changing situation. Your librarians should be able to provide current advice.

Consultancy Agreement

There are sometimes occasions when you could be asked to perform a consultancy service for another organization. Your institution will almost certainly require you to complete an agreement for this. Payment will probably need to be made directly to your organization. You may be able to arrange with your institution for the monies generated to be made available for your research.

The consultancy agreement should cover the following:

- Commencement and completion dates
- Milestones
- Contact details
- Services to be provided
- Deliverables
- Key personnel
- Client duties
- Ethics required
- Payment
- Expenses
- Insurances

References—Agreements

Follow Follow these links for useful templates:

[1] Australian Group of Eight (Go8) universities' MIA can be found online at: https://research.unsw.edu.au/document/nhmrc_go8_mia_2016.docx.

[2] Material transfer agreement template UK. https://www.mrc.ac.uk/documents/pdf/brunswick-material-transfer-agreement/.

[3] Macquarie University Publication Agreement Options. http://www.mq.edu.au/about/campus-services-and-facilities/library/copyright/publication-agreement-options.

4.4 Developing Your Study Methods

Project Lightning needed to recruit a large number of study participants and tried out a range of recruitment avenues. Some worked better than others; some didn't work at all and needed to be abandoned. Study staff and investigators knew what was happening at any one time, but when it came to writing up there was only a rough collective notion of the avenues tested. No one knew about all of them. Certainly no one had evidence of exactly what was done when and why, because records were inadequate.

So what happened? Hours and hours of linking together spikes in enrolments with amendments to ethics approvals, hunting for old copies of study materials at the bottom of drawers, and phone calls to past team members to check their recollections of events. Pieces of the puzzle were eventually cobbled together.

How could this have been better handled?

Checklist

(Tick when completed)

- ☐ Set up project folders on the computer/server, with appropriate team access
- ☐ Write up a project manual/Standard Operating Procedure (SOP)
- ☐ Distribute the protocols to the team
- ☐ Create a contact list and study log
- ☐ Set up a method to file correspondence
- ☐ Plan team meetings
- ☐ Diarize reviews of your SOP
- ☐ See study document templates at the end of this chapter

4 RUNNING THE STUDIES

Introduction

There is simply nothing more important in research than good organization. Bright ideas for that next research step are important—almost essential—but capturing the day-to-day steps you take in carrying out that brilliant research idea is vital, or the whole project is in danger of becoming wasted effort and wasted money. It is a rare project that has sufficient funds to do it all again. There are no projects that can be written up for successful publication without sufficient documentation.

Institutions the world over are littered with failed projects. These projects haven't necessarily failed because the research ideas were bad but because the steps taken in the research were not appropriately documented and the ideas were lost. Research "breakthroughs" that cannot be repeated are no good to anyone.

There are four basic steps to take.

- Step 1: create a study protocol
- Step 2: follow the protocol
- Step 3: ensure that study staff also follow the protocol
- Step 4: know where the study documentation can be found and amend it when your procedures change.

This all sounds obvious, but failure to follow these simple, commonsense steps is probably the greatest cause of project failure.

With respect to day-to-day research activity, every member of the team, whether it is a team of one or of ten should work as though they are about to go on long leave. Today's efforts should be written up before you go home, and in a way that requires no further explanation to a new reader.

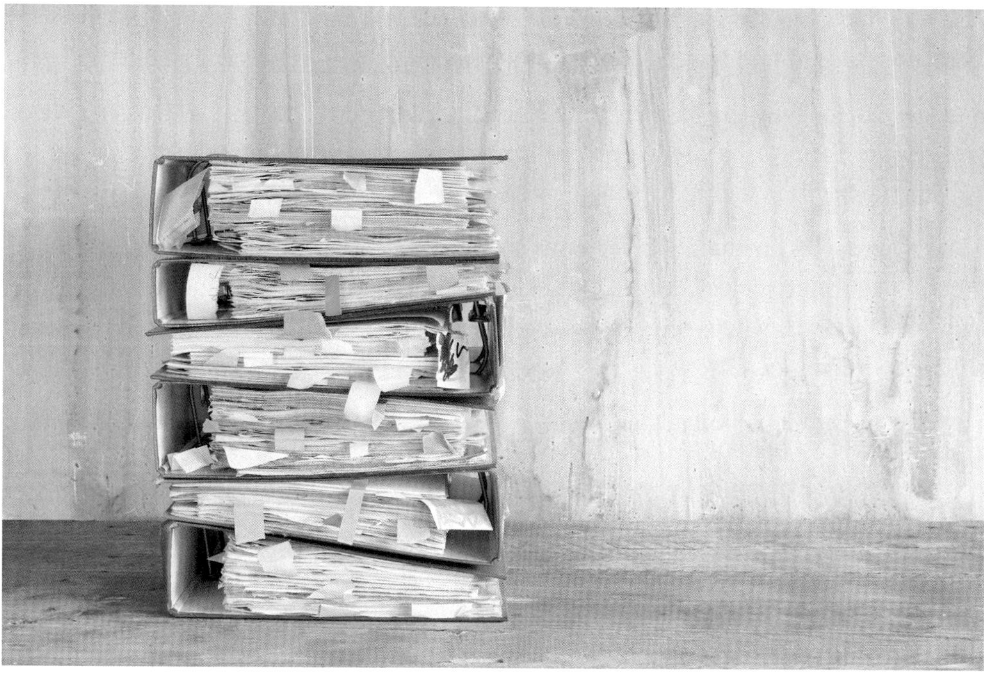

Image Credit: Stack of messy file folders by thomas-bethge/iStock

Development of Study Manual/Standard Operating Procedures

The study manual or SOP provides guidance for the day-to-day management of the project and a means of maintaining centralized records.

It is obvious, then, that all staff need to have access to the manual or SOP. Keep it on the server where it will be accessible to all and will be routinely backed up.

It is very important to maintain meticulous records of the progress of your research. Again, this might be obvious to some, but sadly, as mentioned earlier, universities are crammed with the ghosts of projects where findings are unable to be published or, worse, results that cannot be reproduced because the right records were not kept.

Why keep these records? The time will come when you are writing up the methods for your project. "When did we decide to change the questionnaire?" "Why did we do that?" "Whose idea was it?" "When did we change to the new reagent?? Was that about money, or about availability? Was it because it was better, or were we made to make the change?"

Four years on, when your project staff are different and you can't quite remember the whys and wherefores, a record of these small details will be invaluable.

You must develop a study log and templates for all your record-keeping, and instruct your team how you require them to be used. This information needs to be maintained (and consistently reviewed and updated) in the study SOP.

A good SOP provides instructions for consistent project procedure implementation and data collection. It details the project's organization, operations, data management, and quality control, including management, where relevant, of participants and clinical sites. The SOP should also record incomplete, unsatisfactory, or unsuccessful project outcomes.

You may like to use the templates at the end of this chapter as a starting point for your study documents.

There are a few simple steps to take, *starting on day one*.

Set Up a System on the Computer

- Establish an electronic filing system on the computer network accessible to all project staff
- Set up folders for each broad purpose
- Where necessary for study confidentiality, limit access to those folders
    - Establish a "paper trail," electronic or paper, for recording access permissions to project folders
- Establish standards for file naming that are followed consistently. If everyone in your team uses a different document-naming protocol, it can create chaos. (See further detail in Data Storage and Management in Chapter 4.5.)

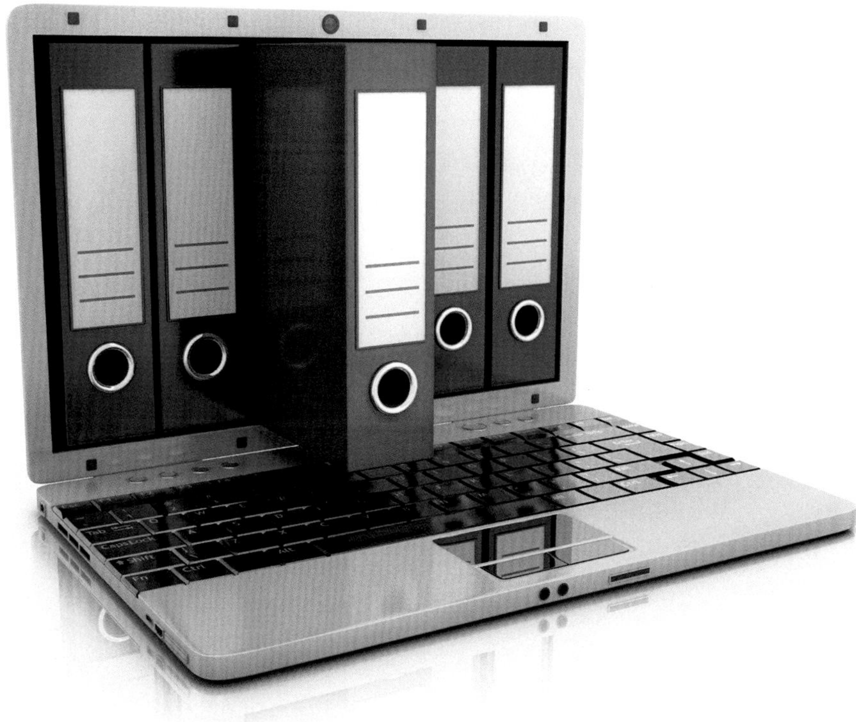

Image Credit: Laptop 3d and files by vladru/iStock

Contacts List

Keep a contacts list! To many this might seem like practical common sense, while to others it seems unnecessary. You know where Joe is, right? Well, you might forget. Not only that, but someone else might need to contact Joe one day when you are not around. Write it down and make sure the others can find it too.

It makes sense to maintain a record of contact details of all the people involved with your project and have it available to all your team members. Be conscientious about updating it every time there is a change. This includes contact details for home and work for your own team members.

This little practice will save you so much time in the long run.

Log Activity

Keep a daily log of project activity. This is used to record the day's major activities, informal issues, or required actions. It acts as your project diary. Often your entries might be a record of thoughts, conversations, and observations. There may be more than one daily log for your project as other team members might keep one too. In a laboratory, this would be your laboratory book.

The daily log can take a number of formats, including a document or a spreadsheet, a desk diary or log book, an electronic diary/calendar/task lists, or an entry in a project management tool. Whichever it is, do the following:

- Provide sufficient detail for your entries to be understandable later (a short note might make sense at the time, but will it in several months' time?)
- Always include a date
- Think about who should have access rights to the daily log (e.g., should the daily log be visible to everyone working on the project?). This, of course, will depend on the nature of the information you include

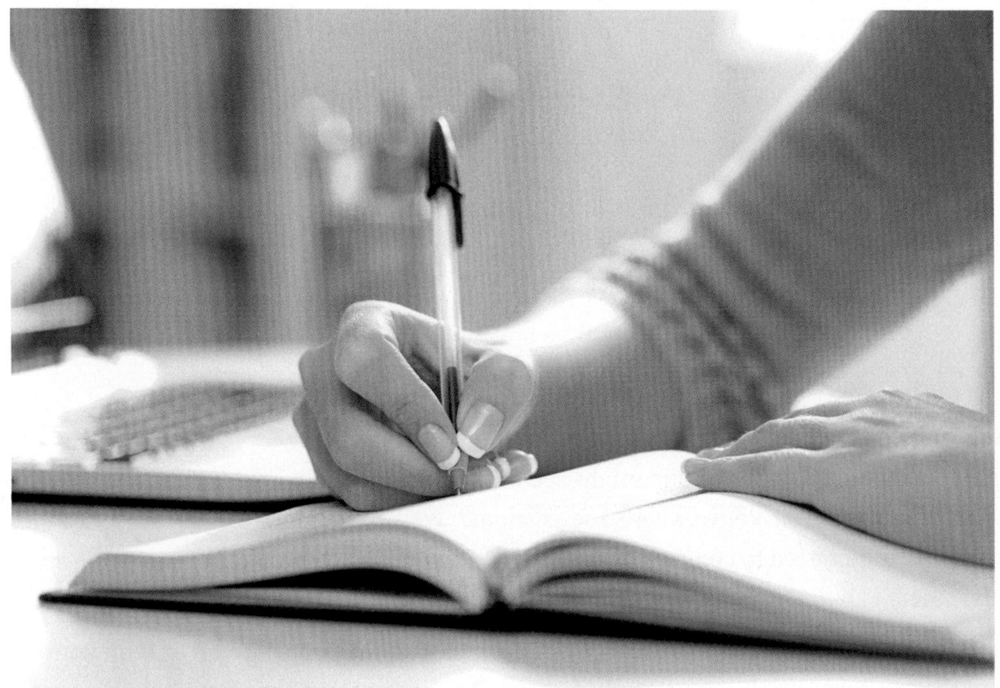

Image Credit: Writing in an agenda by AntonioGuillem/iStock

Similarly, you should keep a phone log, a record of project-related phone calls, again noting the date and their general purpose. Note if they were from, for example, study participants, co-investigators, or your funding body.

If your study is one that causes you to have interaction with the general public, you should log these calls. If you are receiving many calls on the same topic, it will save much effort if you develop a set of frequently asked questions. Place the questions and their answers on the project website—thus reducing the number of calls—and also keep the answers handy by the phone so that you can be sure that all staff are giving consistent responses.

File Correspondence

- File study correspondence, both paper and electronic. If you are a paper person, put them in a folder in chronological order. If you prefer electronic filing, scan the paper copies and keep in a folder, labelled by date as well as subject.
- File study emails. "Print" an email trail as a pdf, and keep it in a folder, labelled by date as well as subject. Don't forget to save the attachments as well.

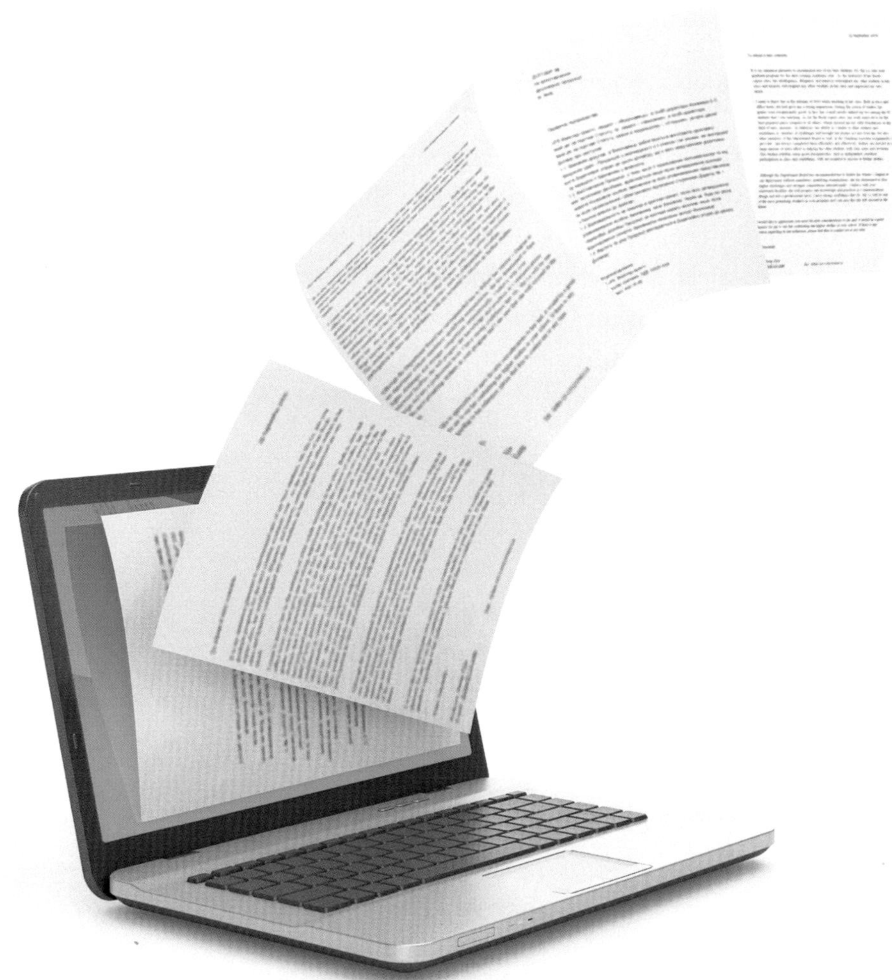

Image Credit: Uploading documents from laptop by Model-la/iStock

4 RUNNING THE STUDIES

Study Meetings

- Hold regular study meetings. Set an agenda and record minutes of decisions. There may need to be more than one type of regular meeting for each project/program.
- Specify a chair for each meeting and define the chair's responsibilities, which might include the following:
  - Room booking
  - Meeting reminders
  - Distribution of agenda and later minutes
- File the agenda and minutes electronically in a specific place accessible to all study staff. (See Chapter 4.8 for further detail about meetings.)

> The steps taken above are the stepping stones, which together begin to form the SOP for your study.

The SOP will grow as the project grows. It is imperative to record all the "How to's" for the project, from day one, so that you have both a record of how things should be done and also a method to follow if you are unlucky enough to have changes in your project staffing. All project methods need to be recorded so they can be clearly understood and can be reproduced by any staff member. They will be there as a record at the end of your project when you write up your project methods.

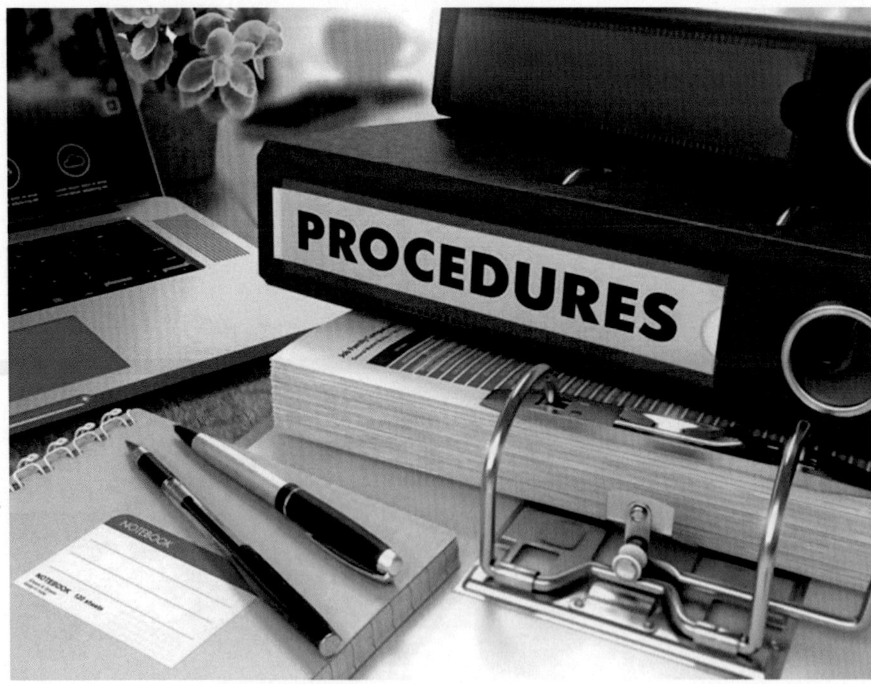

Image Credit: Procedures by ESB Professional/Shutterstock

The minute you have your documents finalized, you will want to change them. It is how the world works. Adopt—and adhere to—standard version control practices. Rename the new version and file a copy of the previous version in a particular archive folder. Keep a list of your versions and the date they came into use.

Important!! Be sure to note the alterations to your SOP in your daily log.

You should diarize a quick review of the SOP every month to ensure that it matches what you are actually doing. Have a more detailed review every quarter. You will be amazed how things change.

Laboratory Protocols

Many laboratories keep a master collection of laboratory protocols, which is available either electronically or in print and is updated periodically. Laboratory protocols are rarely the type of records you need to store for the long term, but it can be very useful to have the master collection available. It is much easier to write a new protocol when you have a previous one as a guide.

Using Laboratory Books

Like the daily log mentioned earlier, which applies to general projects, your laboratory book provides a daily record of activity in the laboratory. Every single person working in the laboratory should have one and should keep it up to date. It provides the following record:

- Experiments that worked and, importantly, those that didn't
- Equipment used
- Timing of activities

In its simplest form, laboratory records allow your work to be reproduced by others. These records should allow you, and others, to re-create your work and reproduce your results, thus validating your work.

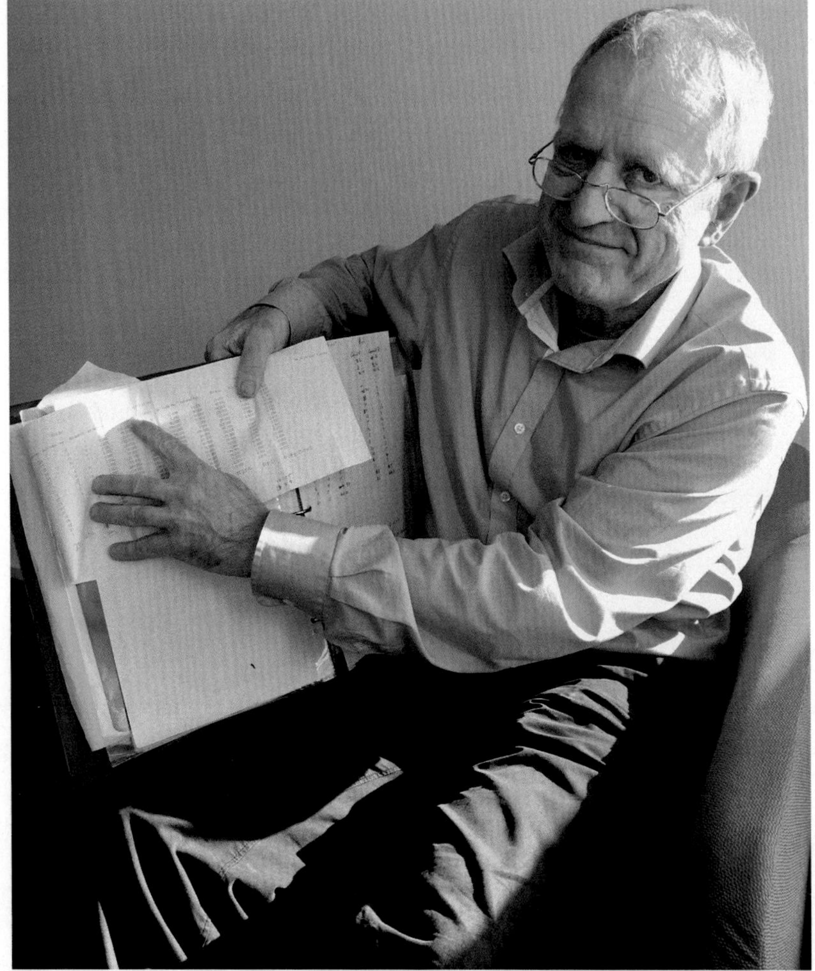

Image Credit: Prof David Vaux points out a pivotal moment recorded in his 1987 lab book/Walter and Eliza Hall Institute

Apart from providing you with a record of project knowledge when it comes to writing up, your laboratory notebook also provides you with the following:

- Evidence to prove that you have met your contractual responsibilities
- A record if you are defending or applying for patents
- A system which helps you avoid fraudulent record-keeping
- Opportunity to give appropriate credit to all members of the team

When you have a requirement for good record-keeping in your laboratory, you are teaching your team good laboratory practice. Good record-keeping teaches people to put their thoughts into words and to make a record of their hypotheses. Importantly, your laboratory books also provide you with a record of tests that didn't work and avoids replication of those failures down the line. It provides you with a pathway to follow when tracing where you might have made an error.

An outline of good practice for hard-copy versions of laboratory notebooks is provided in Table 4.4.1. The principles apply just as well for electronic notebooks.

TABLE 4.4.1 Good Practice for Laboratory Notebooks

- Use a permanently bound book, making consecutive signed and dated entries. When appropriate, have the entries witnessed by an independent person.
- For logs generated by computer, you can use a loose-leaf notebook and paste copies of the logs in, but pages must be consecutively numbered (using a sequential page-number stamp), dated, and signed.
- Each entry should be able to stand on its own to permit others to reproduce the work.
- Try to organize material with consistent sections and headings.
- Identify and describe reagents and specimens used, for each entry.
- Identify sources of those materials as specifically as possible (e.g., reagent manufacturer, lot number, purity, expiration date).
- Enter serial numbers and calibration dates for each instrument.
- Use proper nouns for items, not abbreviations.
- Write all entries in the first person, and be specific about who did each element of the work.
- Explain nonstandard abbreviations.
- Use ink and never obliterate original writing, just strike a line through a mistake; never remove pages or portions of a page.
- If a page is left blank or a space within a page is left blank, draw a line through it.
- Permanently fix any attachments (such as graphs or computer printouts) to the pages of the notebook with glue; date and sign both the notebook page and the attachment, signing over the boundary where possible.
- Give a full outline of new experiments, including their objectives and rationale.
- Include factual, not speculative, summaries of progress and findings from time to time.
- Enter ideas and observations into your notebook as soon as you can. It is also useful to summarize discussions from laboratory meetings or topical suggestions made by others, citing the person(s) by name.

Attribute Adapted from Making the Right Moves [1].

While many people find it easier to jot something on paper while they are on the run, electronic laboratory notebooks (ELNs) do everything their handwritten forebears do—and more. They make life easy because you can search and you can organize and re-organize your material. You can link your notebook to analytical software and can usually download and store data directly. Many ELNs also offer secure access for multiple users and for remote users. Choosing the right ELN for your laboratory requires homework. Make sure that the one you choose not only has all the functions you want but is also compliant with the legal requirements you need to meet.

The information contained in your ELN is very important. It is a good idea to print out a hard copy from time to time, as part of your backup plan.

Like other study records, laboratory notebooks should be kept for the life of the project and for a period of at least five years beyond. Completed laboratory books should be marked clearly with name and time period and stored securely. A person who leaves the laboratory must leave their laboratory notebook behind. With appropriate permission, a person leaving the group might take a copy of the laboratory book to their new position, but never let them take the original. A laboratory book whose entries relate to anything that has been patented should be kept by the principal investigator beyond the life of that patent, plus six years.

References—Developing Study Methods

[1] Howard Hughes Medical Institute, Burroughs Welcome Fund, 2006. Making the Right Moves: A Practical Guide to Scientific Management. http://www.hhmi.org/developing-scientists/making-right-moves.

Further Information

The NIH Manual of procedures provides excellent, very detailed document templates with which you can manage the most complex of projects:

https://www.nidcr.nih.gov/research/toolkit/Documents/mop_template_v6_22DEC2014.dotx.

https://www.nidcr.nih.gov/research/toolkit/Documents/SOPTemplate_Approved20101001.doc.

http://www.nidcr.nih.gov/Research/toolkit/#startup3.

For version control guidelines:

http://www.nidcr.nih.gov/Research/ToolsforResearchers/Toolkit/VersionControlGuidelines.htm.

https://www.nidcr.nih.gov/research/toolkit/Documents/Protocol_Amendment_Summary_Changes.doc.

For lab notebooks:

MIT Department of Mechanical Engineering also provides good lab notebook instructions at http://web.mit.edu/me-ugoffice/communication/labnotebooks.pdf.

Electronic Lab Notebooks:

http://postdocexperience.scienceblog.com/2012/11/19/electronic-lab-notebooks/.

The 9 Best Electronic Lab Notebooks (ELN) Review for Your Research:

http://splice-bio.com/the-7-best-electronic-lab-notebooks-eln-for-your-research/.

Associated Documents—Developing Your Study Methods

4.4.1 Project Daily Log

Date	Main Activity, Problem, Event or Comment	Results

4.4.2 Phone Call Log Template

DATE	FIRST NAME	LAST NAME	CALLER PHONE	CALLER EMAIL	REASON FOR CALL	FOLLOW UP REQUIRED

4.4.3 Study Contacts List

SALUTATION	FIRST NAME	LAST NAME	EMAIL	PHONE	INSTITUTION	POSTAL ADDRESS

4.4.4 Agenda

Project Name:

Project Manager:

Agenda for the meeting scheduled *<Day> <Date> <Month><Year>* to be held from *<Start time> – <End time>* in *<Room>, <Campus>*

---

1. **Attendance:** *List members*

2. **Apologies:** *List apologies*

3. **Minutes from the Previous Meeting**

4. **Matters Arising from the Previous Meeting**

5. **Agenda item 1 –** *Add item*

6. **Agenda item 2 –** *Add item*

7. **Agenda item 3 –** *Add item*

8. **Agenda item 4 –** *Add item*

9. **Agenda item 5 –** *Add item*

10. **Other Business**

Next meeting: scheduled for <Day> <Date> <Month><Year> to be held from <Start time> – <End time> in <Room>, <Campus>

4.4.5 Minutes and Actions Template

Project Name:

Project Manager: **Minute Taker:**

<Day>, <Date> <Month> <Year>, <Meeting Room>, <Building>, <Campus>

1. Attendance	
Name	Title
Name	Title
Name	Title
Name	Title
Name	Title
Meeting Commenced at <Time> pm and concluded at <Time> pm	
2. Apologies	
Apologies were noted from *<names>*	
3. Item	
	Action Item 1 *<Name/s>*
4. Item	
	Action Item 2 *<Name/s>*
5. Item	
	Action Item 2 *<Name/s>*
6. Item	
	Action Item 2 *<Name/s>*
7. Other Business	
	Action Item 2 *<Name/s>*

Next Meeting: *<Day>, <Date> <Month> <Year>*

4.4.6 Study Suppliers List

SALUTATION	FIRST NAME	LAST NAME	COMPANY	EMAIL	PHONE	PRODUCTS PURCHASED	POSTAL ADDRESS

4.4.7 Emergency Contacts List

FIRST NAME	LAST NAME	EMAIL	ALT EMAIL	PHONE	ALT PHONE	NEXT OF KIN/PARTNER	NEXT OF KIN PHONE

4.4.8 Project Timeline Template

TASK	JANUARY	FEBRUARY	MARCH	APRIL	MAY	JUNE	JULY	AUGUST	SEPTEMBER	OCTOBER	NOVEMBER	DECEMBER	JANUARY
STUDY MEETING													
COLLABORATOR MEETINGS													
FUNDING DUE													
REPORT DUE													

4.4.9 Standard Operating Procedure

Title: **Insert Title**	Version Number: <#>	Effective Date: **<DATE>**	Page 1 of 2

Revision History		
Version No.	**Effective Date**	**Description**

Template instructions (to be deleted upon use):

This template has all necessary styles embedded. Please use only those styles included in the document. Do not reformat anything, as this may affect the styles.

There are additional explanatory text and sample headings included for your convenience. Modify as appropriate during implementation.

Note it is often helpful to include images, diagrams or computer screenshots to demonstrate the instructions..

Approved By: **Date:**

INSERT NAME AND TITLE HERE, Signature above

4.4.9 Standard Operating Procedure

Title: **Insert Title**	Version Number: <#>	Effective Date: **<DATE>**	Page 2 of 2

1 Purpose

Instruction: Include a simple statement regarding why you are writing this document. It may also be helpful to describe the purpose of the subject matter in the SOP.

2 Scope

Instruction: This describes to whom or under what circumstances (or both) the document applies.

3 Definitions/Acronyms

Instruction: If the definition is standard (accepted throughout the Industry) and published, cite the publication (or website).

3.1 First term: Definition of first term. (Citation, if applicable)

3.2 Second term: Definition of second term. (Citation, if applicable)

4 Procedures

4.1 Heading 2

4.2 Heading 2

- Example bullets
- Example bullets

4.1.1 Heading 3

4.1.1.1 Heading 4

5 References

Instructions: List all citations and references to other documents/tools. If none, include "None" herein.

6 Appendices

Instructions: Use appendices sparingly. If forms or other items are included as appendices, consider identifying them as EXAMPLES if it is acceptable to edit them when they are used. If no appendices are included, delete this section

END OF DOCUMENT

4.5 Data Storage and Management

Bella liked to keep her files on her desktop. She didn't like the idea of others being able to access them. She didn't understand that the institution's daily backup didn't include those desktop files. You know what is coming next, don't you? The computer died, and away went two years' worth of work. Silly, silly Bella.

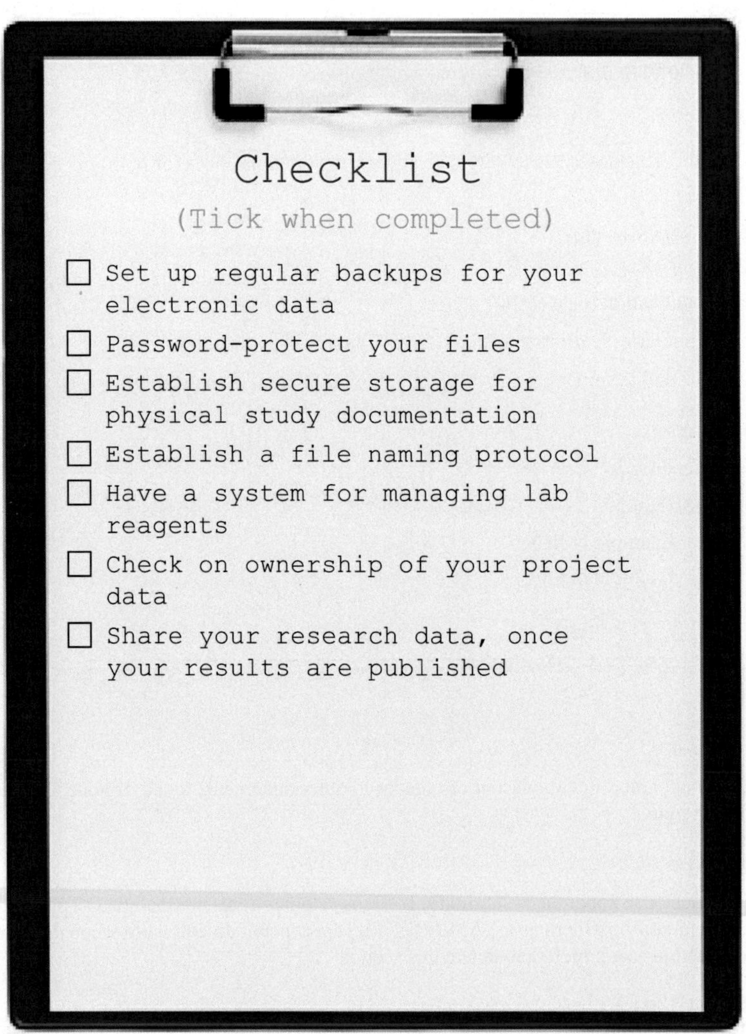

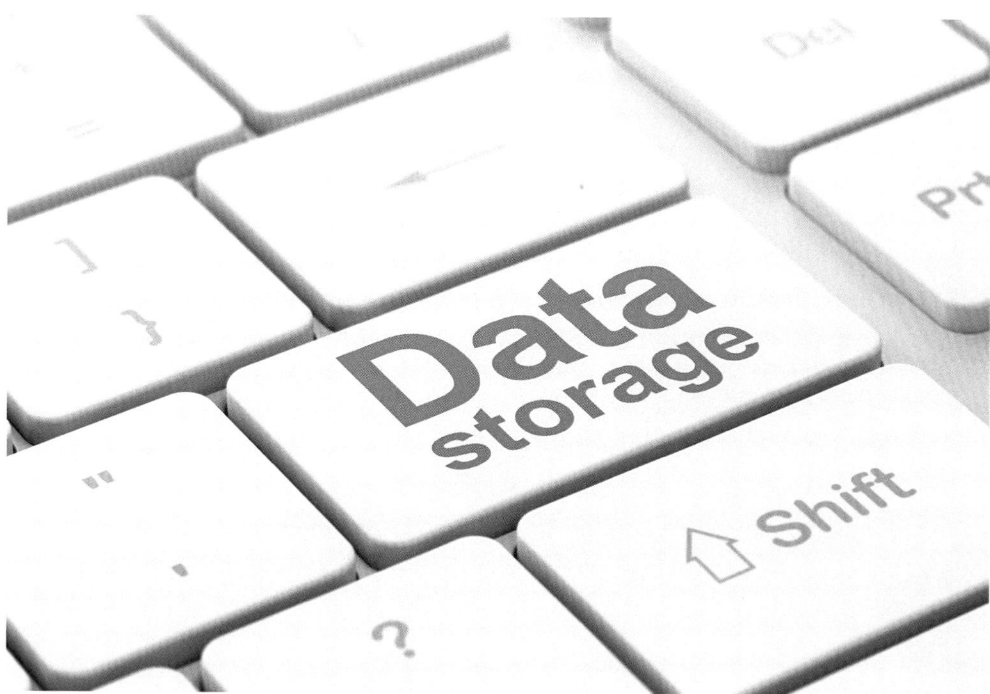

Image Credit: Data concept by Maksim Kabakou/Shutterstock

This is a chapter that really shouldn't have to be included in this book. It would have been covered when you studied "Common Sense 101" because it sets out the most basic of the rules for good research practice. Those same basic rules are rules very commonly broken. Read on.

Proper data management and record-keeping are essential components of good research management. They make your research efficient and, at the same time, help you create documentation of your research results.

In these days of the "cloud" we no longer have to worry about our ability to store data (except perhaps in fields such as genomics and bioinformatics); however, there are still many important aspects of data management to think about.

You will generate both research records and data during the course of your research project. The University of Melbourne Policy on the Management of Research Data and Records [1] defines research records as: "...documents containing data or information of any kind and in any form (including both paper-based and electronic format) created or received by an organization or person for use in the course of their work and subsequently kept by that organization or individual as evidence of that work, or because of the informational value of the data that such documents contain. Records associated with the research process include correspondence (including electronic mail as well as paper-based correspondence) ; project files; grant applications; ethics applications; technical reports; research reports; master lists; signed consent forms; and information sheets for research participants."

Good record-keeping during the life of your research project is imperative for the protection and management of your IP. Your records can also provide evidence in the case of a patent application and will provide justification if your research records are called into question.

You could even be audited by your institution or your funding body during the life of your project. You must be able to provide almost immediate access to all the data requested by an auditor.

Record management goes beyond just knowing where the data are. It includes the collection, retention, storage, and ultimate disposal of research data and primary materials after the specified retention period.

Research data must be retained according to the periods specified in your code of practice or according to archives and records legislation. You should be sure to determine and plan for the retention period required for your research data during the planning phase of your project.

In general, the minimum retention period for research data is five years post-publication; however, the actual period may vary depending on the local jurisdiction, the discipline and type of research, other institutional policies, and the requirements of funding bodies or commercial partners. Some examples of time periods are as follows:

- Research data should be retained for 15 years or more for most clinical trials
- Research data for areas such as gene therapy (e.g., patient records) must be retained permanently
- If the work has community or heritage value, research data should be kept permanently, preferably within a national collection
- If results from research are challenged, all relevant data and materials must be retained until the matter is resolved
- Research records that may be relevant to allegations of research misconduct must be kept according to the terms of the resolution of the matter.

Secure Storage

You are expected, often required, to store all data in a secure manner. Electronic data have particular requirements to ensure privacy is maintained. As part of your research protocols you may have made the undertaking to an ethics committee that data would be password. Often this may be due to the sensitivity of some data that may need to be stored in an encrypted form.

In addition to privacy and security, you also need to consider using a durable format for storing your research data. Durable formats are those that will be usable for at least the lifetime of the project and for the duration of any legislative and/or funding agency retention period.

For digital research data, you should adopt file formats that are widely used and accepted as best practice within the researcher's discipline or another user community.

Consider, too, the long-term availability of, and support for, any hardware and software used to create and manipulate research data. When setting up your systems, think about the following:

- The likely time that the hardware and software will be available
- The level of technical support available now and likely to be available in the future

Where there is a reliance on specific software, store the programs and any related documentation with the research data, assuming the terms and conditions under which you bought or licensed the software permit you to do this. It is surprising how quickly the landscape changes; you could be left with data safely stored yet completely inaccessible.

It is becoming common for international funding agencies to require a formal data management plan as part of the funding application process.

There are several online resources to help you develop your own data management plan, including the following:

- Data Management Manual, Australian National University [2]
- Research Data Planning Checklist, Monash University [3]
- The Australian National Data Service [4] provides a number of useful guides on research and research data management

Your data management plan is a valuable resource. Make sure you retain a copy of the data management plan for your own records and use it as a discussion document when talking to collaborators, service providers, and research administrators.

It is good practice to write an analysis report at the completion of a major analysis or project. This will save an enormous amount of work for someone else later, when they are trying to understand "how did he do that?" See the form for a Completed Project Analysis in Closing your Project at the end of Chapter 6.5.

Backing Up and Storing Your Data

First and foremost, back up your data. We all know someone who has lost "everything," whether that everything is from their PC that died, their phone which was left in a taxi, or every bit of project information on a lost USB drive. There is simply no excuse for not having one or more backups, preferably real-time backups that can be accessed from anywhere. Set yourself up so that you have backups happening automatically, without having to think about it. Consider the following:

- Cloud storage
- A USB drive backed up every week or two and stored at home
- An external drive making a continuous copy
- Continuous backup when in Wi-Fi mode
- Old-fashioned paper copies

Your institution almost certainly backs up all data on a daily basis. This is all very well, but not if you store your information on your desktop, lap top or on your personal drive. This is not a risk worth taking. Put your data onto the server. If you are anxious about others looking where they shouldn't, create password protection for your documents. Then record the password somewhere safe!

Prepare for the worst. What if your institution has a fire or if you break your leg and you can't get in to work? Do you have copies of your data backed up to the cloud or on your laptop? Broken leg time could be the perfect time to write up your next paper.

Muchmore and Duffy [5] provide a list of excellent options for modern day cloud storage and file-sharing options for your research data.

Be aware that if you are storing your data in the cloud, and your data contains personal, private, or confidential information, there could be difficulties if your cloud is hosted in another country that has less rigorous privacy compliance requirements than yours.

File Naming

You need to establish standards for file naming that are followed consistently. If everyone in your team uses a different document-naming protocol, it can create chaos.

Decide on a consistent system for the file names of electronic and paper documents, as well as for the identification of samples and specimens. Use it for everything that your team catalogues and stores. Table 4.5.1 summarizes the recommendations of the University of Leicester's advice for good research data management [6].

TABLE 4.5.1 Naming Files and Folders

Always order the elements in a file name in the most appropriate way to retrieve the record.
Keep file and folder names short, but meaningful.
Avoid repetition and unnecessary words in file names and file paths.
Use capital letters to delimit words, rather than spaces.
Include numbers in a file name as a two-digit number rather than one, i.e., 01, 02...99, (unless it is a year or another number with more than two digits).
Include dates "back to front," and use four digit years, two digit months, and two digit days: YYYYMMDD or YYYYMM or YYYY or YYYY-YYYY.
If including a personal name in a file name, give the family name first followed by the initials.
Avoid using common words such as "draft" or "letter" at the start of file names, unless doing so will make it easier to retrieve the record.
The file names of correspondence should include the name of the correspondent, the subject, the date, and whether it is incoming or outgoing correspondence.
The file name of an email attachment should include the name of the correspondent, the subject, the date, "attch" (indicating an attachment) and an indication of the number of attachments sent with the covering email.
The version number of a record should be indicated in its file name by the inclusion of "d" (for draft) followed by the version number (sometimes v and number are used).

Adapted from University of Leicester Recommendations.

Include dates in the format YYYYMMDD. They will be easy to find and appear chronologically.

Don't use excessively long folder and file names—there may be problems when backing up, restoring, or copying data.

Physical Storage

As mentioned earlier, original study records and data must be retained throughout the life of the study and beyond. Sometimes these will be in paper format. Consequently, you must plan to either digitize your paper records or store them, like your electronic data, for at least five years beyond the end of the project, in a safe place. Ensure that you keep appropriate records of the storage location(s). It is essential that the storage location is secure and provides an environment where the records will not deteriorate.

Managing the Laboratory's Reagents

Your laboratory's reagents are another form of research data. It is important to have a system in place for keeping track of reagents that are used in your laboratory.

Keep records of the reagents used and store the reagents themselves somewhere easily accessible. Use a database or an excel worksheet to keep track of these items. Your team members will have records in their own laboratory notebooks, but ensure that everyone in the laboratory updates the central database regularly.

When people leave the laboratory, have them place their unique reagents in storage boxes and document their location.

You will also need a reliable tracking system for the sharing of reagents, noting requests of reagents from other sources and transfers of yours to other laboratories. See Chapter 4.3, for detail about MTAs.

Research Data Ownership, Access, and Sharing

Questions regarding ownership of research data can be very complex and can cause enormous difficulties. Many of these issues can be avoided by thinking ahead and by clear communication between all collaborators before a project starts. It is a really, really good idea to take proper advice from your legal team about ownership of research data if there could be any possible difficulty.

You must consider ownership of both IP and the actual research data.

During your project preparation, you will identify the background IP, the IP to be generated in the project, the background research data, and the research data to be generated. This list should be documented and updated as the project progresses. This is particularly important for a cross-institutional project. You should remember that the ownership of the project's research data may be influenced by the funding or contractual arrangements for your research project.

Before your project starts you should consult your legal advisors to understand the arrangements in place regarding the ownership of the data you will generate during the course of your research project.

Note that staff and students may have different ownership rights from one another regarding data produced in the course of research.

Case Study

This is complicated but is representative of real-life situations.

> *In the UVW Study, a large epidemiological study, researchers may apply to access the study's questionnaire data for their own, separate project. Let's call a hypothetical project Project Orange. These UVW data become background research data for Project Orange. The research data generated by addition to and manipulation of the original data belong to Project Orange during its active phase, during which it has exclusive use of the data.*
>
> *After completion and publication of results, the Project Orange research data must be shared with the UVW Study. As the UVW Study is a collaborative resource, all data collected as part of it will, after a defined period of exclusive use, become available for use by other researchers in approved research projects.*
>
> *The researcher(s) own all IP rights in the data and materials collected by Project Orange and must grant the UVW Study an irrevocable, transferable, non-exclusive, sub-licensable, and royalty-free license to use, copy, and modify any data or materials that result from Project Orange.*

A related consideration is who has the right to use the data generated in a research project? Does it belong to the researcher or the institution? It can be very complicated when a researcher leaves an institution for elsewhere. Does she get to take the data with her? Who owns it? If she is still going to work on the project, can she take it with her? May she have a copy? Are your research students able to take the data they generated during the course of their study with them when they leave?

The answer to all these questions is "Sometimes, yes, sometimes no." It depends on the arrangements that have been made. In some unfortunate cases, the answer might be no on all fronts, and the researcher has to walk away from her project.

In many cases, these problems are resolved by permission to grant not ownership, but a license to use the data elsewhere.

Don't leave resolution of these sorts of issues to the last minute or you might find yourself leaving your data behind. It is much better dealt with in advance, preferably at the very beginning of your project.

Research Data Sharing

In the past, researchers did their very best to keep all research data secret, whereas in modern times it is recognized that making your research data available to others has many benefits. These include the following:

- Greater exposure of your research which may be useful for obtaining grants or getting published
- Increasing citations of your published work
- More opportunities for forming research collaboration across disciplines and with international researchers

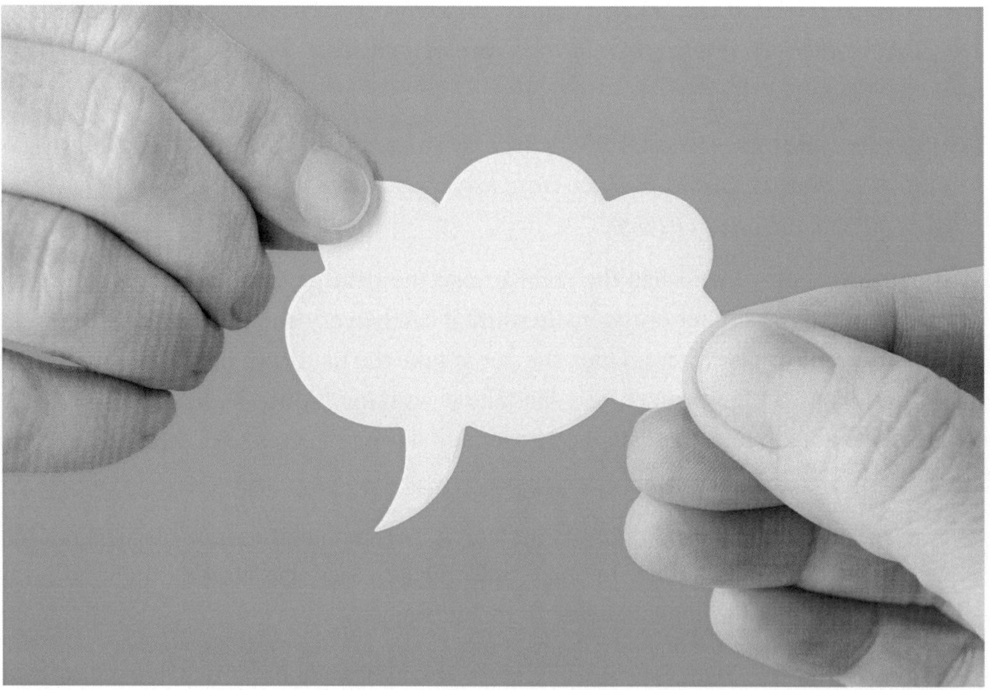

Image Credit: Sharing thoughts and information by mrPliskin/iStock

Piwowar [7] demonstrated that publicly available data were significantly associated with a 69% increase in citations, independent of journal impact factor, date of publication, and author's country of origin. They concluded that this correlation between publicly available data and increased literature impact may further motivate investigators to share their detailed research data.

Nowadays in many countries, researchers and institutions are also required to make data available to others. Research codes of practice require that research data should be made available for use by other researchers unless this is prevented by ethical, privacy, or confidentiality matters. Furthermore, many funding agencies require researchers, where possible, to make data publicly available within a specified timeframe, generally through deposit in an institutional or discipline-specific public repository.

Some journals also require researchers to make the data used in the publication available to interested persons. The Nature Publishing Group [8], for example, state "authors are required to make materials, data, code, and associated protocols promptly available to readers without undue qualifications."

Before you share data, whether during a project or after it is finished, you need to make sure that you have considered, and preferably taken independent legal advice about, the implications of doing so, with respect to terms of data and IP ownership and ethical requirements like privacy and confidentiality.

References—Research Data

[1] University of Melbourne Management of Research Data and Records Policy (MPF1242). http://policy.unimelb.edu.au/MPF1242.

[2] Data Management Manual, ANU. http://anulib.anu.edu.au/research-learn/research-data-management/managing-your-data.

[3] Research Data Planning Checklist, Monash. http://www.monash.edu/__data/assets/word_doc/0011/157772/datahdrchecklist_doc.doc.

[4] The Australian National Data Service (ANDS). http://www.ands.org.au/.

[5] Muchmore, M., Duffy, J., February 2017. PC News. http://au.pcmag.com/storage-devices-reviews/3696/guide/the-best-cloud-storage-and-file-sharing-services-of-2017.

[6] University of Leicester website. http://www2.le.ac.uk/services/research-data/organise-data/naming-files.

[7] Piwowar, H.A., Day, R.S., Fridsma, D.B., 2007. Sharing detailed research data is associated with increased citation rate. PLoS One 2 (3), e308. https://doi.org/10.1371/journal.pone.0000308.

[8] Nature Publishing Group. http://www.nature.com/authors/policies/availability.html.

4.6 Understanding Intellectual Property

A group of international collaborators engaged a contractor to write some software code for their model. An agreement had been made between the collaborators, but there was no agreement for the contractor who, to make matters extra complicated, happened to be the partner of one investigator. Recipe for disaster.

At the end of the project everyone, including the contractor, expected to own the IP. This was not the understanding of the principal investigator. There was blood on the floor!

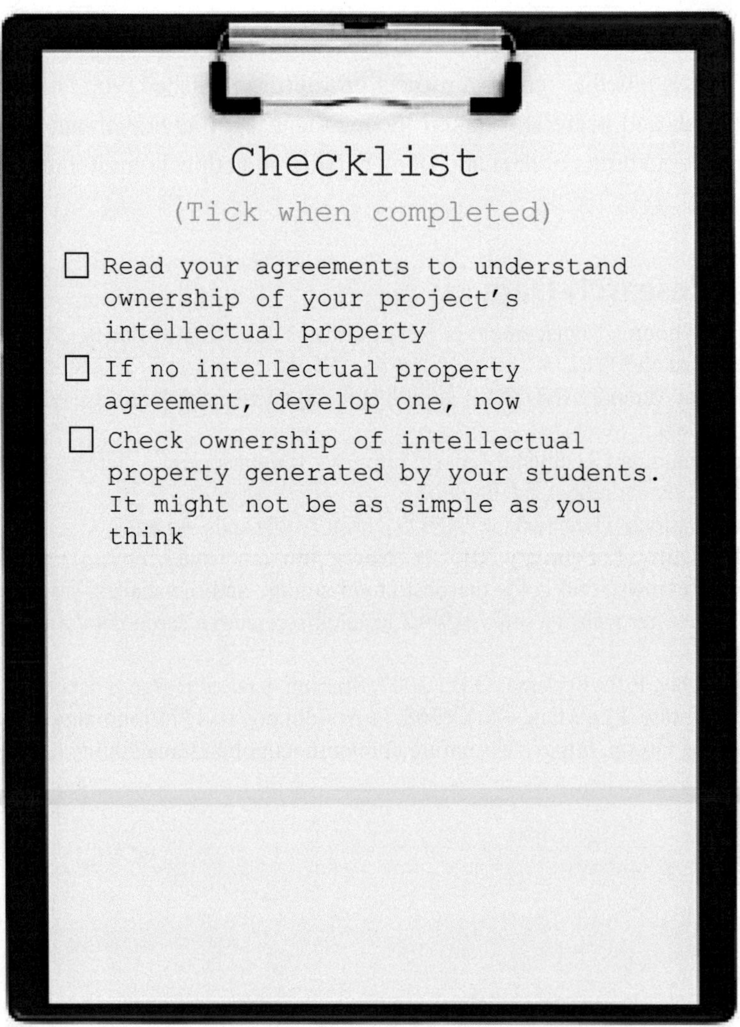

IP is described as "property rights that exist over the practical application of the creations in your mind." It has been mentioned on numerous occasions earlier in this book but is intentionally repeated in case the way you are using the book has not brought you to it already. It matters enough to merit a chapter of its own.

In the workplace, IP includes rights relating to scientific discoveries, industrial designs, trademarks, service marks, commercial names and designations, inventions and from activity in the industrial, scientific, literary, or artistic fields. The employer is the owner of all IP created by the employee in the course of work, unless a specific agreement has been made to the contrary.

Why Does Intellectual Property Matter in Research?

Once an idea is tangible, you can protect it. In research, the need for protection might arise when you take IP into a collaboration and later when new IP has been developed. You will want to state your ownership of what went in and will usually agree that the result of the collaboration is jointly owned. It is very important to discuss this at the beginning of the project, not at the end.

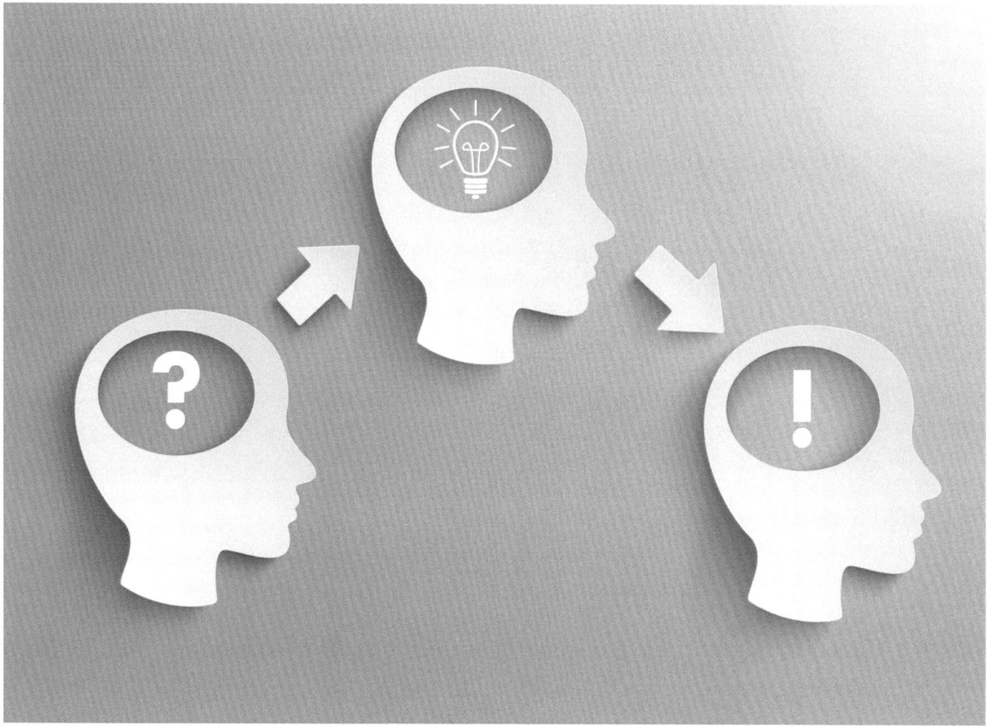

Image Credit: Three white heads by Alexander Limbach/Shutterstock

Generally speaking, IP generated at work belongs to your employer. It is, however, common practice to agree that IP brought into an agreement between two or more collaborating institutions remains the property of those institutions, while outputs generated together are shared equally.

In academic circles this can provide difficulties if you change institutions, and you must be aware that "your" work outputs can be regarded as "their" outputs. It is likely that this is specified in your employment contract.

There is one major exception to this in academia, which is the PhD thesis, the content of which usually belongs to the student. This may result in some confusion if the student is simultaneously employed in the same area of research.

Where collaborators are involved, particularly from other institutions, there should be formal agreements in place to decide the ultimate ownership of any IP. (See Agreements Chapter 4.3).

Some Intellectual Property Definitions

- *Background IP* is IP brought into the project by individuals or collaborators.
- *Project IP* is any knowledge that is created through running the project—including research outcomes, data, publications, products, techniques, or expertise. The IP produced will often tie in with the designated research targets, but research can throw up unexpected results, and thus unexpected IP.
- *Commercialization* of IP occurs when IP has potential commercial. If it is new, has value, and could be applied in a manner that people would pay for, then it may represent a commercial opportunity.

University policies typically dictate the sharing of any profits arising from the commercialization of IP. This is a complex legal issue. The opportunities and issues associated with potential commercialization should be approached and agreed upon by all parties before the IP and potential commercialized output is produced. Commercialization offices in universities should be able to assist with this process. See Chapter 7.6 for further information about commercialization.

Intellectual Property and Students

If you have a student in your team, you need to remember that that student is not an employee of your institution and is therefore not bound by the same obligations as your staff members. Therefore if you need the student to be bound by the same sorts of IP and confidentiality obligations as your staff to protect your project, you will need to have an agreement put in place between the university and the student. The form of this additional arrangement will vary from institution to institution. Check with the university to see what arrangements can be made.

References—Intellectual Property

A very good source of broad information on IP, "IP - Your Business Edge", has been put together by the Australian Government. https://www.ipaustralia.gov.au/tools-resources/interactives/ip-your-business-edge-issue-01-2016.

4.7 Managing your Project Budget

Bert's project ran out of money. It was quite simple really—he didn't keep a record of how much was being spent. Early in the project he gave permission to someone else in the team to do the ordering, but he never took any serious notice of the invoices as they came past. Certainly not enough notice to have an idea of how the costs were mounting.

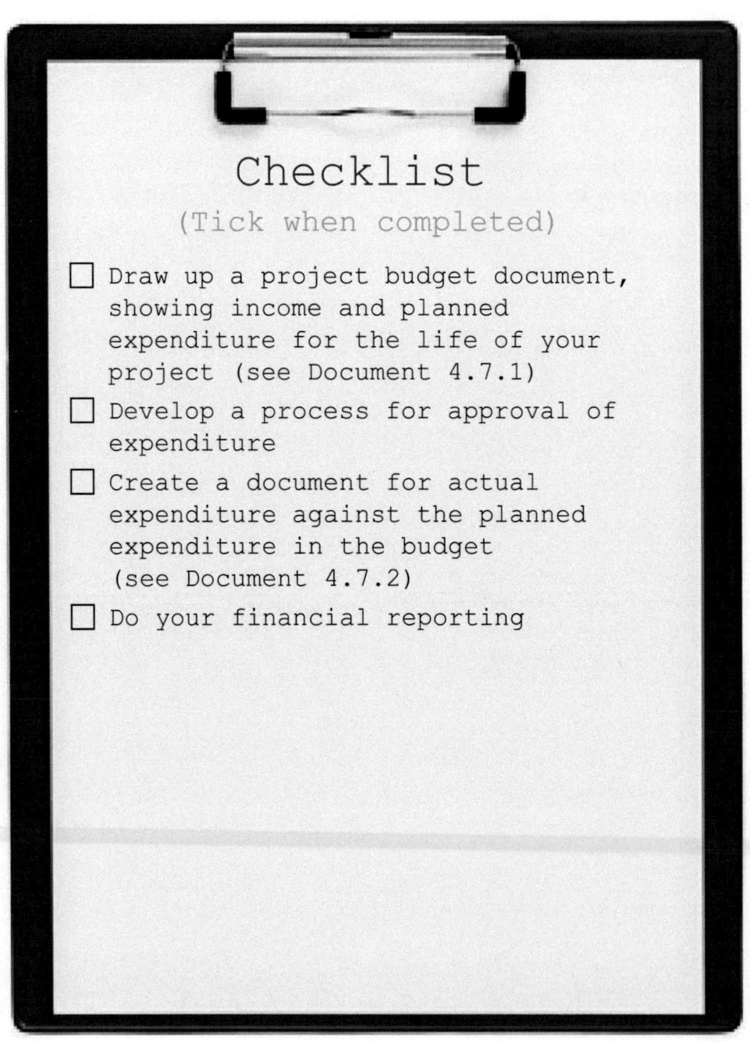

Once your project is funded, you must do your best to conduct the project within the agreed budget. The very first step is to have a copy of your budget. Use Document 1.6.1 Grant Application Budget Template at the end of this chapter to create your budget document if you do not already have one.

Just as for your household expenditure, you need to keep an eye on what you have spent, and keep enough in reserve for the future. You can't spend what you haven't got. There is many a project that has died halfway through because the funds were not administered properly.

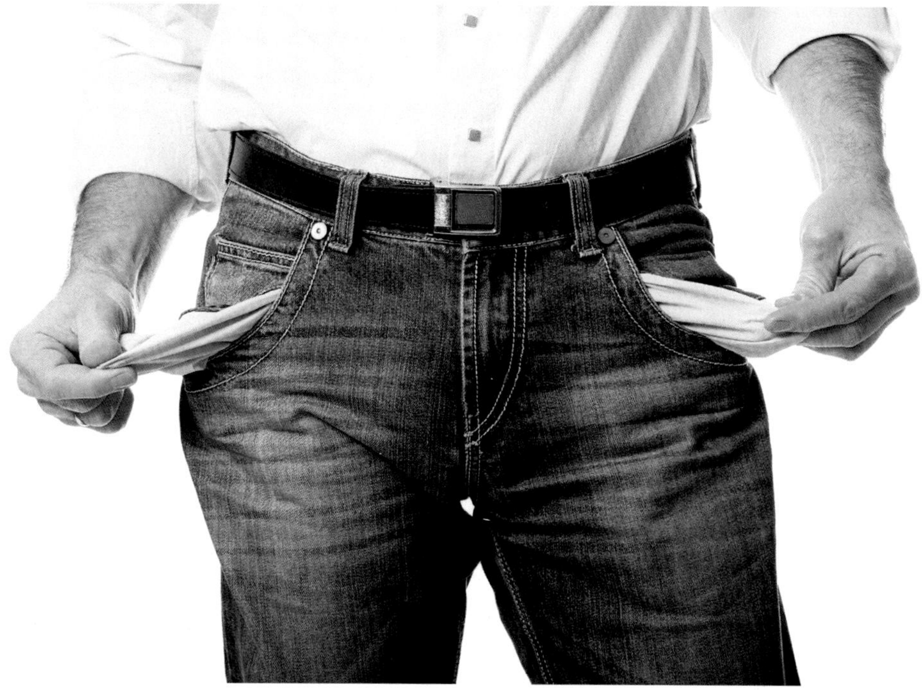

Image Credit: Man showing his empty pockets by PhotoMediaGroup/Shutterstock

Even though payments are being made by your institution, and they are keeping account, you should maintain your own record of all your expenditure, against budget. If you update a simple spreadsheet every month, you will be less likely to get nasty surprises. Not only can you see when you have spent too much but you can also keep an eye on where you are underspending and make wise use of extra funds. You may wish to use Document 4.7.2 Actual Expenditure versus Budget Template to monitor your expenditure.

This simple record will also be of great assistance when you come to report back to your funding agency.

Methods for Managing Project Expenditure

The following are five steps for to successful planning and controlling a project budget:

- Develop an overall budget plan to allocate your resources for the life of the project
- Set up a system for recording all financial transactions
- Have a system for reporting actual expenditure against the planned budget
- Understand the likely costs for the whole life of the project
- Have the ability to re-forecast when there is change from your initial intentions

Your budget plan will be developed at the beginning of the project, taking into account the full detail of what you intend to do during your project and when you intend to do it. This plan, prepared in the project planning phase (See Chapter 2.11) should ensure you have the resources to complete your research, including staff, consumables, equipment, and the use of facilities. Once you have built your full budget plan you can allocate your actual resources to your budget, thus setting the limits for your expenditure.

Plan Around Expenditure Timing

You must work out the likely timing for expenditure when planning your budget. This is especially relevant if your funding will come to you in parts, e.g., one year at a time, or one quarter at a time. You can't spend it if it hasn't arrived yet.

Salaries are relatively easy to plan, being month by month, but will all the project staff start on day one? Will each person always be full time or will loads change? Think about when you are likely to want to attend a conference? At what point will you need to pay for your data or your special software?

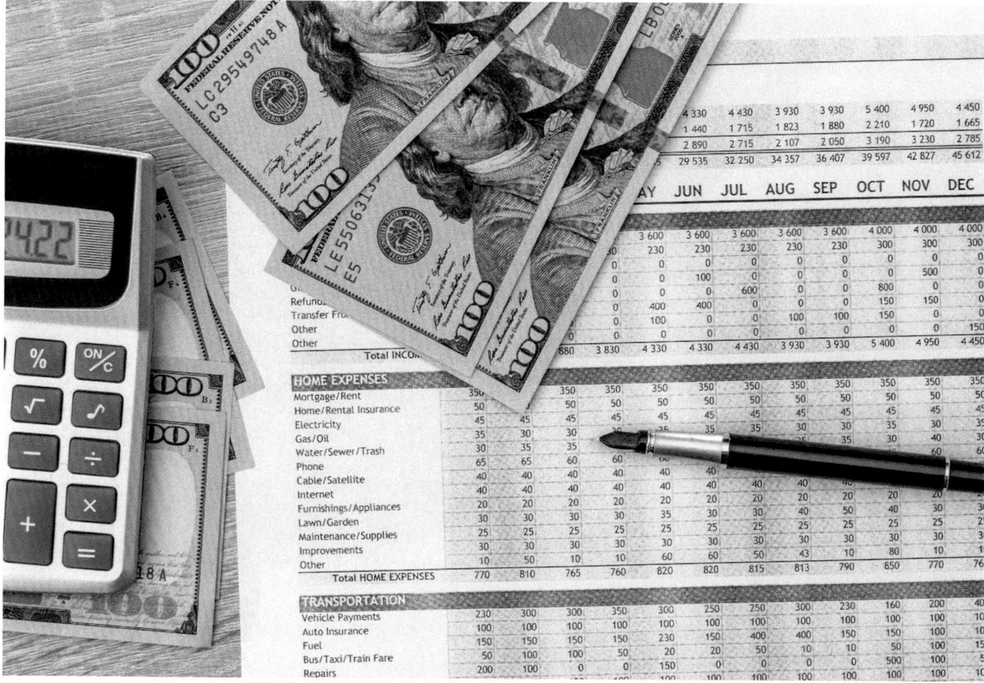

Image Credit: Analysis of the annual budget by RomanR/Shutterstock

Day-to-Day Management of Project Funds

In a small project, it is likely that you, as chief investigator, will be the only person with power to approve project expenditure. If your project is larger, or has collaborators from a big department or different faculties in the university, there may well be a need for more than one person to have permission to authorize spending from your project account. You should limit the number of people with authority to sign for expenditure to maintain control. Be sure, though, that anyone who is authorized to spend your project's money has a clear understanding of the procedures and of how much they might spend.

Establish a system to record expenditure approval—and use it even if you are the only possible signatory. This "system" could be as simple as signing and dating an invoice noting the specific budget section or cost account from which the money should come, prior to payment. The expenditure should also be recorded on your project expenditure document. A more formal system could require a cover sheet specifying invoice number, service provider, date, amount, and budget line. Whatever method you choose, keep a copy of the documentation either in paper form or electronic in a specific place, not in a pile in your in tray or the back of your car.

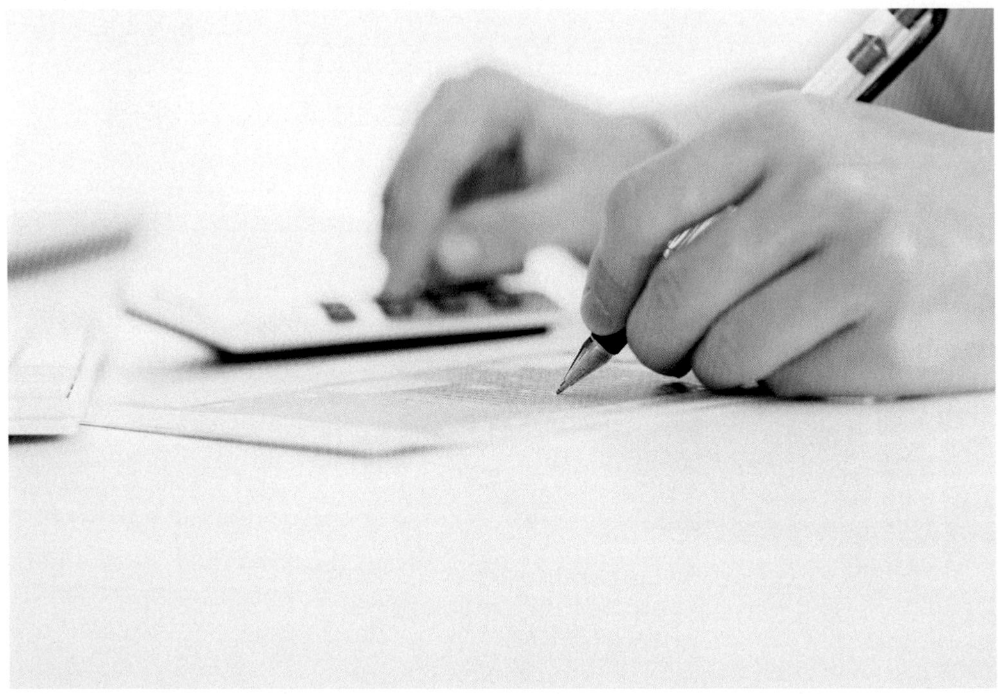

Image Credit: Caclulating expenses by fotostorm/iStock

Budget Review and Reporting

You should diarize a review of your expenditure every month, checking actuals against budget. If variance starts to creep in, correct it with a re-forecast.

Even if you are tracking on target, it is a good idea to also regularly review your costs to see whether they can be brought down, so that money might be made available for something else. Consider whether you could buy in bulk, change to a different supplier, or even share costs with another project.

It is vital to have a good reporting system which does the following:

- Identifies variances by subject heading
- Provides an explanation for the variance and/or of its rectification
- Shows actuals to date versus budget to date

It is most important to understand your budget reporting system, even if you do not personally handle the day-to-day expenditure. As lead investigator, you are the person responsible. Without a good reporting procedure, you could place your project in serious jeopardy. Mishandling your budget could have far-reaching consequences for your reputation and the reputation of your collaborators and your institution.

Managing Expenditure at Other Institutions

Where a project has collaborators from different institutions, it is usual to organize for the monies to be sent from the funding agency to the principal investigator's institution, from which it will sent to where they will be spent. This would be specified in your collaborator agreement (see Chapter 4.3). The investigator at each site should keep a record of expenditure against budget and should report regularly to the rest of the team. It is usual for the investigators at other institutions to provide an annual acquittal report to the lead investigator.

Making Changes to Your Budget

During the life of the project you may have to re-allocate funding that was planned for, say, salaries to equipment or equipment to reagents. You are usually permitted to do this (depending on the arrangements with your funding agency), as long as you don't spend more than you have available. If you decide to alter the allocation of funds, make a dated note at the bottom of your spreadsheet explaining why you have re-allocated expenditure. In many cases, you will need to seek formal approval from your funding body before making this change.

Amazingly, sometimes there is money left over, and funding bodies may require the return of their unspent funds. This situation might have arisen because all the project costs that should have been allocated to your project have not in fact been charged. An example could be where add-on costs for staff have been picked up by the university instead of by the project. Be aware that this budgetary error will end up as an expense for your university, which could have been avoided.

Tips for Managing When You Don't Receive Your Full Amount

It is unfortunately fairly common for a successful grant applicant to receive significantly less money than was applied for. Managing the budget becomes much more difficult! Unless you can source some other pots of money to fund aspects of the project, this will often result in your objectives being curtailed.

If you fail to find extra money, don't try to complete the original project objectives with the reduced funding. If you prepared your budget accurately in the first place, then you will not be able to deliver everything you promised to the required standard on your reduced income.

As you can't do everything you had undertaken to do with only 60% of the budget, you must work out how to deal with the problem. If there is no other source of funding, you will need to re-work the project plan, taking into account the reduced budget, and inform the granting agency.

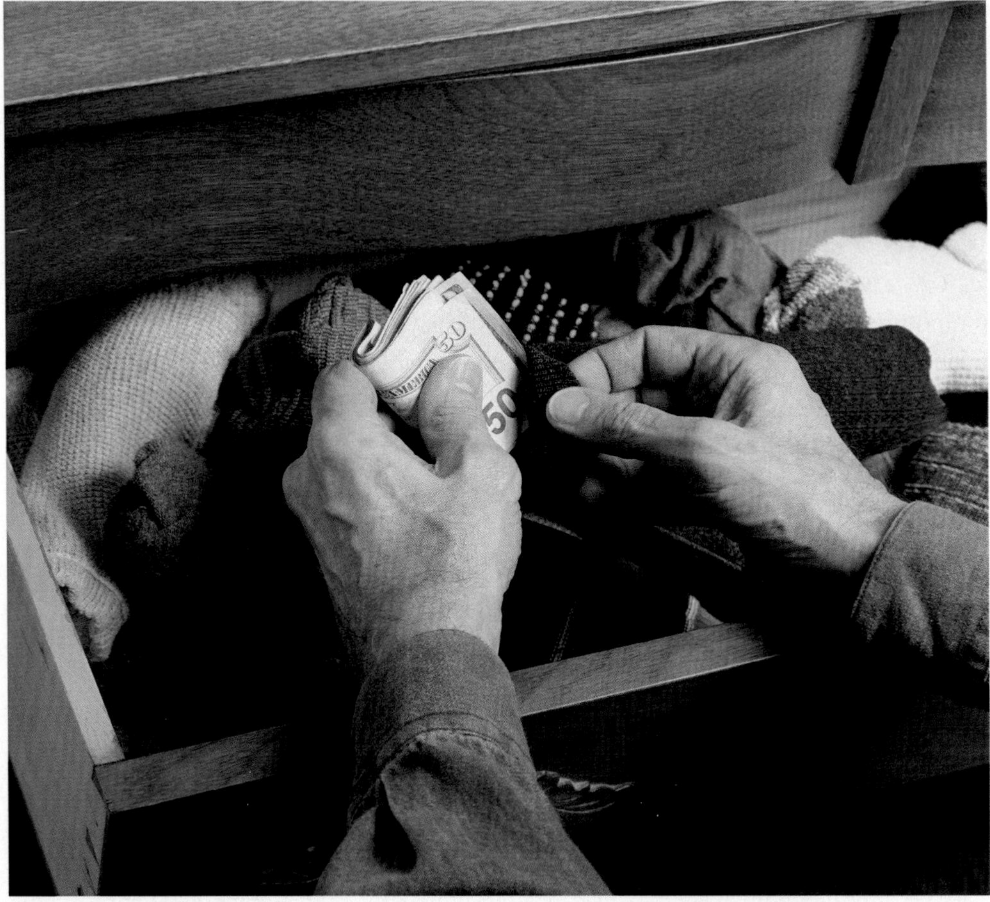

Image Credit: Man hiding cash in sock drawer by Ken Tannenbaum/Shutterstock

In summary, in the case of receiving reduced funds, you could do one of four things:

- As a first step, you can try to find some more money. Your university might have some discretionary funds.
- Form a collaboration with another organization or investigator who would have a vested interest in the success of your project and who has the funds available to carry out the tasks.
- Reduce your project's aims, and correspondingly reduce costs. If you take this track, you must advise the funding body. They need to know about, and approve, changes to your project and why they have been made. If following this option, you could treat the project as a pilot study, which will provide results to help you attract further funding.
- Apply funds from your consulting account, if you have one.

Beware of another trap for the unwary, which might be set by your institution. Many universities have a policy of taking a percentage of your grant funding for overheads. The $100,000 you had earmarked for salaries could suddenly become $80,000 after they take their cut, before you have even engaged someone for a position. Obviously it is best to see if this applies at your university before submitting your application. You might need to ask for more in your budget.

Financial Reporting

During the life of your project, you will be responsible for financial reporting for your project. This reporting will include annual progress financial reports and "acquittal" or final financial reports; financial reports may also be required for audits.

Progress Reports

Your research office will usually be responsible for sending progress reports to your funding body, but as lead investigator you will have to check to see they are correct and provide reasons for any variance from the original agreement.

Acquittal or Final Reports

A report is always due at the end of the project. This report explains expenditure during the life of the project. The funding body will usually require certification from your institution that the funds have been spent in accordance with the terms and conditions of your funding agreement.

This report is usually submitted via the research office on a standard form. Funds will usually have to be spent—acquitted—by a time that will have been specified in your deed of agreement. This final report is prepared only after all project expenditure is complete, usually within two months of the completion of the project.

Audits

Funding bodies may request an audit of your project expenditure at any time. You should always be in a position to comply with such a request. Using your monthly budget documentation, you should be able to offer an explanation of all expenditure and variation against budget and provide the auditors with appropriate records.

Seeking Additional Funding

Times are tough all over the world, and they are becoming tougher. Learn to look outside the obvious for funding sources. For small pots of money try to find the following:

- Travel grants
- Equipment grants
- Young investigator grants
- PhD scholarship—for a student for your team

Look too for opportunities available from the following:

- Support groups for a particular area of research
- Smaller trusts and foundations with an interest in your cause
- Local Rotary or other community service groups that might have a member who is a champion for your cause
- Family members or work places of people who suffer from "your disease"

You can even try crowd funding. This is tempting, but realistically you are unlikely to be successful! It is definitely worth a try if it is not going to take too much of your time.

> The best place to look is among people or organizations with a vested interest in the successful outcome of your research.

Associated Documents—Managing Your Project Budget

4.7.1 Operational Project Budget

		Year 1													Year 2	
	Budget	Jan	Feb	Mar	Apr	May	Jun	Jul	Aug	Sep	Oct	Nov	Dec	YTD Total	Jan	and onwards
Staff Costs																
Salary Person 1	**1,20,000**	10,000	10,000	10,000	10,000									40,000		
Oncosts Person 1	**21,600**	1800	1800	1800	1800									7,200		
Salary Person 2	**45000**				5000									5,000		
Oncosts Person 2	**8100**				900									900		
Training					1000									1,000		
														0		
Conference Fees	**4000**													0		
Travel and Accommodation	**1000**													0		
														0		
Consultants Fees	**3000**															
Software purchase	**1800**															
Software licencing or annual support																
Data Fees	**1500**			1500												
Data Storage														0		
														0		
Consumables	**30,000**													0		
														0		
Equipment Purchase	**10,000**													0		
Equipment service and maintenance	**1,000**													0		
														0		
Volunteer costs	**500**													0		
Volunteer Travel														0		
														0		
Publication Fees	**3000**													0		
														0		
Telephone	**1500**													0		
Stationery	**500**													0		
Printing														0		
Postage, Freight and Courier	**500**													0		
Meeting Costs	**1000**													0		
Total	**254000**	11800	11800	13300	18700	0	0	0	0	0	0	0	0	54100		

4.7.2 Actual Expenditure vs Budget Template

		Year 1													Year 2	
	Budget	Jan	Feb	Mar	Apr	May	Jun	Jul	Aug	Sep	Oct	Nov	Dec	YTD Total	Jan	and onwards
Staff Costs																
Salary Person 1	**1,20,000**		10,000	10,000	10,000									40,000		
Oncosts Person 1	**21,600**	1800	1800	1800	1800									7,200		
Salary Person 2	**45000**				5000									5,000		
Oncosts Person 2	**8100**				900									900		
Training					1000									1,000		
														0		
Conference Fees	**4000**													0		
Travel and Accommodation	**1000**													0		
														0		
Consultants Fees	**3000**															
Software purchase	**1800**															
Software licencing or annual support																
Data Fees	**1500**			1500												
Data Storage														0		
														0		
Consumables	**30,000**													0		
														0		
Equipment Purchase	**10,000**													0		
Equipment service and maintenance	**1,000**													0		
														0		
Volunteer costs	**500**													0		
Volunteer Travel														0		
														0		
Publication Fees	**3000**													0		
														0		
Telephone	**1500**													0		
Stationery	**500**													0		
Printing														0		
Postage, Freight and Courier	**500**													0		
Meeting Costs	**1000**													0		
Total	**254000**	11800	11800	13300	18700	0	0	0	0	0	0	0	0	54100		

4.7.3 Completed Budget - Project Thunderstorm

Project Thunderstorm Budget		Year 1	Year 2	Year 3	Year 4	Year 5	Total
DIRECT RESEARCH COSTS							
Second Yearly Research Symposium							
	10 Travel Scholarships - Research Trainees	5,000	5,000	5,000	5,000	5,000	25,000
	International Speaker	-	7,000	-	7,000	-	14,000
	Venue Costs - Refreshments , Audio Visual etc.	-	5,000	-	5,000	-	10,000
		5,000	17,000	5,000	17,000	5,000	49,000
Management Committee Meetings							
	Travel and Accommodation	8,000	8,000	8,000	8,000	8,000	40,000
	Venue Costs and refreshments	1,000	1,000	1,000	1,000	1,000	5,000
	Parking , Taxis and Transfers, Subsistence	1,000	1,000	1,000	1,000	1,000	5,000
		10,000	10,000	10,000	10,000	10,000	50,000
International Advisory Board Forum							
	Venue Costs and refreshments	1,000	1,000	1,000	1,000	1,000	5,000
	Parking , Taxis and Transfers	500	500	500	500	500	2,500
		1,500	1,500	1,500	1,500	1,500	7,500
Travel Scholarships - Trainees							
	Interstate/Overseas Training	8,000	-	8,000	-	8,000	24,000
		8,000	-	8,000	-	8,000	24,000
Translation & Education							
	Consumer Forum	5,000	-	5,000	-	5,000	15,000
	Patient self-management resource development	5,000	10,000	5,000	2,500	2,500	25,000
	Web portal development	10,000	10,000	-	-	-	20,000
	Webinar series	-	-	7,500	-	-	7,500
		20,000	20,000	17,500	2,500	7,500	67,500
Website & Blog Development/Maintenance	Website design and activation (including for ACTIoN)	5,000	-	-	-	-	5,000
	Maintenance Costs	1,000	1,000	1,000	1,000	1,000	5,000
		6,000	1,000	1,000	1,000	1,000	10,000
	SUB TOTAL DIRECT RESEARCH COSTS	50,500	49,500	43,000	32,000	33,000	2,08,000
SALARIES AND ADD ON COSTS							
	Manager (0.5 FTE) - PSP-3	18,415	36,831	36,831	36,831	36,831	1,65,737
	Clinical Trial Coordinators (each at 0.2FTE)						
	Site 1	-	13,397	13,397	13,397	-	40,191
	Site 2	-	13,397	13,397	13,397	-	40,191
		-	26,794	26,794	26,794	-	80,382
	Translation and Patient Initiatives Coordinators						
	Site 1	-	20,000	20,000	20,000	-	60,000
	Site 2	20,000	20,000	20,000	3,333	-	63,333
		20,000	40,000	40,000	23,333	-	1,23,333
	PhD Stipends						
	Student 1	-	26,824	26,824	26,824	-	80,472
	Student 2	-	26,824	26,824	26,824	-	80,472
		-	53,648	53,648	53,648	-	1,60,944
	Lab Staff						
	Lab position 1	27,912	33,495	33,495	33,495	33,495	1,61,890
	Lab position 2	27,912	33,495	33,495	33,495	33,495	1,61,890
		55,824	66,989	66,989	66,989	66,989	3,23,780
	Post doctorate Fellows (2years)						
	Fellow 1	-	29,464	29,464	14,733	-	73,662
	Fellow 2	36,831	36,831			-	73,661
		36,831	66,295	29,464	14,733	-	1,47,323
	SUB TOTAL SALARIES	1,31,070	2,90,556	2,53,726	2,22,328	1,03,820	10,01,499
RESEARCH FACILITIES							
	Consumables incl. courier	26,193	29,771	10,670	5,968	-	72,602
	Storage Costs	7,200	7,560	7,938	8,335	8,752	39,785
	Plasticware incl tubes	6,738	7,782	17,793	1,560	-	33,872
	Metabolomics/proteomics/scientific analysis	-		50,000	50,000	50,000	1,50,000
	SUB TOTAL RESEARCH FACILITIES	40,131	45,113	86,401	65,863	58,752	2,96,259
	GRAND TOTALS	2,21,701	3,85,169	3,83,127	3,20,190	1,95,571	15,05,758

4.8 Project Meetings

At Institute Boris, meetings were long, boring, and disorganized. There was usually a standard agenda, but no one stuck to it. Minutes weren't taken, so no one could be held accountable when actions weren't followed up. The staff stopped turning up, and anyone who came was usually ill-prepared and disengaged. These meetings for the sake of meetings were a complete waste of time.

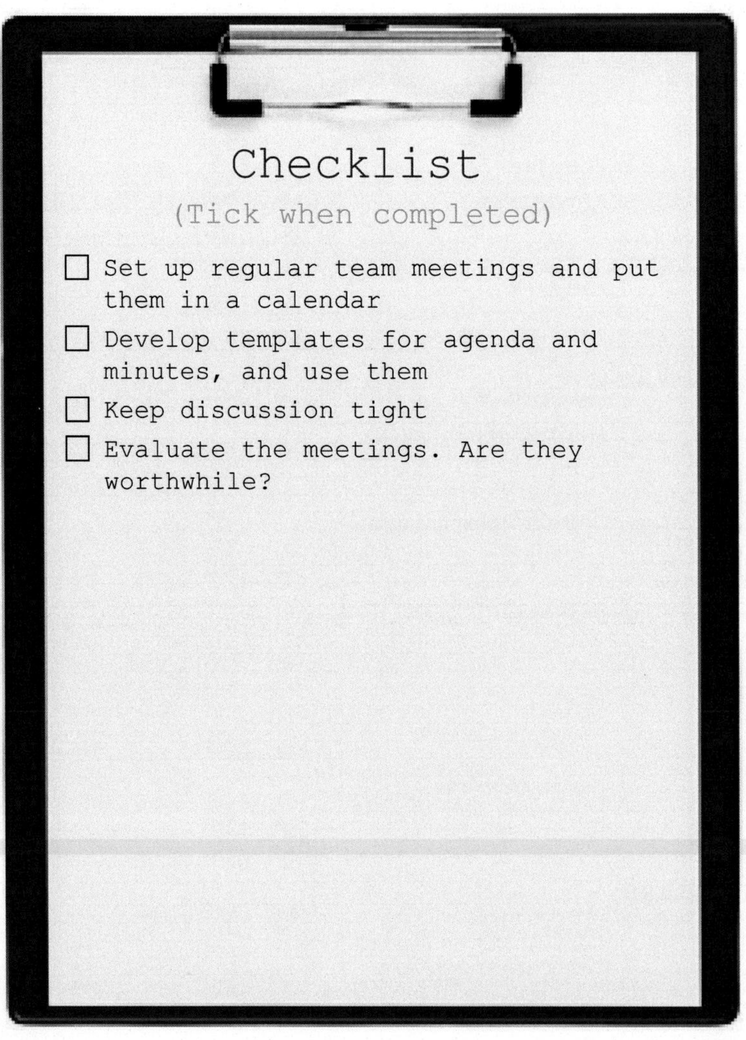

Projects typically involve a lot of meetings. Between meetings for project teams, individual project streams, advisory committees, and other "as required" meetings, you could have many meetings per month.

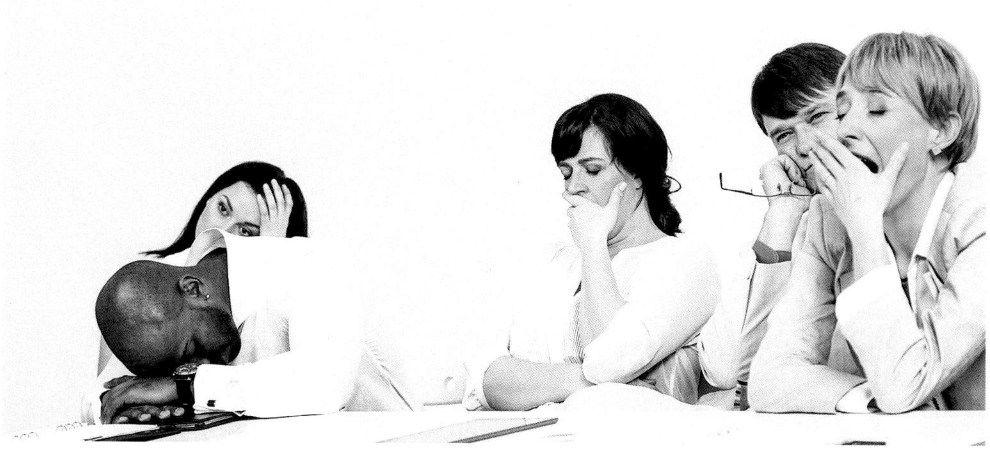

Image Credit: Boring seminar by lovro77/iStock

> Meetings should be outcome driven, and not be meetings for the sake of meetings. They should have a clear purpose. The duration should be minimal—not a default time of 30 or 60 minutes.

The following good meeting practices will save a lot of time, money, and boredom:

- Schedule regular recurring meetings
- Always prepare, circulate, and stick to an agenda
- Take and distribute minutes. Note action items and establish in your team a practice of following them up and reporting back at the next meeting
- Expect attendees to be on time, ready, and prepared
- Keep the meeting on track
- Keep it relevant
- Start and finish on time
- Take five minutes at the end to review the meeting's effectiveness and outcomes

❹ RUNNING THE STUDIES

A good meeting document template helps you deliver a good project and should include the following:

- Dates of this and the previous and next meetings
- Attendees
- Apologies
- Acceptance of minutes
- Actions arising
- Risks
- Issues
- Impending milestones
- Other topics of interest

See templates for meeting minutes and agenda at the end of Chapter 4.4.

4.9 Marketing Your Research to Your Stakeholders

Professor Ian Frazer is a perfect example of a research scientist who knows how to sell his dream. He has, as the co-inventor of the HPV vaccine (among other triumphs), of course, achieved enormous success. Ian's work has led to groundbreaking advances and has saved countless people's lives, but there was a time when he wasn't famous.

Ian's skills for explaining his research are exemplary. When addressing an audience, he explains what he is doing now, and lays emphasis on what comes next. He is simply wonderful at explaining why it matters. Even though Ian is heading up laboratories brimming with funding, he tries to never miss an opportunity to explain why he needs more.

Ian has helped save the world from the consequences of HPV infection. Now he is onto skin cancer, and who knows what next. You can be sure that he will keep his stakeholders in the loop.

Checklist

(Tick when completed)

- ☐ Diarize reporting to your stakeholders
- ☐ Create a newsletter for those stakeholders, send updates regularly
- ☐ Use social media to talk about your project
- ☐ Visit your stakeholders
- ☐ Arrange visits to your institute

You've got your funding, you have your plan, you just want to get on with your work. No need to be telling anyone about what you are up to until it is all finished and you have something to say. Right? *Wrong!!!*

Research dissemination is much more than publications. It should start right at the beginning of your project, and shouldn't finish until long after the project end. There are sections for publishing and presentation in later chapters, but your research dissemination should begin along with your project.

It is very important to keep your stakeholders in the loop about your progress, right from the start. They have believed in you and the research idea you are working on enough to invest in it. They have offered you time, money, and belief in your cause. It is very much in your interest to keep them in the loop about how you are getting on.

You need to market your research and why it matters. Your stakeholders want to know the following:

- Why is it important?
- How are you spending your time and money?
- What difference is it going to make?
- How is it going to benefit them?

If you are the recipient of external funding, you will be aware that you have to submit an annual progress report. This other sort of reporting serves a different purpose, and, in the end, the principal beneficiary will be you.

Whichever category the stakeholders fall into, it is a wise investment of your time to tell them about your work. You know why you are doing what you are doing, but they need to be reminded, especially about *why it matters* and *how the outcome is going to make a difference.*

Consider your target audiences and their viewpoints. These might include the following:

- Funding bodies
  - Are they spending my money wisely and well?
  - Are they doing what they said?
  - Will they finish on time?
- General public
  - Are they going to find a cure?
  - Is this going to make my life better?

- Research participants
  - How are they using my information?
  - When are there going to be results?
  - Did what I do help anyone?
- Your colleagues in your institution
  - How does this work fit with the organization's strategy?
  - When will they be finished?
  - Is there anything relevant to my work?

Here following are some easy ways to report to your stakeholders.

Email a Newsletter

Set up a template that makes it easy to send out a quarterly email newsletter. Focus on the following:

- What your project is about
- Why it matters
- What you are doing now
- What you are doing next

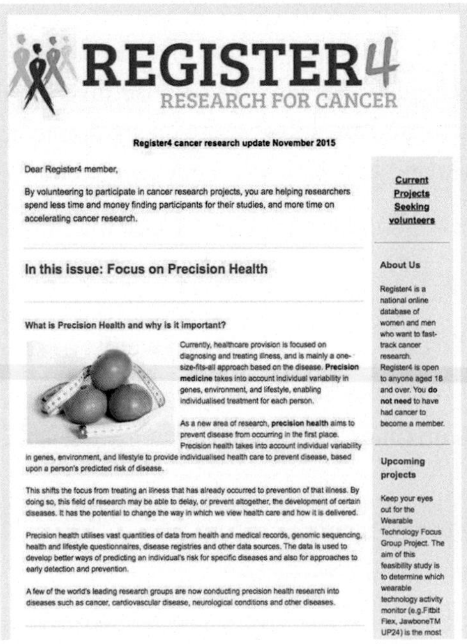

REGISTER4
RESEARCH FOR CANCER

Register4 cancer research update November 2015

Dear Register4 member,

By volunteering to participate in cancer research projects, you are helping researchers spend less time and money finding participants for their studies, and more time on accelerating cancer research.

In this issue: Focus on Precision Health

What is Precision Health and why is it important?

Currently, healthcare provision is focused on diagnosing and treating illness, and is mainly a one-size-fits-all approach based on the disease. **Precision medicine** takes into account individual variability in genes, environment, and lifestyle, enabling individualised treatment for each person.

As a new area of research, **precision health** aims to prevent disease from occurring in the first place. Precision health takes into account individual variability in genes, environment, and lifestyle to provide individualised health care to prevent disease, based upon a person's predicted risk of disease.

This shifts the focus from treating an illness that has already occurred to prevention of that illness. By doing so, this field of research may be able to delay, or prevent altogether, the development of certain diseases. It has the potential to change the way in which we view health care and how it is delivered.

Precision health utilises vast quantities of data from health and medical records, genomic sequencing, health and lifestyle questionnaires, disease registries and other data sources. The data is used to develop better ways of predicting an individual's risk for specific diseases and also for approaches to early detection and prevention.

A few of the world's leading research groups are now conducting precision health research into diseases such as cancer, cardiovascular disease, neurological conditions and other diseases.

Current Projects Seeking volunteers

About Us

Register4 is a national online database of women and men who want to fast-track cancer research. Register4 is open to anyone aged 18 and over. You **do not need** to have had cancer to become a member.

Upcoming projects

Keep your eyes out for the Wearable Technology Focus Group Project. The aim of this feasibility study is to determine which wearable technology activity monitor (e.g.Fitbit Flex, JawboneTM UP24) is the most

Pop in a couple of pictures. People like to read about people. Include a profile of someone in your team and describe them and their interests away from work.

Write your news very simply, concentrating on using lay terminology if your audience is the general public. With your simple template sent by email, the cost is only your time.

Encourage your recipients to send your newsletter on to other interested parties. You never know where an email might end up so be sure to remember to include the following:

- The name of your institution
- Your contact details
- A provision to subscribe and unsubscribe

Talk About Your Work on Social Media

Post regularly on social media. It's cheap, easy, and gets an immediate response.

> *"Social media just has to be part of your day. It will shine arc lights on the work you have produced."* @SimonChapmanAO [1] - 9797 Twitter followers (and growing).

See more about using social media in Chapter 1.9.

Visit Your Stakeholders

Take every opportunity to address your corporate sponsor. For your talk use slides with few words and lots of images. Remind them why you are doing what you are doing. Thank them and remind them that they are helping you make a difference.

Have Stakeholders Visit You

Also take opportunities to invite your stakeholders to your workplace. A 30 minute tour around a laboratory is worth every bit of time "wasted" as your stakeholders get to feel a sense of ownership. Never underestimate how much this matters, especially if you find later on that your project needs more time or money.

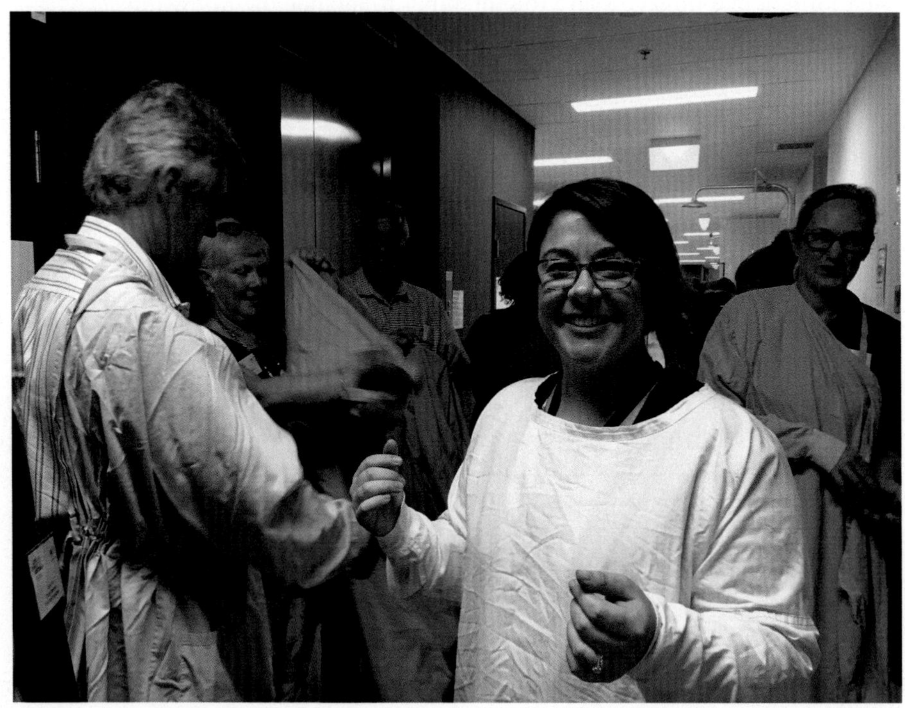

Keep Your Research Participants Updated

If your project involves collecting data from people, do them the courtesy of keeping them up to date. People who feel involved in your work will be proud of their contribution and proud of you. This leads to good publicity, and may well lead to more participants (if they recruit their friends and families), and to further investment.

Consider sending out a brief quarterly project update (or newsletter as previously mentioned) to all participants about your research progress.

An added benefit of regular communication is keeping track of participants who move about. If they feel responsible to you, they will advise you about their change of address or other circumstances.

If you need further funding at any stage, the relationship you have built up may make them feel inclined to help when you need it.

> *Remember to include this further contact in your ethics application and ask participants to consent to receiving updates.* Collect the participant's email address right at the start of the project. Email provides an invaluable means of "free" and rapid contact.

Campaign Monitor is an example of an excellent tool for email dissemination and can be used to track the progress and opening rates of your messages.

Keeping members of the community in the loop about your research is becoming increasingly important. If you want to increase your chances of getting further funding, or winning that sought-after fellowship, you will have to demonstrate that you are reaching out to the community. It is now a requirement to include community engagement in your CV. *Include the stakeholder engagement activities described on your CV.*

Keep Your Website Updated

Setting up a project website was discussed in Chapter 1.9. Remember to upload your newsletters and copies of or links to your social media to the website. Include photographs of the site visits. All these methods contribute to making your project alive, real, and relevant.

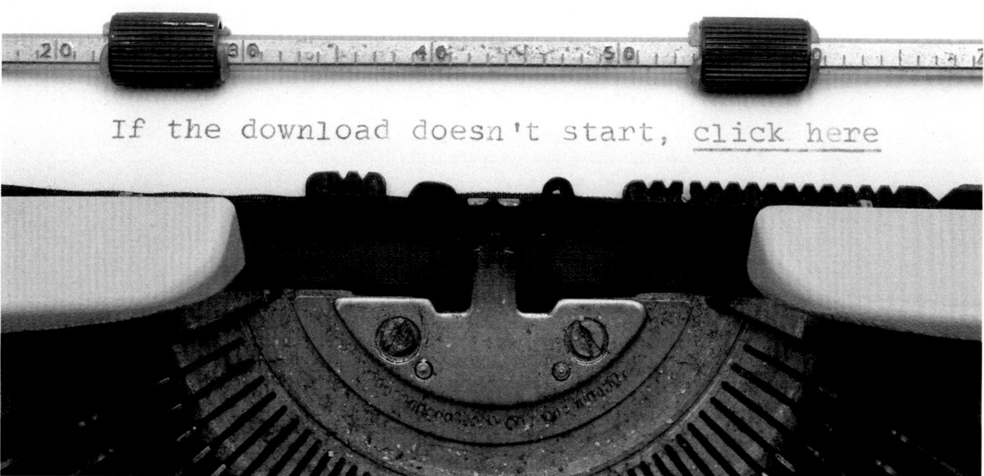

Image Credit: If the download doesn't start, click here by luoman/iStock

References—Marketing Your Research to Your Stakeholders

[1] Chapman, S. Get people talking: using social media to promote your research, University of Sydney Library. http://libguides.library.usyd.edu.au/c.php?g=508217&p=3475813.

4.10 More About Marketing—Communication Planning

The Rainbow Society raised funds for children in need. Some of those funds went to support research into the outcomes of their placement programs. Needless to say the Rainbow Society were interested in the answers. In spite of being the principal stakeholder, and the keeper of the treasury, they were unable to make the researchers understand the importance of feeding back to the community. Their requests for regular newsletters fell on deaf ears and many supporters lost interest in their cause.

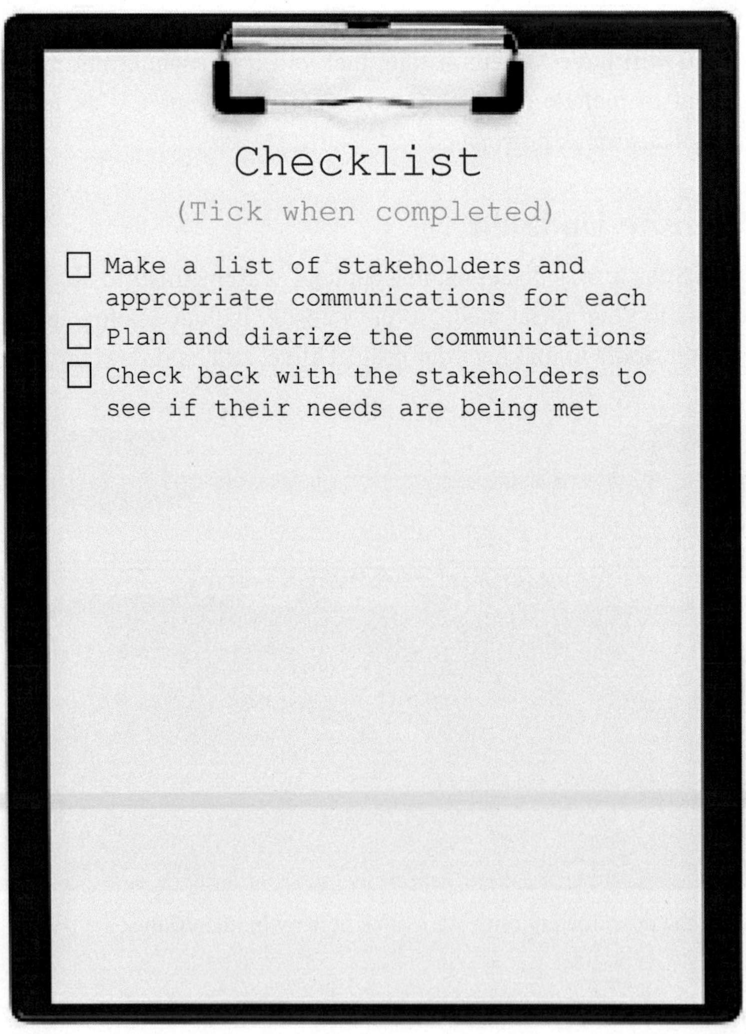

It is important to have a communication plan for your project and to develop it up front. This is not an afterthought to be tacked on reluctantly at the end. As mentioned in Chapter 4.9, you need to be communicating with your stakeholders throughout the life of the project and at the end when you publish its results.

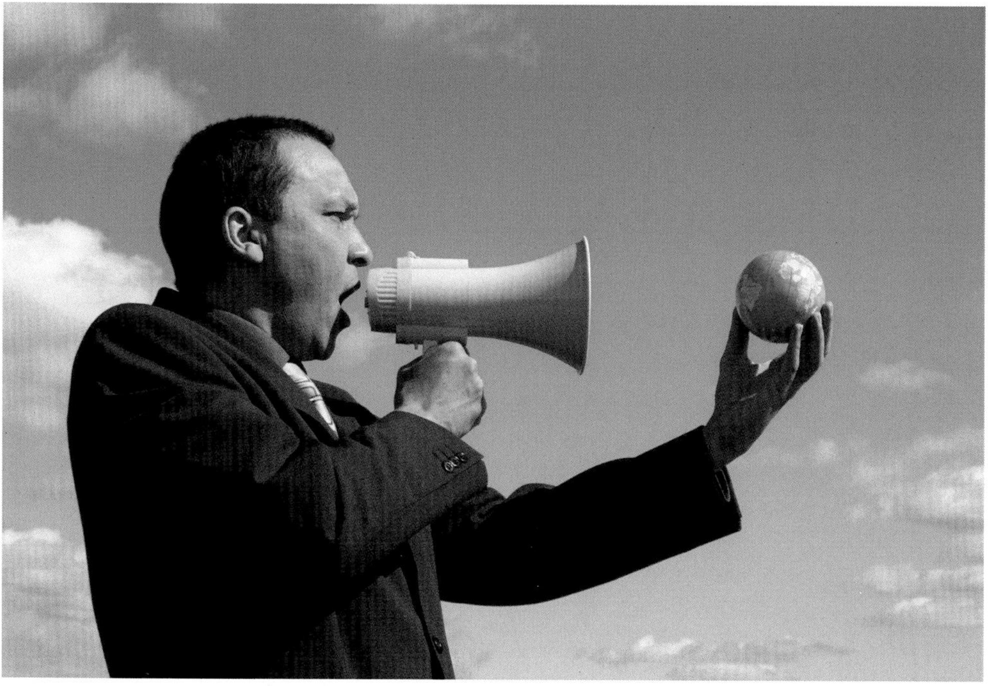

Image Credit: Calling the world by redmal/iStock

Stakeholders for a communication plan should include the following:

- Your funding body
- Your university
- Collaborators
- The whole research team
- Mentors
- Ethics committee/institutional review board
- Study participants
- Suppliers

❹ RUNNING THE STUDIES

Use your communications to market the benefit of your project and the strengths of your team to your stakeholders.

It may sound obvious to include the whole research team; however, there are many surprising instances where one half of a project team doesn't know what the other half is doing, particularly if they are at different institutes. Remember to give everyone a regular report. This effort will not be wasted. Not only does it perform the useful task of keeping the rest of the team up to date but it will also provide you with useful background material when the time comes to write up your project.

You may also consider putting updates on your website or, if appropriate, having your media department prepare a media release when there has been an achievement of note. It is also worthwhile to write a regular study newsletter and send it out by email whether as an attachment or by electronic direct mail. This sort of regular communication builds engagement with your project and gives stakeholders a sense of ownership. It provides yet another way to enhance your reputation.

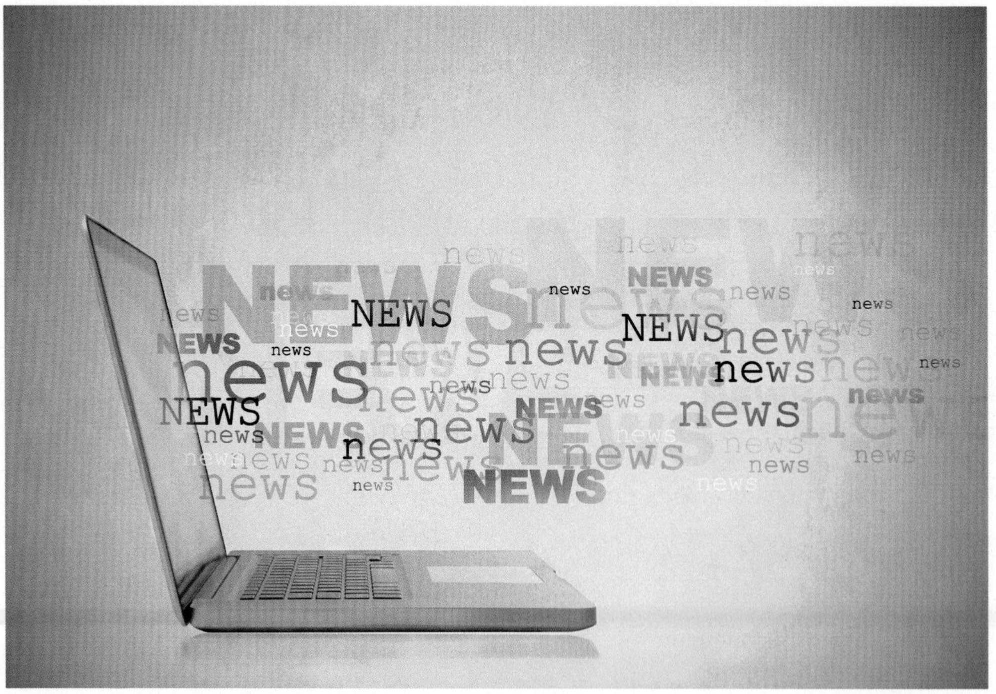

Image Credit: Laptop with the word news coming out of the screen by Ollyy/Shutterstock

You may wish to use the Communications Plan Template 4.2.2 at the end of Chapter 4.2 to map out your regular reporting and other stakeholder communications throughout the project. Similar information can be found in Table 4.10.1.

TABLE 4.10.1 Project Communications Plan Template

Stakeholder communication	Objective	Type of communication	Frequency	Level of communication	Individual(s) responsible
Funding agencies	Demonstrate project progress for continued funding	Progress report	Annually	Scheme/Project manager	Research leader
Research managers/ administrators					
Ministerial assessors and reviewers					
Auditors					
Collaborators—industry (business development, legal, academic)					
Collaborators—academic (inside the institution, outside the institution)					
Internal administration—host institution and other institution—executive					
Internal administration—host institution and other institution—administration					
Internal administration—host institution and other institution—legal office					
Internal administration—host institution and other institution—HR					
Internal administration—host institution and other institution—finance					
Internal administration—host institution and other institution—marketing					
Project staff and students					

4.11 Equipment and Consumables

Jeff and Marty decided to buy the equipment for their new laboratory secondhand. What a deal! They would save thousands. Unfortunately, when the whizz bang machine broke down, they discovered it was not only out of warranty but the parts also weren't available either. Someone was going to have to track them down overseas and the lead time for delivery was months.

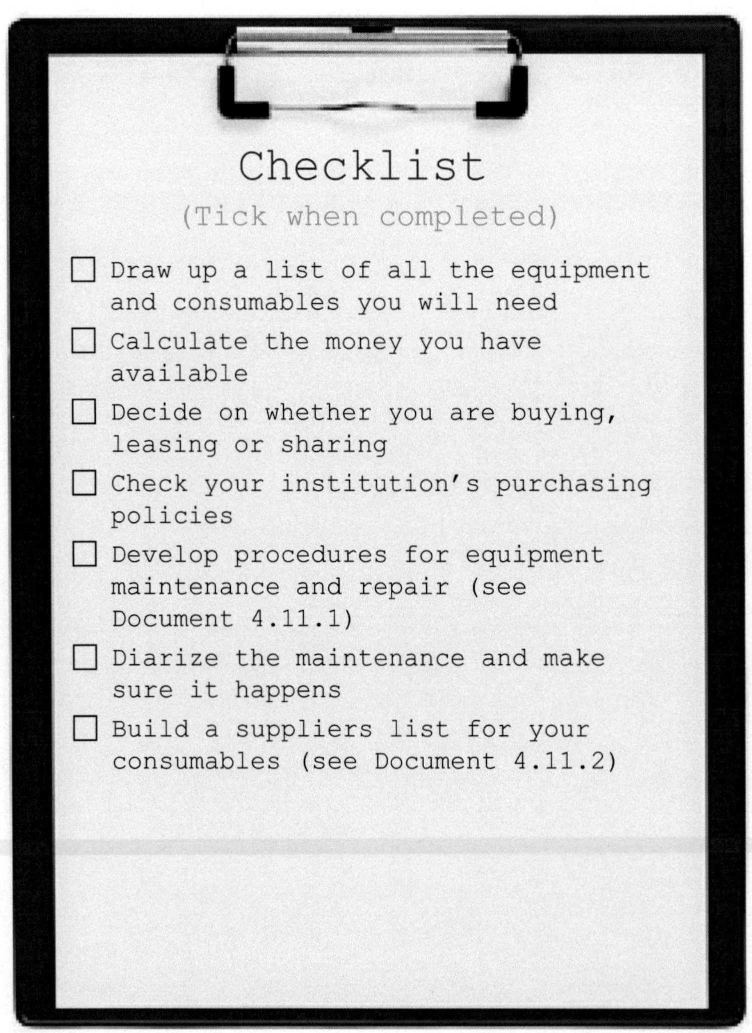

Planning for Your Equipment

Trying to work out what you need in the way of equipment and consumables can be daunting, especially the first time. Remember that you are not alone here: this has all been done before by your colleagues. Start by asking advice from them.

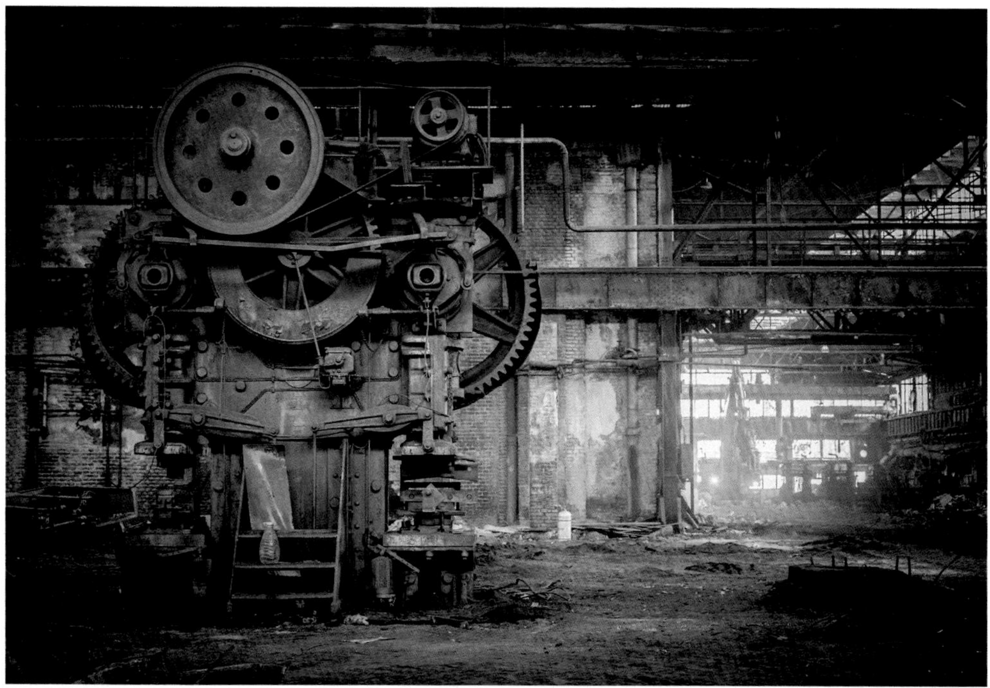

Image Credit: Abandoned metallurgical factory by Momente/Shutterstock

Your institute will have relationships with preferred suppliers, and you might, in fact, be required to go through them.

Start with the big picture. Draw up a complete list of equipment and consumables you expect to need for the life of the project. Then work out the money that will be available to pay for it and when you will have access to that money. Now you are ready to source it, deciding whether you are buying, leasing, borrowing, or sharing.

You are likely to want to buy, but before you go ahead, do consider the possibilities of sharing equipment. Provided that you can manage a sensible roster for access, sharing an expensive piece of equipment can save a very significant chunk of project costs. You will benefit from having access to others who use the equipment, and you will be able to share knowledge about how to use it, as well as sharing the costs of maintenance and cleaning.

In a similar vein, investigate whether you can reduce your set-up costs by accessing stored furniture and fittings that are being held by the university. Think about whether equipment such as computers or printers (if indeed you have to provide them) should be hired or leased.

Equipment Procurement

Do Your Homework

Take the time to do your homework before you go ahead to buy or lease each piece of your planned equipment. Check the costs, and the price of any additional parts you might require. Investigate, too, the cost of servicing of one type of machine compared with a rival brand and the expected response times for those service providers. If you plan to lease your equipment, check to see if servicing or parts or particular service providers are part of the deal.

Do consider whether you might be able to manage with good second-hand equipment instead of buying new. If you buy secondhand:

- Will there be a warranty?
- Will you be able to get parts and service?

Before you order your equipment consider the following:

- Which functions are essential and what is not so important? Can you therefore manage with a lesser model?
- Can your needs be simplified?
- Can standard methods and off-the-shelf equipment be used?
- Can the use of the equipment be shared with other research groups? As mentioned earlier, cost sharing has many benefits. Can your department or institution share equipment costs?
- What are the staff cost implications in terms of numbers, training, necessary expertise, etc.?
- Are there any special approvals required?
- Will there need to be building modifications? Will you have to pay?
- Will there be an environmental impact, such as a need for special waste disposal?

Check Procurement Processes

Once you have made the decision to acquire a piece of equipment, make sure you understand the procurement process at your university.

- What is the university approvals process? Is there a tender process, or specified supplier? Who must approve the final decision?
- You must familiarize yourself with relevant policies
- Find out if any specialist training will be required, and who will provide it
- Factor in any foreign currency fluctuations that might affect the costs
- Factor in the consequences of delays before delivery

Note that in most cases ownership of equipment funded by your grant will revert to your institution after the award period ends. If you are the principal investigator and you relocate during the life of the grant, the equipment generally goes with you.

Looking After Your Equipment

It goes without saying that your equipment is valuable, and its smooth working is integral to the team's success. So look after it!

- Use it as it was intended
- Ensure that you stick to the manufacturer's guidelines for servicing
- Have it serviced by a reputable supplier
- Keep a log which records the services and repairs, upgrades or calibrations and quality control checks
- Keep the manual in a sensible place where everyone can find it
- Keep your equipment clean and maintained regularly
- Keep a note of the warranty expiry date
- Teach your team to use it properly
- Diarize the maintenance so it is not forgotten

Your lab's standard operating procedures should contain a section about operation and care of your equipment, and should be accessible to the whole team. See Document 4.11.1 SOP Equipment Maintenance and Repair Example at the end of this chapter.

Someone senior should be delegated to keep an eye on the records for particular pieces of equipment. The stories of the research assistant who accurately plotted the steadily rising temperature of the −80 freezer every morning, and raised no alarm, are true. Diligent junior staff whose lack of understanding (and supervision) might lead to melted and ruined samples are out there in the real world.

Managing Consumables

During your project planning phase, you will have thought about the consumables you will need, and found out where to source them. There is sure to be a prescribed method of ordering at your institute and a list of preferred suppliers or established procurement contracts.

After having sorted this out, plan your likely volume of use and frequency of purchases. There may be merit in buying all you will need of some consumables in your initial purchase, e.g., if the goods need to be from the same batch, or if lead time from order to delivery is very long. There might also be very attractive volume discounts.

More usually, you will purchase your consumables according to need, allowing you to keep in step with your budget. It is good practice to allocate the task of managing general consumables to a team member, or rotate the duty according to a roster, thus exposing everyone to this area of lab management.

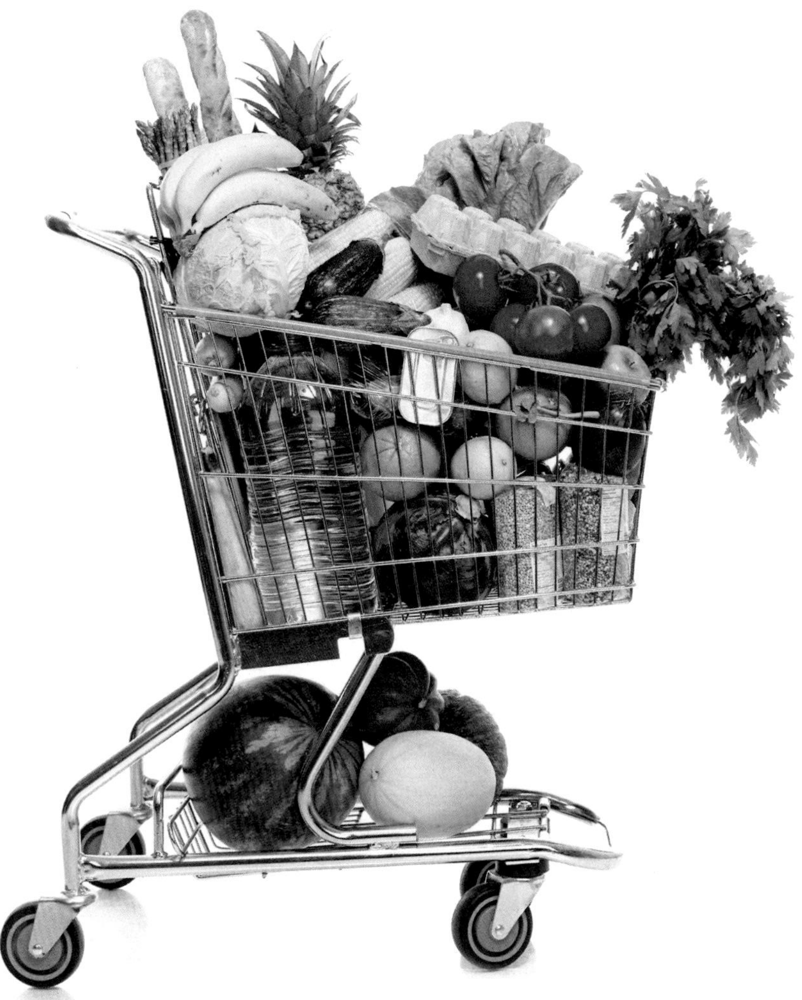

Image Credit: Full shopping grocery cart by Kurhan/Shutterstock

Before the first orders come, consider whether there needs to be any special precautions for storage or handling, and make sure you can meet the needs. Consider, too, whether there needs to be any special training for your team.

It is a good idea to create an order sheet which includes everything you use in the lab, grouped according to supplier. That makes it easy to re-order, and to build a record of how much of every item is being used in a fixed period. See Document 4.11.2 Consumables Purchasing and Inventory Template.

The cost of consumables can get away from you, so be sure to keep an eye on your budget. Pipettes don't grow on trees.

Associated Documents—Equipment and Consumables

4.11.1 SOP Equipment Maintenance and Repair Example

Project xxx	
Equipment Maintenance and Repair	
Version: 1	SOP# 25
Effective Date:	Next Review Date:
Approved by:	**Position/Title:** Laboratory Manager

Contents

1. Scope

This SOP describes the procedure for periodic equipment maintenance and emergency repair of equipment as a result of a breakdown.

2. Equipment Register

A list of all equipment together with serial numbers and purchase dates is found in Appendix I.

3. Equipment Maintenance.

To ensure equipment performs according to pre-determined specifications, they must be maintained according to the maintenance schedule, as set out in Table 1 below. Some routine maintenance is carried out in house according to the appropriate SOP identified in the *Table*. Some equipment requires annual checks and calibrations by external contractors. Contractors should be booked from the contact details provided in *Table 2*. The month of the year when work is to be carried out is indicated. An order for the work should be generated by the purchasing department according to *SOP #24 Purchasing Consumables or Services.* A certificate of compliance should be provided by the contractor after the completion of the work.

Table 1: Maintenance Schedule

Equipment	Maintenance Activities			
	Daily	**Weekly**	**Monthly**	**Yearly**
Forma 907 freezers	Temperature monitoring *SOP#1 Daily Biobank Activities*	CO_2 bottle weight reading refer *SOP#2 Weekly and Monthly Biobank Activities*	De-icing freezers according to *SOP#2 Weekly and Monthly Biobank Activities*	Christmas shutdown maintenance and calibration
Top Safe Biocabinet	Cleaning of cabinet. *SOP#14 Procedure for Cleaning Biohazard and Centrifuges*			Christmas shutdown maintenance and calibration
Eppendorf Centrifuges			Clean according to *SOP#14 Procedure for Cleaning Biohazard and Centrifuges*	Christmas shutdown maintenance and calibration
CO_2 Monitor				Every May CO_2 calibration
Alarm			Alarm Qualification. Refer *SOP #19 Procedure for Alarm Qualification.*	Christmas shutdown maintenance and qualification
Air Conditioning CFI			Three Monthly inspection and service	
Label Printers				Nil maintenance, repair as required
Bar Code Scanner				Nil maintenance, repair as required
Computers				Nil maintenance, repair as required
Printers				Nil maintenance, repair as required

4. **Approved Service Providers**

Table2.

Equipment	Approved Supplier #1	Contact Details for booking service.	Approved Supplier#2	Contact Details
Freezers				
Biocabinet				
Centrifuges			R	
CO_2 Monitor				
Alarm				
Air Conditioning				
Label Printers				
Bar Code Scanner				
Computers				
Printers				

5. **Equipment Maintenance Checklists for External Contractors.**

These are the minimum requirement that should be undertaken by external contractors. The service and calibration specifications are provided in Appendices A-E. Any failure to meet set specification should be communicated to x Manager.

An inventory of manufacturer's manuals is provided in Appendix H.

6. **Emergency Repairs.**

In the event of an equipment breakdown the approved supplier for that service should be contacted. This information is provided in *Table 2.* An order for the work should be generated by the purchasing department according to *SOP #24 Purchasing Consumables or Services.*

In the event of a Freezer breakdown, critical parts are kept in stock to expedite the repair of the freezers. These parts should be provided to the freezer repairers if required. They are itemised in Appendix F and are kept in the ***Equipment Spares*** cupboard. Any part that is used in repairs should be re-ordered from xx.

7. **Storage of Certificates.**

When a contractor completes the maintenance and /or calibration of an item of equipment, a certificate of conformance must be supplied. Upon receipt, these must be checked against Equipment Maintenance Checklists. If satisfactory, forms should be stored at xxx:

8. Appendix A: Freezer Maintenance Checklist.

Check and or perform				Status (pass/fail)
1. Freezer operation and performance history				
2. Electrical safety and continuity				
3. Condition of condenser fans/motors				
4. Clean condenser with compressed air				
5. Cabinet vent vacuum relief port				
6. Condition of electrical wiring and circuit boards				
7. Adjustment of door lock, strike and handle				
8. Seating and condition of door seals				
9. Remove ice build up in cabinet, around seals and thermometers				
10. Back up batteries and charge circuitry. Replace battery every 2 years				
11. Function of alarm system including notification by alarm monitoring				
12. Clean and replace air filter				
13. Check condition/operation of CO2 back up system				
14. CO2 back up cabinet vent and stack. Inspect and clean				
15. Adjustment of door interlock				
16. CO2 back up system set point				
Calibration	**Set Value**	**Actual Value**	**Display value**	**Pass/fail**
Cabinet temperature				
Heat exchanger temperature				
Battery voltage freezer				
Battery voltage CO2 backup				
Line voltage				
Ambient temperature				

9. Appendix B Centrifuge Maintenance Checklist.

Check and or perform				Status (pass/fail)
1. Centrifuge operation and performance history				
2. Electrical Safety and continuity				
3. Motor, motor shaft, trunnion and buckets				
4. Motor brushes and commutator				
5. Motor bearings and rubber mounts				
6. Condition of electrical wiring and circuit boards, and cooling fans				
7. Check lid lock mechanism				
8. Check out of balance control				
9. Key pad user controls				
10. Internal External cleaning.				
Calibration	**Set Value**	**Actual Value**	**Display value**	**Pass/fail**
Centrifuge Speed	1000			
	2000			
	3000			

10. Appendix C Air Conditioner Unit Maintenance Checklist.

Check and or perform				Status (pass/fail)
1. Change evaporator filters every 6 months				
2. Clean condenser fans				
3. Check refrigerant gas levels, check for leaks gas levels				
4. Check all bearings				
5. Check electrics and associated controls to ensure correct operation				
6. Check pipes and mountings to ensure they are vibration free				
7. Check operation of safety controls				
Calibration	**Set Value**	**Actual Value**	**Display value**	**Pass/fail**
Temperature setting				

11. Appendix D: Alarm Maintenance Checklist.

Check and or perform				Status (pass/fail)
1. Check Back up battery voltage. Check charge circuits. Change main battery every 2 years				
2. Check CMOS battery voltage. Change every 5 years				
Calibration	**Set Value**	**Actual Value**	**Display value**	**Pass/fail**
Temperature setting	29 °C			

12. Appendix E CO_2 Monitors Maintenance Checklist

Check and or perform	Status (pass/fail)
1. Calibrate IR sensor to 2% (low alarm) and 3% (high alarm) CO2.	
2. Verify audible and visual alarm	

13. Appendix F Inventory of Freezer Spare Parts

An inventory of freezer spare parts is maintained at the biobank. These can be found in the cupboard labelled **FREEZER SPARE PARTS at xxx.**

Item Code	Description	Quantity	Unit Cost	Total Cost
xx	Micro Board	1		
xx	High Voltage Board	1		
xx	Axial Fan Motor	2		
xx	Single Door switch	1		

14. Appendix G Inventory of Equipment Manuals

These manuals were provided by the manufacturer and accompanied the product

These are kept in a filing cabinet in the Biobank Office marke*d **Equipment Manuals***

Equipment	Manual Number
Freezers	1
Biocabinet	2
Centrifuges	3
CO2 Monitor	4
Alarm	5
Air Conditioning	6
Scanner	8
Printer	9

15. Appendix H Inventory of Assets

Asset	Model	Date of Purchase	Location	Serial Number
Freezer1 (next to garage door)			I	
Freezer2				
Bar Code Scanner				
Centrifuge 1				
Biological safety Cabinet				

4.11.2 Consumables Purchasing and Inventory Template

PRODUCT DESCRIPTION	PRODUCT NUMBER	PRICE	QUANTITY	SUPPLIER	EMAIL	PHONE	WEBSITE	POSTAL ADDRESS	QUANTITY ORDERED	QUANTITY TAKEN	USED BY	DATE

4.12 Study Participant Recruitment

The Women's Study aimed to better understand the issues confronted by menopausal women, and the way they dealt with them. The invitation sent in the mail to randomly selected, appropriately aged women, made it clear what the study was about. This was a subject dear to the hearts of the women targeted. The phones rang continually for three days, the mail bags were full, and the recruitment target was achieved in record time: mission accomplished! If you are lucky enough to have questions about something people want to talk about, it is a great advantage. Try to make your study sound inviting to your target market.

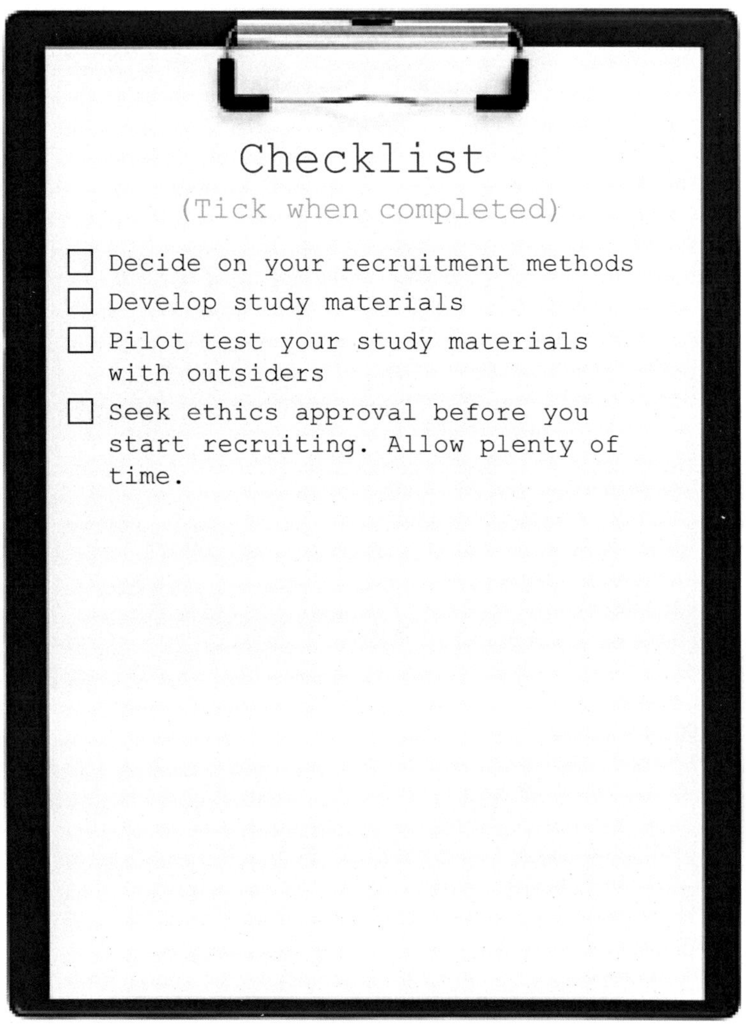

❹ RUNNING THE STUDIES

Recruitment of participants is a major focus for studies that involve participation of human subjects. It can be time consuming and costly. Delays are common, and often take the researchers by surprise. They can be so wrapped up in their topic, they are surprised that everyone eligible doesn't want to take part, and immediately.

The case above is from a project for which it was unusually easy to recruit. The reason it is included is that it is a case where the people the investigators were trying to talk to immediately saw the request was relevant and interesting to them.

The first steps will always be to design study materials supporting the recruitment: information sheets, consent forms and then perhaps a questionnaire (See Chapter 4.13).

Make sure your project information is clear, easy to read, and makes your project sound interesting. People respond well when it is something about *them*. They love to talk about themselves. Make your document talk to *them*, make it relevant to their lives and address their concerns.

It is essential that before you have your first interactions with your study subjects, you request and receive your ethics approval.

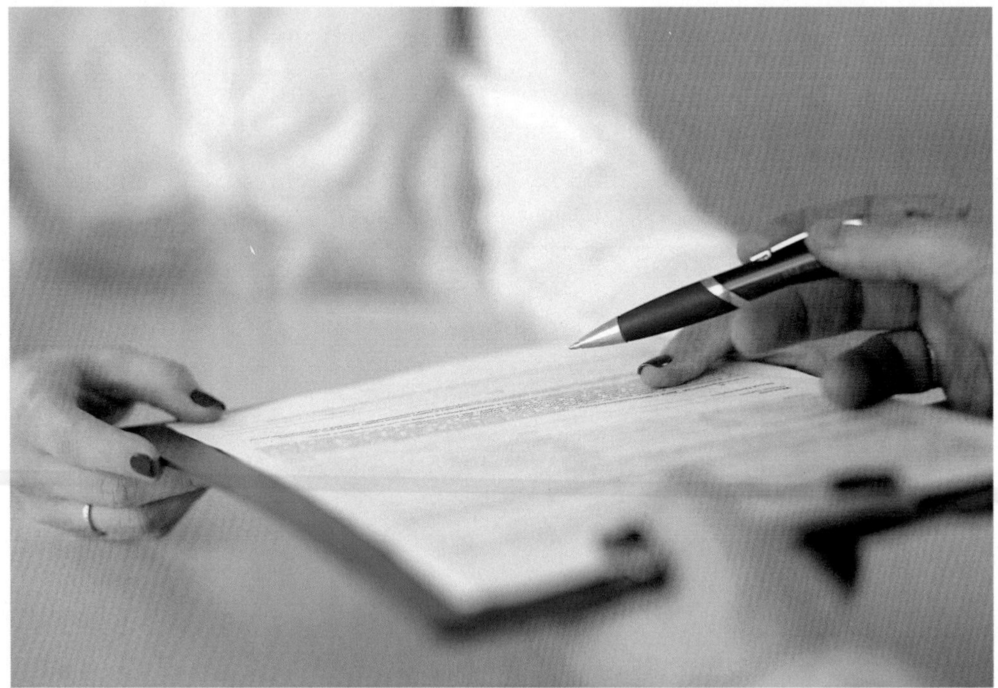

Image Credit: Clipboard on a medical uniform, by Micolas/Shutterstock

Where to Find the Subjects?

At last you are ready to start recruiting. It is often beneficial to begin with a pilot study in order to make sure your study materials are as good as you think they are, that you are getting the sorts of answers you hoped for, and that you can actually find the people you need.

Recruitment via Collaborators

The first step, and most logical, is to collaborate with people who have access to the population in which you have interest. If you are looking at a medical condition, approach the specialist clinicians, or the hospital where the patients are treated. Consider, too, any support organizations where the target people might be members.

If you want to interview people about housing, try partnering with government agencies working with housing. If your project is going to provide information which is useful for the service provider, they might be keen to be part of collecting it, so saving you costs and recruitment time.

Recruitment via Agencies Routinely Collecting Data

Depending on the laws in your country which define access, you might be able to arrange recruitment by obtaining access to people via the electoral roll, via hospital admissions data or records of pharmaceutical use.

In Australia, for example, it is possible, though time consuming to arrange, to recruit people to approved studies through a third party, via Medicare and the Clinical Cancer Registries. Study subjects might also be invited into studies through the Electoral Roll. An extraction from the list can be requested for the number of participants required, the age range and geographic distribution. You need to request the numbers based on your likely response rate.

Similarly, it is sometimes possible to obtain de-identified data for individuals via Medicare or the Pharmaceutical Benefits Service.

Check to see if these opportunities are available in your country. Whatever the avenue selected, allow plenty of time to negotiate. There are many hurdles to be overcome on the way.

Self-Recruitment

Many a study comes undone because it is too difficult or too slow to recruit study participants. Often, for example in a clinical trial, or an epidemiological study which relies on participants who are both representative and randomly selected, it is of vital importance to adhere strictly to criteria and random selection. Sometimes, though, recruitment methods don't need to be so strict, and your study is able to request people to nominate themselves.

Apart from advertising or putting up posters in the hallway, or pulling strangers in from the street, there are some easy ways you might consider, with minimal costs.

Recruitment via Related Channels

If you are working on a health related study, think about seeking assistance from the people who are already dealing with your target audience. This could include health insurance companies, hospitals, support groups. They might well be interested in your results and will be keen to help you. It could also be of value to them to be seen to be assisting research. Ask them to place an advertisement in their newsletter or on their website, or add a mailer in their planned post.

There are some organizations which collect lists of people who are interested in assisting unspecified research projects which relate to a particular cause. Vanderbilt University Recruitment Innovation Centre [1] provides access to consented potential participants who are people who have attended the University medical facilities. Register 4 [2] in Australia has a similar list of people interested in helping cancer research.

Consider, too, the organizations which might benefit from being seen to assist you and your research. The power supply company, a target for criticism as costs go up, might distribute leaflets with its mailings thus helping its image by showing the community it is providing philanthropic support for a good cause.

Recruitment via Your Website

People are, by definition interested in themselves. It is actually very easy to get them to answer questions about themselves because they like to see how they fit in with others. Slant your request to them accordingly. Make the request about them, not about you.

"Do you suffer from diabetes?" will work much better than "we are looking for people with diabetes".

"Do you live in Green County? Are you older or younger than xx? Will be more successful than "we are looking for people over 65…"

Make it easy. Place a link to the recruitment questions you need to ask within your text, and before you know it you will have your initial answers in your database.

Recruitment via Electronic Direct Mail

The same principles apply for electronic direct mail as above, but be careful with your email header. Make it eye catching, and about them. "May we feature you?" "Would you like to…"?

You will receive a better response if you can personalize the email, so, if you have it, include their name in the message.

If it is appropriate for your study, broaden your reach by inviting people to share your request by email or social media.

Recruitment via Social Media

Never under-estimate the power of social media. If you are lucky, this will really get going fast. More likely, it will just provide a straightforward, easy to manage mechanism. Provide a link from your post to your website and proceed as above. Email the request and encourage sharing. Send it out on Twitter and FaceBook.

You can post and re-post your message. Set a schedule in a social media broadcasting system like Hootsuite so that you can set and forget.

Don't Recruit at All—Use Another Study Population

Sometimes it might be possible to conduct your research on a population which has already been recruited into an ongoing longitudinal study. It is worth approaching the investigators of one of these large studies and asking if your questions are relevant to their purposes, and whether you might approach their population or a subset of it.

Note that these study subjects might have become "expert" and bias could be introduced.

Recruitment in Specialist Populations

There are special rules of engagement for recruitment in some specialist populations. This includes the following:

- Aboriginal and Indigenous people
- Children
- Immigrants

The key to success in research within any specialist communities is communication. As part of your planning for ethics approval, prepare your messages about what you are doing and why it matters, then seek assistance from influencers within the group concerned. Never go in with the view that "it is for their own good, they will be better off". You don't yet know whether your cause matters to them, and if it does, how much it matters. They might have priorities higher up their list.

Aboriginal and Indigenous People

Conducting research, indeed collecting information, about Aboriginal and Indigenous populations needs to be handled with the greatest sensitivity. There have been just so many studies where researchers have waded in, boots and all, to ask bossy well-meaning questions, give poorly considered “answers” to on-going problems and left the scene leaving a trail of destruction behind them. This is not the way to go about conducting ethical research in any minor population group.

As specified in the Australian Code for Responsible Conduct for Research [4], but mirrored in many other countries with Indigenous peoples, it is essential that the heritage, diversity, cultural property and knowledge of the Indigenous peoples or communities to be involved will be recognized, valued and respected in research. The Australian Guidelines for Ethical Research in Australian Indigenous Studies [3] state that it is essential that Indigenous people are full participants in research projects that concern them, share an understanding of the aims and methods of the research, and share the results of this work. At every stage, research with and about Indigenous peoples must be founded on a process of meaningful engagement and reciprocity between the researcher and Indigenous people. It should also be recognized that there is no sharp distinction between researchers and Indigenous people. Indigenous people are also researchers, and all participants must be regarded as equal partners in a research engagement.

The first step, then, to successful research within a minority group is consultation within that community. It is vital to share your ideas and hear the views of representatives of the group, and to follow their suggested paths. This consultative approach will almost certainly lead to initial delays in your project, but will result a successful outcome in the long term.

It is usually necessary to seek additional, or special, ethics approval for conducting a study within an Indigenous population. Again this will be a time consuming process, but it is entirely necessary. Much can be achieved with the support of the communities behind you. You can be certain that very little will be achieved without it.

It is recommended that you consult the Australian Guidelines for Ethical Research in Australian Indigenous Studies [3], or equivalent in your country, prior to beginning planning for research involving Indigenous peoples.

It is important to remember that your language may well not be the language used by your study participants. Consider translating your study materials or having special additional material to support your requests. Again, these materials should be developed in consultation with the peoples or communities to be involved in the research.

Culturally and Linguistically Diverse and Immigrant Communities

The same principles as above apply to research within culturally and linguistically diverse (CALD) communities or immigrant groups. These people are often important research subjects as they might carry a disease or an infection common in their home country, but rare or at least less prevalent in their adopted country.

An example is people with hepatitis C infection, which is prevalent in south and eastern Asia who have migrated elsewhere. Many people who are carriers of this infection are unaware of either the infection, or its potential consequences, which include a greatly increased likelihood of developing liver cancer. Many carriers of hepatitis C have left their Asian communities and are re-settled all over the world where they are of great interest to medical researchers.

Members of CALD communities might also be targeted by health authorities because language and educational barriers prevent them from taking up opportunities for preventative health messages, screening or immunization.

There are likely to be cultural sensibilities within minor population groups of which you are not aware. Getting off on the wrong foot will hinder your research, and that of others, for years to come.

Again, a consultative approach will be best. Tread gently, and take advice from community leaders. Seek assistance from people within the community to spread the word and to explain the requirements.

If you have the budget available, it will be worthwhile providing translated study materials for the immigrant groups. Take the time to have proper translations made, by recognized accredited translators. Check them with the community leaders. If you find that there are cultural sensitivities relating to the research, consider making the sensitive aspects of your research optional. It is better to receive limited input from a particular cultural group than receiving no input at all because some of your questions cause offence.

An example of this sort of sensitivity could be a questionnaire which included questions about sexual behaviors which would be quite inappropriate in many cultures. If "I would prefer not to answer" is a valid response to the sensitive questions, then you stand a better chance of getting responses to your other questions.

Children

Research involving children comes with a separate set of requirements. This will usually require consent from a parent or guardian, as well as from the child. It is likely that there will be special procedures required by your ethics committee, such as attendance of an observer and/or time constraints for an interview.

References—Study Recruitment

[1] Vanderbilt University Recruitment Innovation Centre. https://trialinnovationnetwork.org/home-page/recruitment-innovation-center/.

[2] Register 4. http://www.register4.org.au/.

[3] AIATSIS, 2012. Guidelines for Ethical Research in Australian Indigenous Studies, (Australian Institute of Aboriginal and Torres Strait Islander Studies), revised second ed. http://www.aiatsis.gov.au/_data/assets/pdf_file/2290/ethics_guidelines.pdf.
[4] The Australian Code for the Responsible Conduct of Research (under review) Public Consultation Draft November 2016. https://www.nhmrc.gov.au/research/responsible-conduct-research/review-australian-code-responsible-conduct-research.

Further Reading

Ablett, S., Pinkerton, C.R. 2003. Recruiting children into cancer trials–role of the United Kingdom Children's Cancer Study Group (UKCCSG). British Journal of Cancer, 88 (11): 1661–1665.

Barker, J., Weller, S. January 1, 2003. "Is it fun?" Developing children centred research methods. International Journal of Sociology and Social Policy, 23 (1/2): 33–58.

Campbell, A. 2008. For their own good: Recruiting children for research, Childhood 15 (1): 30–49.

Coday, M., Richey, P., Thomas, F., Tran, Q.T., Terrell, S.B., Tylavsky, F., Miro, D., Caufield, M., Johnson, K.C. April 2016. The recruitment experience of a randomized clinical trial to aid young adult smokers to stop smoking without weight gain with interactive technology. Contemporary clinical trials communications, 15 (2): 61–68.

Hughson, J.A., Woodward-Kron, R., Parker A., Hajek, J., Bresin, A., Knoch, U., Phan, T., Story, D. May 26, 2016. A review of approaches to improve participation of culturally and linguistically diverse populations in clinical trials. Trials, 17 (1): 263.

Kayrouz, R., Dear, B.F., Karin, E., Titov, N. May 2016. Facebook as an effective recruitment strategy for mental health research of hard to reach populations. Internet Interventions, 31 (4): 1–0.

National Institute of Mental Health. 2005. Points to Consider about Recruitment and Retention while Preparing a Clinical Research Study. https://www.nimh.nih.gov/funding/grant-writing-and-application-process/recruitment-points-to-consider-6-1-05_34848.pdf.

Thornton, L., Batterham, P.J., Fassnacht, D.B., Kay-Lambkin, F., Calear, A.L., Hunt, S. 2016. Recruiting for health, medical or psychosocial research using Facebook: systematic review. Internet Interventions, 31 (4): 72–81. www.sciencedirect.com/science/article/pii/S2214782915300166.

UN (United Nations). 2007 United Nations Declaration on the Rights of Indigenous Peoples. https://www.un.org/development/desa/indigenouspeoples/declaration-on-the-rights-of-indigenous-peoples.html.

UNESCO. 2003 Convention for the Safeguarding of the Intangible Cultural Heritage, UNESCO, Paris. http://unesdoc.unesco.org/images/0013/001325/132540e.pdf.

WIPO (World Intellectual Property Organization). 2006a The Protection of Traditional Cultural Expressions/Expressions of Folklore: Revised Objectives and Principles. (Document Code WIPO/GRTKF/IC/9/4), WIPO, Geneva. www.wipo.int/edocs/mdocs/tk/en/wipo_grtkf_ic_9/wipo_grtkf_ic_9_4.pdf.

WIPO. 2006b The Protection of Traditional Knowledge: Revised Objectives and Principles (Document Code WIPO/GRTKF/IC/9/5), WIPO, Geneva.

4.13 Designing a Questionnaire and Accompanying Study Materials

The investigators for the LIGHT Study worked out their questions, but spent limited effort on the design of the questionnaire. It was a dog's breakfast. The font was difficult to read, there was too much text on each page, and it was altogether an unfriendly document. Recruitment was difficult. Along came an expert with a sales and marketing background. "Make the questionnaire look inviting and people will start to read it and understand", she said. She was right.

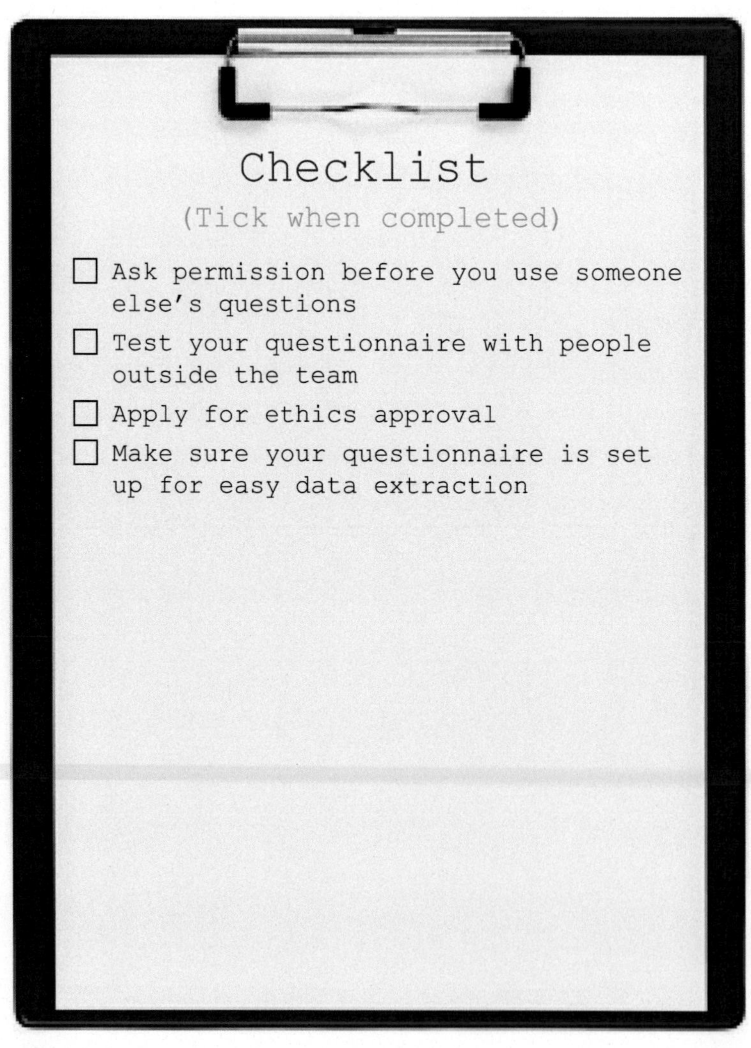

As this book is about managing research, not conducting it, it is assumed you know which questions to ask.

In addition to selection of the actual questions, though, there are two important considerations when designing a study questionnaire and its accompanying documents. They are

- Readability and clarity for the study participant
- Ease of extraction of answers

There have been many studies whose materials have failed these simple tests.

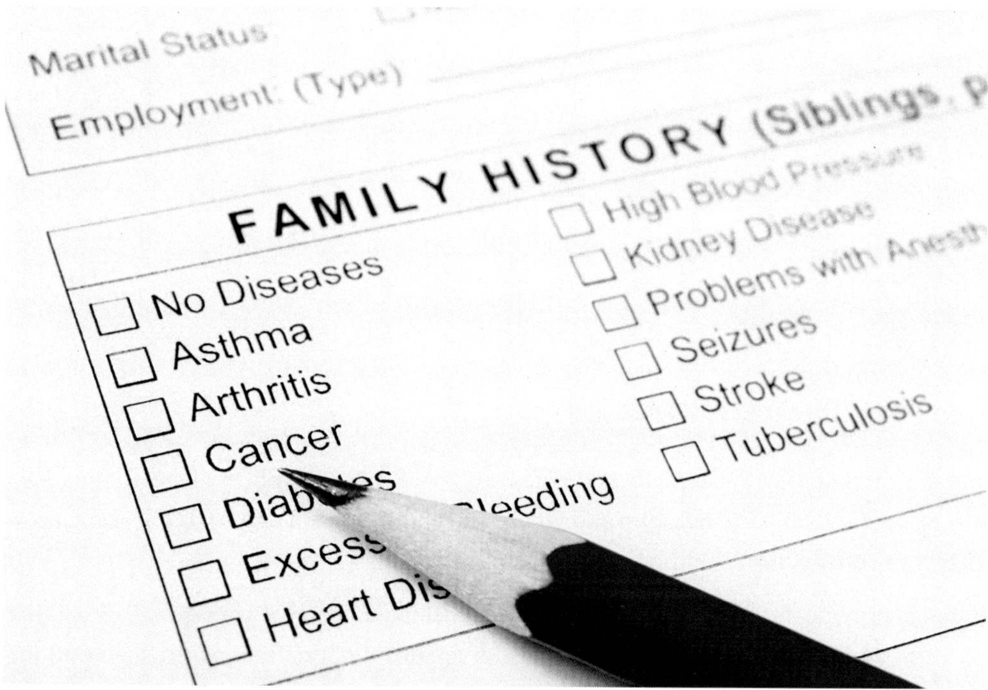

Image Credit: Medical information by Aleksandar Grozdanovski/Shutterstock

Check Readability

You will almost certainly be too close to the topic to evaluate the readability yourself. Try to look with outside eyes. Is it easy to read? Is the font clear? Will they know that they have to turn the page (paper version) or go to a next page (on line)? Are the compulsory sections appropriately marked?

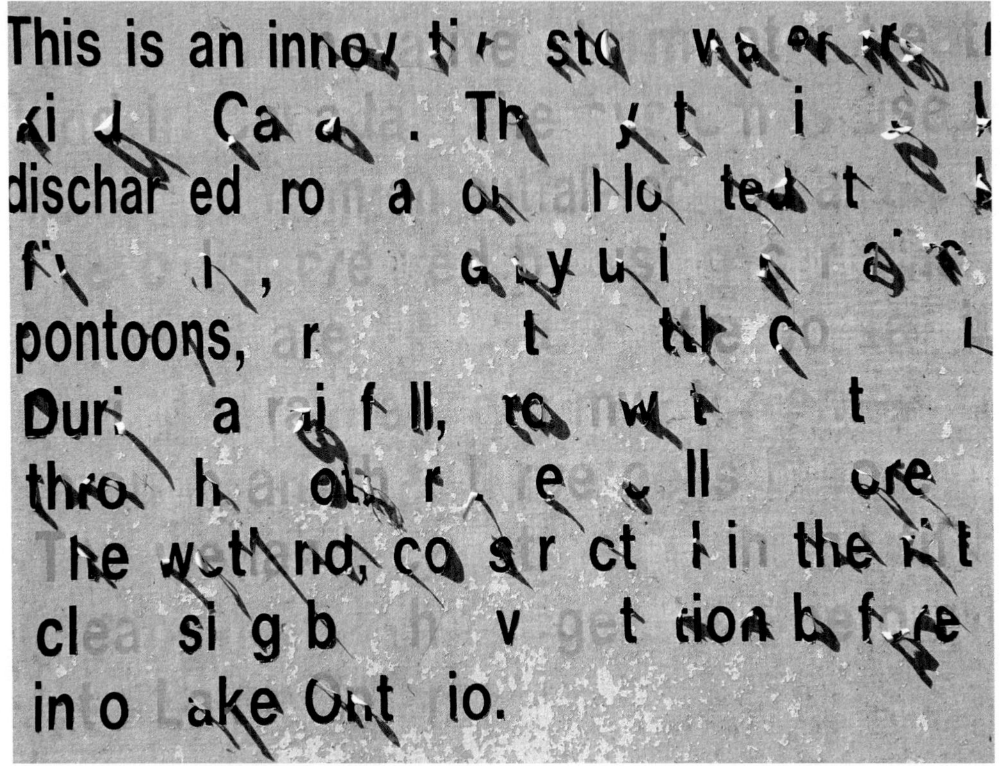

Image Credit: Time Erases by double-P/iStock

Test your questionnaire with people outside the team, preferably members of the public, and make sure they understand both the question and what sort of answers are required. The same applies to accompanying consent forms and information sheets.

As mentioned previously, cultural differences might mean that some of your questions might cause offence. If so, and if they are still to be included, give consideration to making them optional.

A common problem is not leaving sufficient space for free text answers. Do you have enough room?

Test, test, and test again. If you are doing this on-line then test from different platforms and from both desk top and mobile versions.

Last, if you are recruiting in populations where literacy might not be high, or where people speak a different language from you, consider making a special version with more pictures than words or a version in the other language(s).

Set Up for Extracting the Data

The other common problem is inadvertently creating a questionnaire from which it is difficult to extract the data.

Paper questionnaires can be designed to be machine read. This is relatively easy if you have check box answers, but is harder to manage where answers can be free text. Data entry is time consuming and expensive. It might be possible to offer lists of multiple-choice answer options instead of free text, if suitable.

While you won't need data entry for free text answers to on-line questionnaires, interpretation of the answers can still be problematic. Imagine the number of ways people can spell (or mis-spell) the names of common pharmaceuticals, or describe the nature of exercise they have done in the past week. You have to be able to interpret these answers consistently so that apples are apples, not oranges. You can set up rules so that the system queries, say, a mother who says she breast-fed a baby for five years when the answer was meant to be five months, but it is troublesome to have to go through and correct the spellings of countries of birth when they could have been on a drop-down list.

A researcher will often seek to use previously validated questions, which is good practice. It is useful to try to build consistency in questions used within your own institution. There are cases where there is value in comparing responses to the same questions across different projects.

Remember to seek approval to use a question or questions derived from another group's work. There will be value for the "owner" of that question in agreeing, so you are unlikely to receive a negative response, and you might gain a valuable collaborator.

4.14 Project Reporting

Investigator Helen was awarded funding for a two-year grant. Her research did not go as planned, and she veered off in a different direction. Unfortunately, she neither reported back to the funding body about her change of plans, nor completed reports about her progress (or lack of it). When she finally got in touch and asked the organization to support her new direction, her grant was terminated and remaining funding withdrawn.

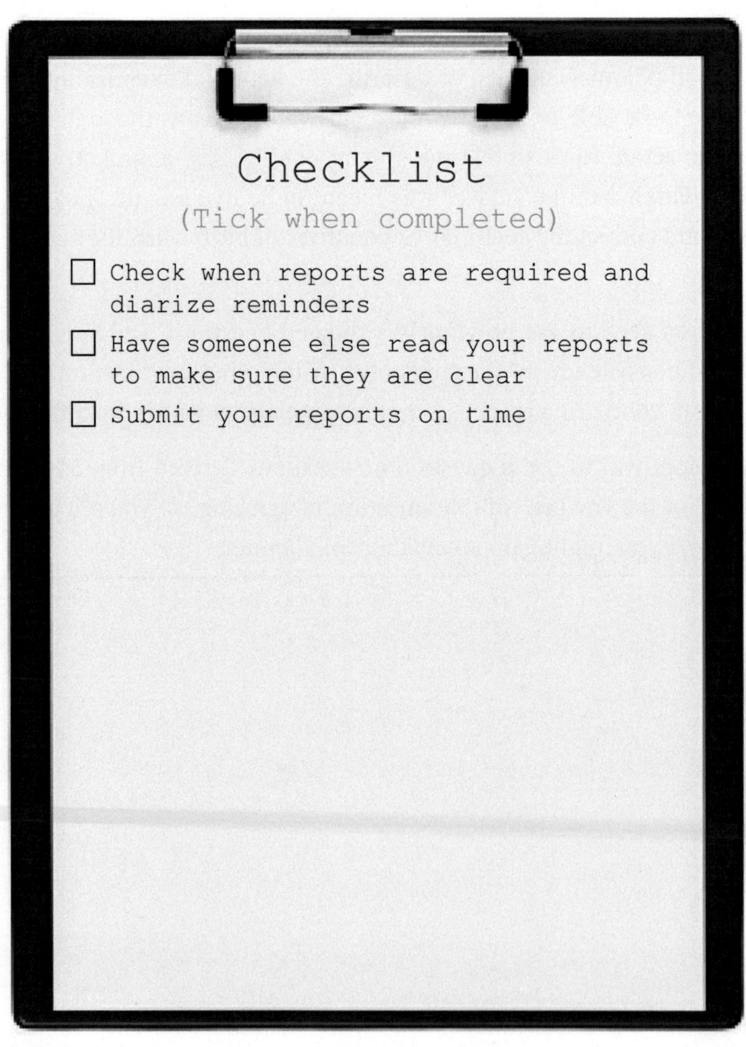

Reporting is one of the realities of life, and is often resented.

Try to think with the approach from the viewpoint of the person you are reporting to. Understand that there is a good reason for reports. Your reports are probably due to your funding body or your institution. If you want them to support you, you need to tell them what you are doing with their money and resources, and they need to know why your work matters. They also want to know how you are progressing.

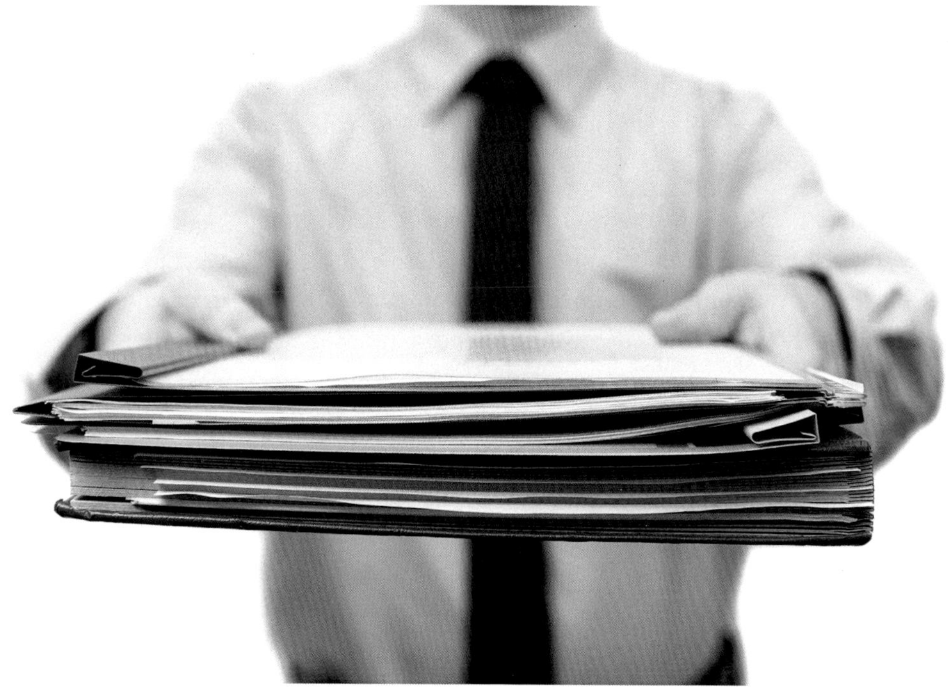

Image Credit: Senior manager is giving a lot of work by Bacho/Shutterstock

Instead of treating reporting as an unwelcome task, take this view:

- Reporting gives you an opportunity to tell them what you are up to
- You can talk about your successes
- You can provide a reason for delays
- You can tell them why it matters
- When you are preparing your report, you can take a step back and look in from the outside, and see where you are going, and where you have been
- The text you use for your report can probably provide the backbone for a later publication

So, report when you are asked to, preferably before the deadline. It will stand you in good stead.

Before you start writing, contemplate your audience. Your readers might not be subject area specialists, and certainly they are not as close to your specific subject as you are. If they are not from your field, use simple language. Don't try to blind them with science, be careful not to bore them or make them confused.

Reporting to Your Funding Body

Your agreement with your funding body will probably specify the nature of the reports required and the times at which they will be due. Make a note in your calendar to prepare these reports and be sure to submit them on time.

The funding body's focus will be on determining whether their money is being spent as agreed, and whether they are receiving the appropriate outcome for their investment. They will be hoping for success stories, or for confirmation that something "works" or equally that it doesn't. Wise investment on their part helps them generate more funds in the future—possibly for people like you.

Reporting to Your Ethics Committee

As with the funding body, your ethics or institutional review board approval probably sets out a requirement for regular reporting. In this case, your committee will probably require annual reports from investigators on your progress and on any ethical problems encountered. They will review whether the study has been run as projected, and whether the outcomes have been successful.

Ethics reporting is usually a condition of ongoing approval. Take it seriously!

Reporting to Your Institutional Advisory Committee

Institutional Advisory Committees are sometimes appointed to provide advice to the institution about its overall research management, practices and governance.

As for the project advisory committees mentioned in Chapter 4.17, the Institutional Advisory Committee will be made up of senior researchers from elsewhere, and will have specific terms of reference. Their brief will be to audit the institution's research portfolio, and perhaps to audit the ethical compliance of the individual projects and programs.

They are powerful committees and need to be treated with great respect. Reporting is likely to be ad hoc, and might take the form of an audit. Prepare for these committees diligently and, wherever possible, provide answers to all their questions in advance.

Further Reading—Reporting

The NHS Health Research Authority provides information of a fairly standard format for ethics reporting. http://www.hra.nhs.uk/research-community/during-your-research-project/progress-reporting/.

These are further examples of reporting templates and much other useful documentation in the NIH Clinical Researcher Toolkit at: https://www.nidcr.nih.gov/research/toolkit/.

Including this report template https://www.nidcr.nih.gov/research/toolkit/Documents/dsmb_report_template_v5_010215.dotx.

4.15 Risks and Issues

A five-year experiment for genetically modified cotton was wiped out when the crop was affected by spray drift. These things can happen, but why did the researcher not minimize his risk by having half his crop in a separate facility down the road?

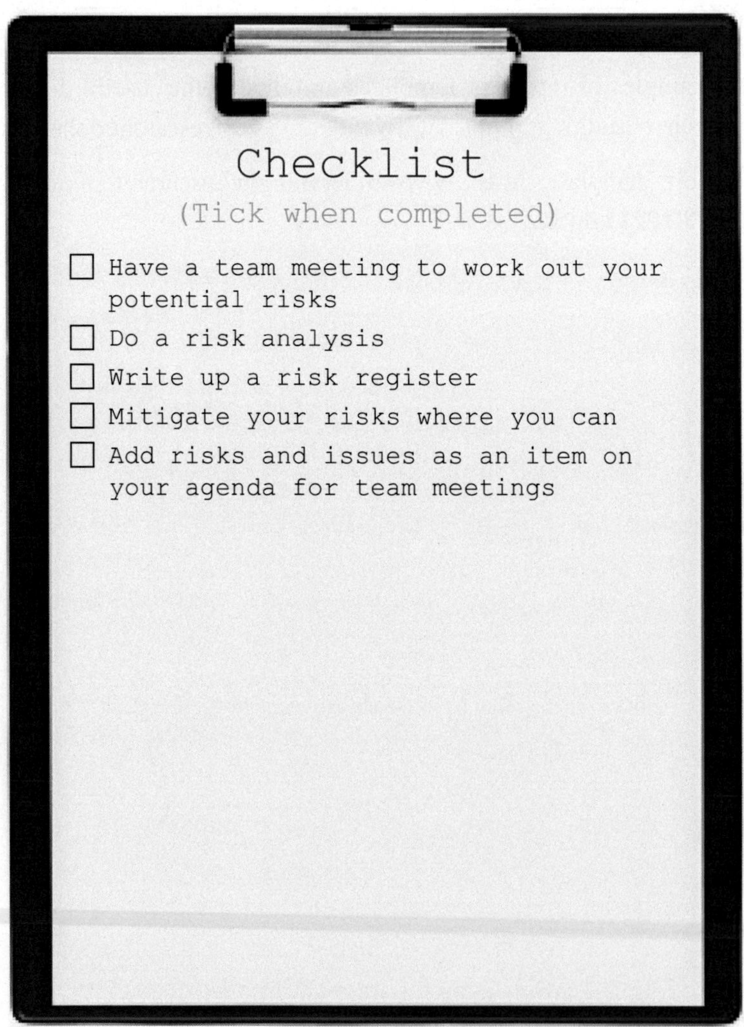
Checklist
(Tick when completed)
Have a team meeting to work out your potential risks
Do a risk analysis
Write up a risk register
Mitigate your risks where you can
Add risks and issues as an item on your agenda for team meetings

Risk

Everything we do in life involves an element of risk, whether it is crossing the road, getting out of bed, or driving a car. Every decision we make, or fail to make, also involves risk. From the time we are tiny babies, we learn to judge risks and make decisions based on our assessments.

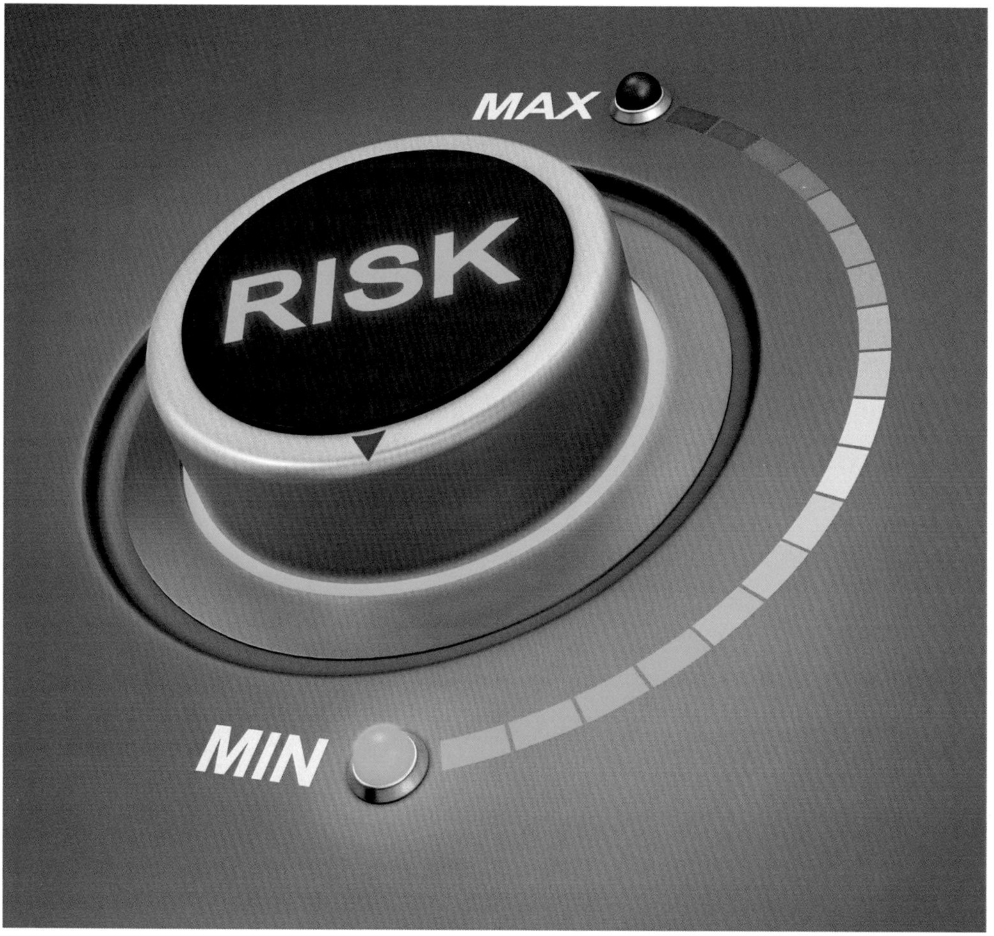

Image Credit: Risk button by Sarawut Aiemsinsuk/Shutterstock

A risk in research is something which might possibly go wrong, and which would harm your project, your institute or your reputation. Your consideration of potential risks at the beginning of the project (and indeed throughout the project) can help you mitigate those risks if you follow up with some good contingency planning.

Risks in a research environment might be any one of the following:

- Reputational risk, to you and the institution, if the project fails
- Financial risk—if the research costs more than expected, if the monies are not managed properly, or simply if there wasn't enough budget in the first place
- Lack of availability of suitable facilities
- Lack of availability of suitable staff
- Loss of key staff
- Ethical risk, if the project is conducted in a way that upsets or harms members of the public or even the research team
- IP risk, if you fail to manage the knowledge you have created
- Risk of loss of data
- Competition—in case your idea is not original and someone beats you to it
- Competition v2—in case your idea is contrary to the status quo, and others actively attempt to prevent you from publishing (unethical behavior, but possible)
- Allowing your research activities to creep out of project scope
- Unsuccessful product—no one is interested and no one wants to publish your work or buy your product
- Changing environment—changes in local politics, government policy, or technology might change everything
- Time delays
- Reliance on others who may not deliver
- Incomplete knowledge of the research area
- Compliance risks
- Legal risks

Risk Management

Risk management is not just for risk managers. It is for everyone working on a project. Risks simply *must* be considered and addressed.

> *A little risk management saves a lot of fan cleaning.*
> Anonymous

Managing risk is a systematic and logical process, which is as much about managing opportunities as it is about managing threats.

Risk management is *everybody's* business.

An example of good risk management practices in operation will be displayed by a pharmaceutical company when they are trialing a new drug. The company will always be aware of the potential of an adverse reaction for trial participants (a risk), however, on the other side of the equation, there is a possibility that during the trials they will discover the drug has a beneficial side effect for a disease or situation which hadn't been considered (an opportunity). In either case, the company will act quickly with the planned follow-up processes they have developed as part of their risk management.

The Risk Management Process

The usual steps of the risk management process are as follows:

- Communicate and consult—with all stakeholders
- Establish the context—identify the situations where you might have concerns
- Identify the risks
- Analyze the risks
- Evaluate the risks
- Treat the risks
- Monitor and review

When you follow the risk management process it will ensure that you maximize your opportunities and minimize the potential losses in your project by giving you a thorough understanding of major risks and possible mitigations.

Risk Identification and Risk Criteria

As a first step, you need to involve the team in identifying your risks and establishing the criteria against which each risk will be evaluated. It is not enough to identify that a project delay is a risk. Will you measure it in weeks or months? If you are collecting images of a particular process, do you need five or a thousand? You can use the Risk Identification Register template 4.15.1 at the end of this chapter to help you record some detail about your known risks.

SWOT Analysis

If you haven't already done so, it may be useful to also conduct a SWOT analysis which will help you identify Strengths, Weaknesses, Opportunities, and Threats for your project as had been mentioned in Chapter 1.4. You can see some sample SWOT ideas in Table 4.15.1.

TABLE 4.15.1 SWOT Analysis Framework

External Context	
Opportunities	**Threats**
• Use your recent findings to develop a new drug for diabetes • Big and growing market	• Competitors—are they already working on this product? • Very long lead time for approval
Internal Context	
Strengths	**Weaknesses**
• Expertise in the new methodology • Expert sales force and customer base to roll it out	• Need to purchase new equipment that is not readily available • Difficult to source appropriately trained additional staff

Risk Analysis

The next step, risk analysis, is essentially understanding the risks. It involves considering the likelihood of the risk occurring, and the consequences if it should occur. You should identify the factors that will influence the likelihood and consequences for each risk and whether risk elements you might come up against can be mitigated.

Using the Risk Assessment Tool below, you can see that a risk which will *almost certainly* happen, but has a *minor* consequence, comes out with a risk rating of *high*. One such risk in a project might be manageable, but multiple high risks would require better planning or better mitigation. If any—or many—elements come up in the high or severe risk area, consider very carefully before proceeding, via the Risk Evaluation step in the risk management process.

Rating	Consequence				
	Insignificant	Minor	Moderate	Major	Catastrophic
Almost certain - controls unsatisfactory to mitigate the risk	High	High	Extreme	Extreme	Extreme
Likely - Controls inadequate to mitigate the risk and require improvement	Medium	High	High	Extreme	Extreme
Possible - Controls reasonable / adequate to mitigate the risk but may still require improvement	Low	Medium	High	Extreme	Extreme
Unlikely - Controls robust and adequate to mitigate the risk	Low	Medium	Medium	High	Extreme
Rare - Controls strong to mitigate the risk	Low	Low	Medium	High	High

Risk Rating Assessment Tool

Rating	Description
Insignificant	Impact can be easily absorbed without requiring management effort
Minor	Impact can be readily absorbed but some management effort is required
Moderate	Impact cannot be managed under normal operating conditions; requiring moderate level of resource and management input
Major	Impact requires a high level of management attention / effort and resources to rectify
Catastrophic	Disaster with potential to lead to business collapse and requiring almost total management attention / effort to rectify

Risk Consequence Legend

Risk Evaluation

The final stage of risk assessment is evaluation of the identified risks. Here you must consider the cumulative effect of multiple risks and whether there have been instances of your types of risk previously. Have they happened before, or have there been near misses? At this point, it becomes a matter of judgment.

Once you have identified your risks, complete a Risk Register, populating it with the specific risks you have identified.

Treat the Risks

At this point, you must do your best to develop and implement appropriate risk treatment strategies to address each of the risks for your project.

Risk Monitoring

You mustn't forget about your risks once your project is underway, even though you have completed your risk assessment. You need to monitor your risks, reviewing all aspects of your risk management on a regular basis and making sure you are still comfortable with your exposure.

You should establish a risk log for your project and invite team members to add to it if any new risks are identified. You should include risks and issues on the agenda for your regular project meetings.

Issues

Issues are different from risks. Issues can be defined as bad things that have happened or are happening within your project. They are often a documented risk that has materialized, e.g., loss of key staff.

You should maintain an issues register to ensure all issues are identified, communicated, understood, owned, and resolved. An issues register should include the items listed in Table 4.15.2 information for each issue.

TABLE 4.15.2 Issues Register Content

• Issue name	• Description	• Raised by
• Severity	• Impact	• Action
• Who is responsible	• Status (open, closed)	• Date closed

Further Reading—Risks and Issues

Meredith, J., Mantel, S. 2014. Project Management; A Managerial Approach, 9th ed. Wiley. HB 436:2004 Risk Management Guidelines Companion to AS/NZS 4360:2004. Available at: www.riskmanagement.com.au.

A brief outline and template for the SWOT process is available at: http://www.businessballs.com/swotanalysisfreetemplate.htm.

Associated Documents—Risks and Issues

4.15.1 Risk Identification Register Template

1.1. Risk Identification

This template includes a brief description of some known risks. Use this template to list your key risks. and their mitigants. You may have other risk groups that are more relevant to your institution or project that will need to be included, such as delays for ethics approval or failure to locate tissue samples.

In this template, pre and post mitigation ratings are required but you could simply present a summary of key risks that level of detail is not required.

1.1.1. Operational Risks

Operational risks are risks that have an impact on the day to day operations of the organisation. These may include Human Resources, Processes, Technology, Safety etc.

Risk Summary	Description	Preliminary Risk Rating	Risk Mitigation Description	Residual Risk Rating

1.1.2. Legal Risks

Legal risks impact the legal position of the organisation.

Risk Summary	Description	Preliminary Risk Rating	Risk Mitigation Description	Residual Risk Rating

1.1.3. Compliance and Legislative Risks

These risks impact the compliance and legislative requirements of the organisation.

Risk Summary	Description	Preliminary Risk Rating	Risk Mitigation Description	Residual Risk Rating

1.1.4. Financial Risks

The risk that the costs of the project will be different from expected.

Risk Summary	Description	Preliminary Risk Rating	Risk Mitigation Description	Residual Risk Rating

1.1.5. Miscellaneous Risks

Other risks that impact the project ability to deliver in some way.

Risk Summary	Description	Preliminary Risk Rating	Risk Mitigation Description	Residual Risk Rating

4.16 Project Advisory Committees

Al said he needed help from outside his collaborator group, so his colleagues agreed, gingerly, to ask some of the really important people in the field for help. Would they sit on the advisory committee? Much to his delight the experts accepted, but then Al let the side down. He was so intimidated by their seniority he was nervous to send project updates, and calling a meeting was way too frightening. Unfortunately, the committee languished and fell apart due to lack of feedback and follow up. Al missed out on freely available great advice.

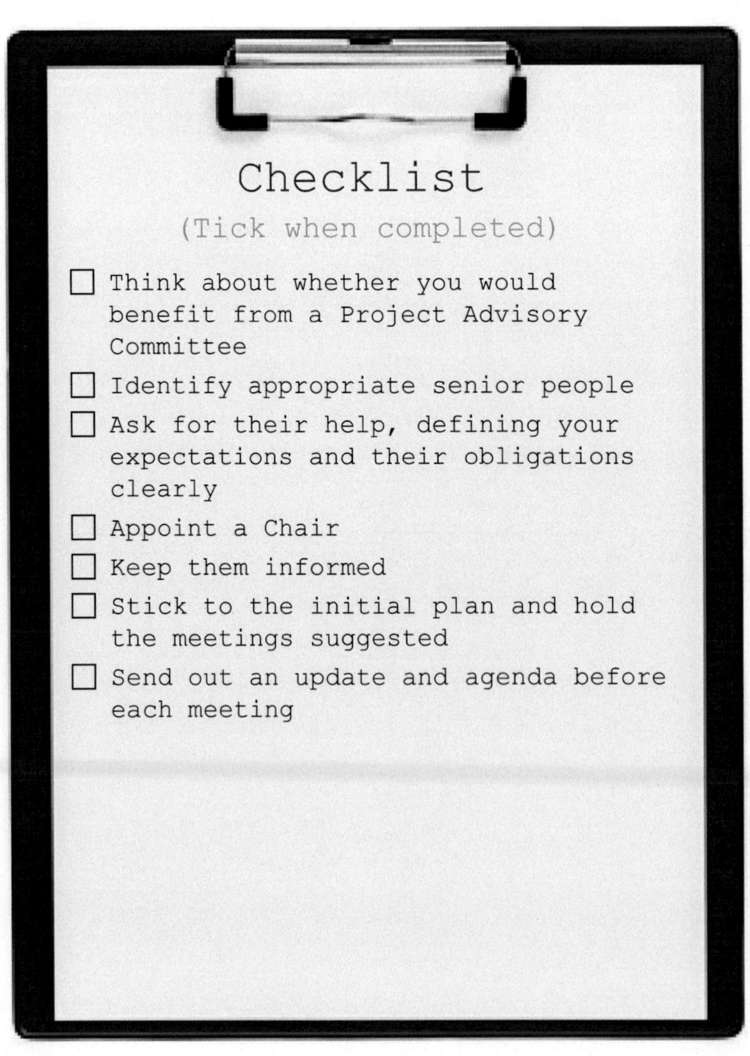

If your project, or projects, will be long-running, it can be very useful to have an advisory committee. The members of this committee will not be your collaborators, or from your institute, but senior people from your field of interest (though probably not from your institution), in a position to give independent, impartial advice.

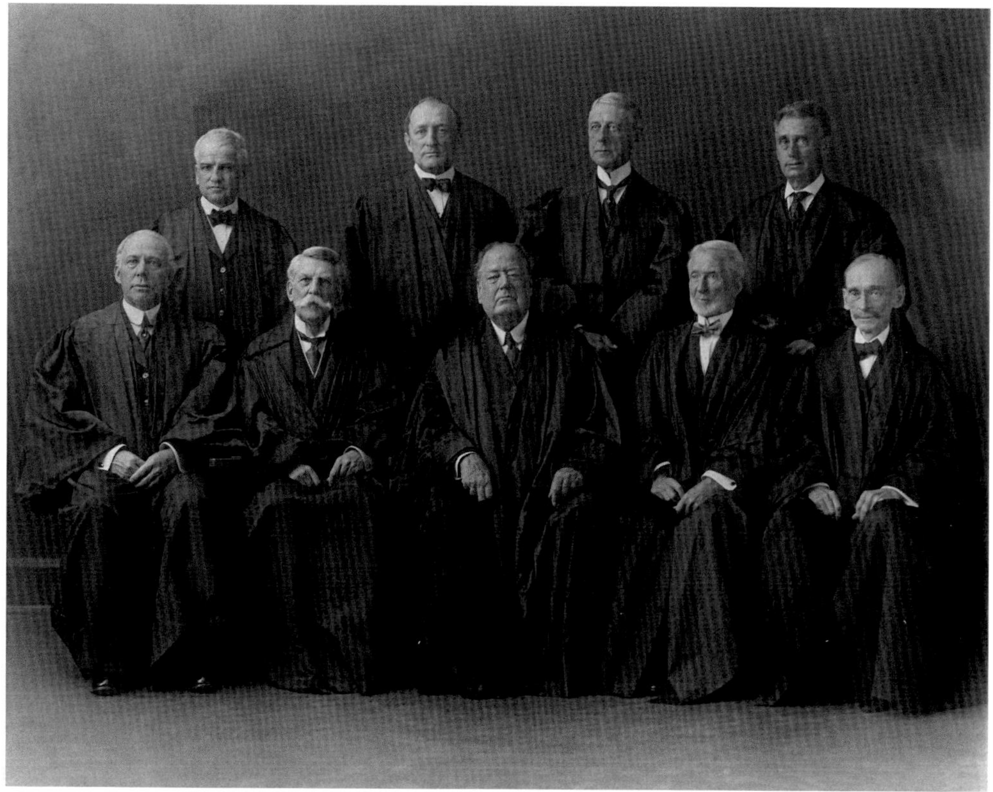

Image Credit: White Court by Everett Historical/Shutterstock

An advisory committee must not be allowed to usurp the responsibilities and authority of the project's investigators. An effective advisory committee, properly composed and structured, can provide non-binding but informed guidance and serve as a tremendous ally in the quest for superior research practices and governance. They can provide a safe environment for investigators to test-drive options before they are forced to make a commitment to move in a particular direction.

Think carefully about your advisory committee's purpose to ensure that it will be structured to maximize its contribution to your project's success. It should have specific terms of reference, an appointed chairman, and a determined meeting frequency. Perhaps set it up so that your advisory committee meets you and your collaborators annually and find out if they might be willing to be consulted as a group by telephone between meetings, if difficulties arise.

As advisory committee members tend not to be continuously involved in the affairs of the project they are called upon to assist, committee members must be provided with suitable information well in advance of their meetings in order to be effective. You should avoid the all too frequent situation where meetings are held with little or nothing distributed in advance. This results in a significant amount of meeting time being taken up in providing background information—and your committee might justifiably lose interest or confidence in your project.

There is probably some benefit to having the chief investigator provide an overall view of project progress at each meeting, but the focus of the meeting should be to obtain feedback from those who, by definition, have been brought in to provide their advice. That advice will be more useful when it can be given after the committee members have reflected on materials delivered in advance, rather than when it is an immediate reaction to information conveyed for the first time at your meeting.

5 PEOPLE MANAGEMENT: FOR YOURSELF AND YOUR TEAM

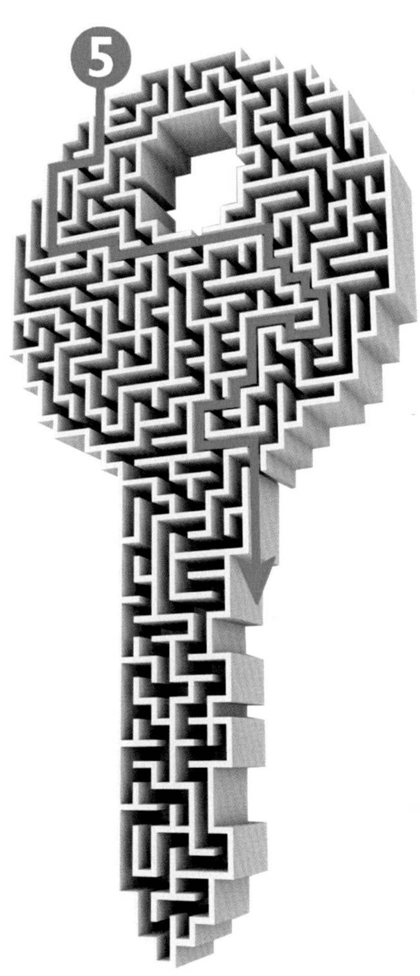

5.1 Finding a Mentor

Why Should You Have a Mentor?

Having a good mentor early in one's career can mean the difference between success and failure in any career.

Lee [1]

If I have seen further than others, it is by standing upon the shoulders of giants.

Isaac Newton

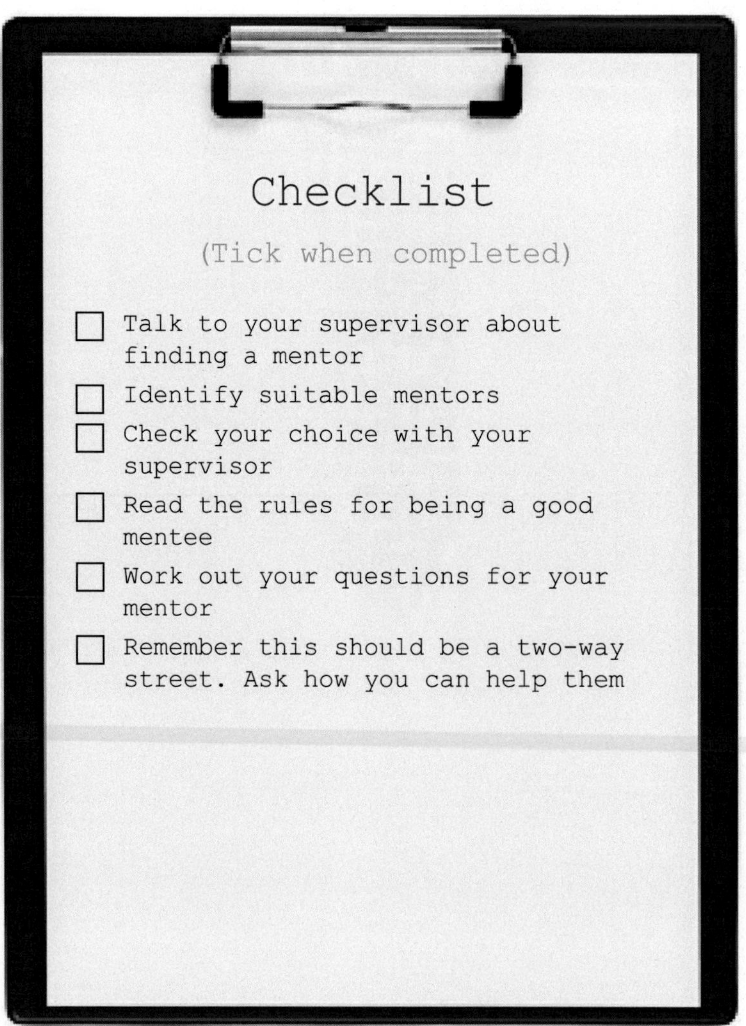

Mentoring is a personal one-on-one relationship between a more experienced or knowledgeable person and someone less experienced. It allows a sharing of knowledge and experience and, importantly, a view from an "outside" pair of eyes. It is a very important practice in academia.

Your mentor is not necessarily the same person as your supervisor (although your supervisor should certainly mentor you, and might remain your mentor forever, long after you stopped working for them).

Established researchers consistently hold the view that their mentors provided them with the best form of support during their research career. They give their mentors credit for having helped them establish good and effective networks, for identifying opportunities for funding or publishing, and for assistance with goal setting. They are consistently grateful for the clear-eyed views that helped them sort out issues with their work. In short, their mentors helped them push their career along. Established researchers also mentioned that they have had numerous mentors along the way, different mentors for different purposes.

> *In his many roles within the university, +++ has never altered his attitude towards students, they remain his core business and he would argue that he has benefited more from this than any of us who he has mentored.*
>
> Lee [1]

On the strength of this, established researchers will usually be glad to offer their services to the next generation. Don't be afraid to ask!

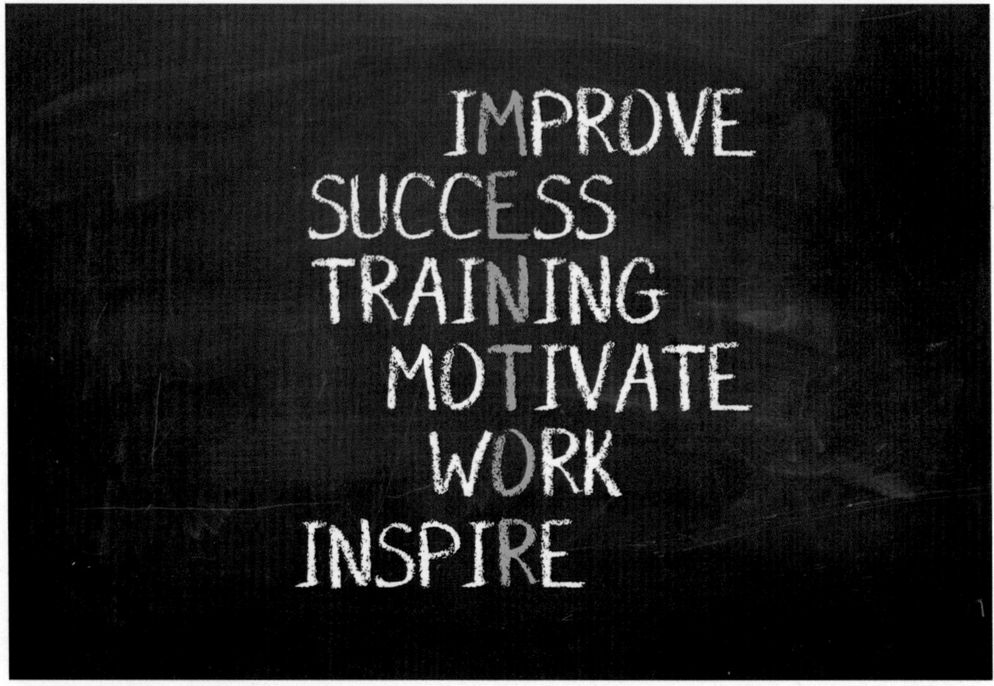

Image Credit: Mentor On Blackboard by rankwolffni/Shutterstock

How Can a Mentor Help You?

A mentor might be required to help you make career choices, might be a senior researcher who can provide background and overview for your specific research area, or might simply be someone with local knowledge who can help you in your early days at your institute. Later in your career you might look for a mentor who can help you with other requirements, such as leadership skills.

In the early years of your career, your mentor is most likely to assist you with the following:

- Reviewing your writing or presentations
- Grant applications
- Getting published
- Career planning—or career change
- Building your network

- Alternate methodologies
- Advice about managing your students

They can also be called upon to help with matters which, strictly speaking, are outside research, but which their greater experience has prepared them for, such as:

- Balancing work and family commitments
- Difficulties with your supervisor
- Coping with cultural transitions after a move from a different part of the world
- Opposing ethnic or gender bias

Identifying Suitable Mentors

Once you have decided you need a mentor—which should be early in your career—you need to find an appropriate person. Realistically, your mentor can come from anywhere. It is geographically helpful if your mentor is from within your university or city, but it is not actually necessary. The fact that the mentor comes from elsewhere automatically means they will be outside the local politics of your institution, which can be a good thing.

A good place to start your search is by asking your supervisor at your institution. Your supervisor might well have an appropriate colleague or collaborator who is known to be someone open to mentoring, and a person who would offer sound advice. Similarly, you could ask for suggestions from your head of school or head of research.

When you are at inter-departmental meetings or even conferences, keep an eye out for senior researchers whose style appeals to you. Introduce yourself and have a conversation. If it feels right, ask around about the person and see what sort of reputation she has. Look up her research profile, track record, and current areas of interest. If all is lining up well, approach your prospective mentor and ask if she would be willing to consider mentoring you. If yes, send in your CV and a link to your profile page so that she can learn a little about you before agreeing. Describe your area of interest briefly and your personal goals.

Remember to discuss your proposed mentor with your supervisor. This is important, so that you are not going behind your supervisor's back. It also matters in case there is a history between them that you would otherwise be unaware of.

Never undervalue the mentoring benefits of a sound relationship with your colleagues with the same level of experience as you. Of necessity, their challenges will be similar to yours. This is a different type of mentorship, but that doesn't make it any less valuable. You can use one another as sounding boards, and learn from one another's mistakes. If you are all having the same problems, there will be power in numbers if you need to take your problem to a higher authority.

Requirements for a Good Mentee

You stand to gain a great deal from a successful relationship with your mentor(s). Having a mentor is not a sign of being at an early stage in your career, and something to get past: it is a sign of great fortune.

You will benefit from having a mentor, or more likely a series of mentors, for the rest of your working days. This is not a situation typical only for science. Many a CEO of a big company will consider herself fortunate to still have a mentor with whom they can discuss their concerns.

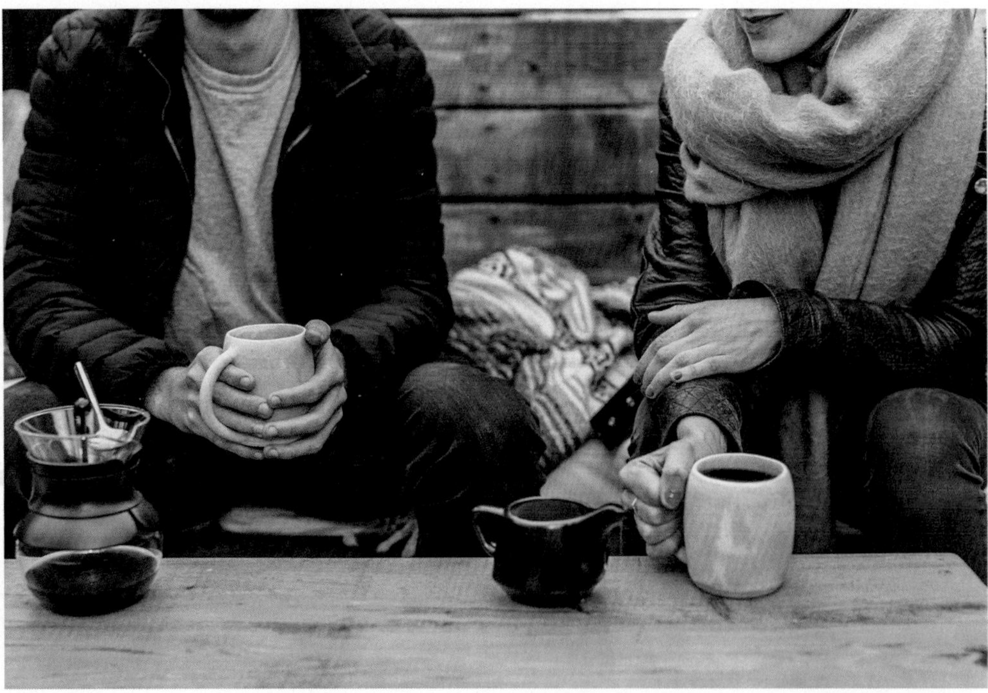

A good mentee will be

- Polite
- Punctual
- Appreciative
- Responsive to the suggestions of the mentor
- Prepared
- Willing to listen to feedback and act on it, or at least reflect on it
- Willing to experiment and try out new processes

Try hard to get to know your mentor, or at least to get to know a lot about her background and experience. When you understand her areas of interest and experience, you will be able to ask appropriate questions that will result in answers derived from their actual experience, not just opinions or best guesses.

The benefits you are likely to derive include the following:

- Sound independent advice, untainted by local politics
- A wider network, as your mentor introduces you to their contacts
- A different approach to the skills and techniques available in your workplace
- Different methodologies
- An opportunity to shadow your mentor for a time
- An independent person to read your written work and offer editorial advice

The following is some extra advice:

- Use your mentor's time effectively. Let her know in advance about something specific you wish to talk about so she can think about it.
- Send work you wish to discuss, or which has been corrected taking into account your mentor's suggestions, ahead of your next meeting. Don't expect your mentor to read it and comment on the spot.
- Try to create a relationship where both parties benefit. Good relationships don't just happen. Think about ways that your mentor could benefit from this relationship too, and find ways to make the most of them for your mentor's benefit.
- Always set the date for the next meeting at the current one—and try to stick to it.

Be open with your mentor, and have frank discussions about your work and plans, and anything which concerns you. This is what a mentor is for.

If the mentoring relationship isn't working out for you, speak up. It might well not be working for the mentor either. Discuss your concerns frankly. The relationship may well mend, or you might agree to part. You might agree to leave out the issue that has been causing difficulty. There is no point in creating resentment or, worse, an enemy.

Once you have a good solid relationship with a mentor, try to keep it up forever. Your mentors will be proud of your achievements because they have helped you toward them. Let them know when you have had a success—be it a new position or a paper published. Your mentors will remain people to whom you can go for a reference or other professional help. The relationship will continue to work for each of you if you allow it to do so.

Ball [2] understands that sometimes it's hard to know how to best use the time you have with a mentor. See Table 5.1.1 for suggestions for a few questions you could pose.

TABLE 5.1.1 Questions for Your Mentor
Can you tell me about your career path? How did you get to where you are?
What would you do differently?
What would you do if you were me?
Could you review my CV and provide a frank assessment of gaps and weaknesses?
Could you help me develop/review my career plan?
What types of outcomes/performance indicators should I be aiming for at my career stage?
What new skills do I need to move ahead?
How can I work smarter?
How should I handle this scenario?
Who else would you recommend I connect/collaborate with? Can you help link me with key contacts/collaborators?
When should I apply for a promotion? Can you help me develop/review my case for a promotion?
Can you suggest some tips for coping with academic knockbacks and rejections?
What professional associations are you involved with? Which would you suggest I become involved with?
What has been your most rewarding accomplishment? What mistakes have you made?
What is the best leadership advice you've received?
What advice would you give on leading a balanced life?
And a killer question that mentors love: How can I help you?

Requirements for a Good Mentor

The outstanding mentors are those that manage to make themselves available when they are needed. Despite their enormous workloads and responsibilities, somehow they make sure their door is always open. They can respond to urgent requests, flick back emails in 20 minutes, read drafts within two days, and be there to listen when the going is tough.

More on this in Chapter 5.3.

References—Mentoring

[1] Lee, A., Dennis, C., Campbell, P., June 14, 2007. Nature's guide for mentors. Nature 447 (7146), 791–797 and Lee, in conversation.
[2] K. Ball, The #1 Key to Academic Success. https://happyacademic.wordpress.com/2017/05/03/the-1-key-to-academic-success/.

Further Reading

Kamp Dush, C., 2016. Advice on Being Advised. Chronicle Vitae. https://chroniclevitae.com/news/1637-advice-on-being-advised.

Rockquemore, K.A., 2014. When It Comes to Mentoring the More the Merrier. Chronicle Vitae. https://chroniclevitae.com/news/326-when-it-comes-to-mentoring-the-more-the-merrier.

The NIH provides valuable information, including a video, on Choosing a Mentor. https://www.training.nih.gov/mentoring_guidelines.

The American Association for the Advancement of Science website ScienceCareers.org has many articles on mentoring. http://sciencecareers.sciencemag.org.

Association for Women in Science features mentoring advice for women in STEM environments. www.awis.org.

5.2 Looking After Your Team

Train people well enough so they can leave, treat them well enough so they don't want to.

Sir Richard Branson

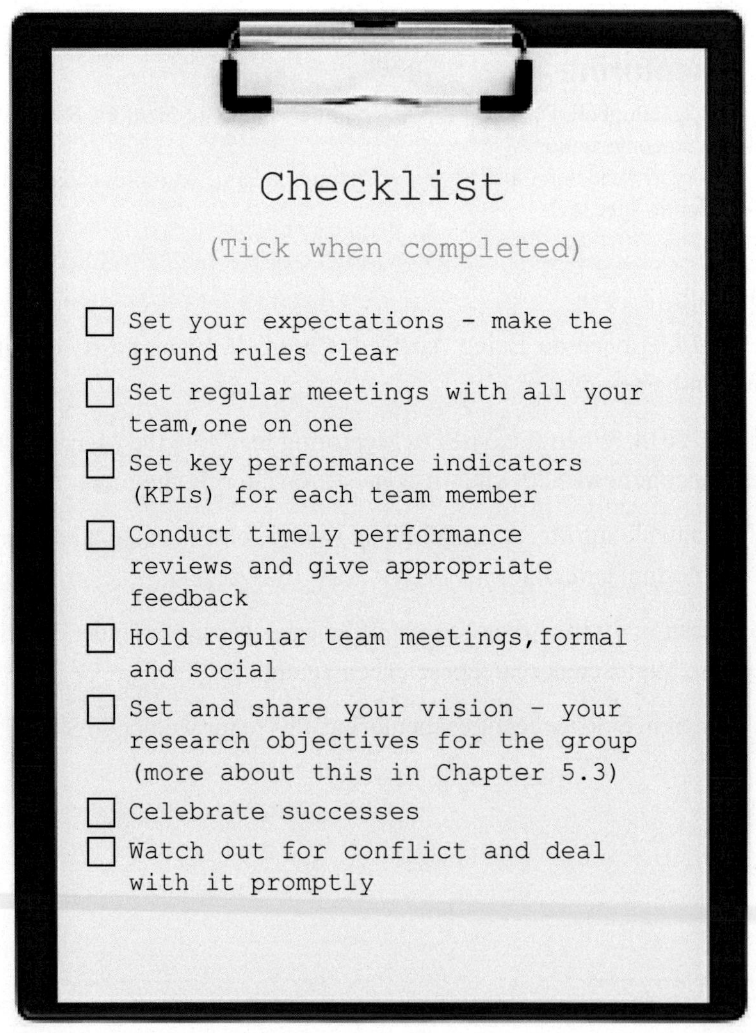
Checklist
(Tick when completed)
Set your expectations - make the ground rules clear
Set regular meetings with all your team,one on one
Set key performance indicators (KPIs) for each team member
Conduct timely performance reviews and give appropriate feedback
Hold regular team meetings,formal and social
Set and share your vision - your research objectives for the group (more about this in Chapter 5.3)
Celebrate successes
Watch out for conflict and deal with it promptly

Checklist

(Tick when completed)

- ☐ Promote collaborative practices - write as a team, hold a journal club or promote skill sharing
- ☐ Offer networking and training opportunities
- ☐ Is your team's knowledge shared? Make sure at least two people know about every process
- ☐ Cultivate a culture of work life balance - and that includes you

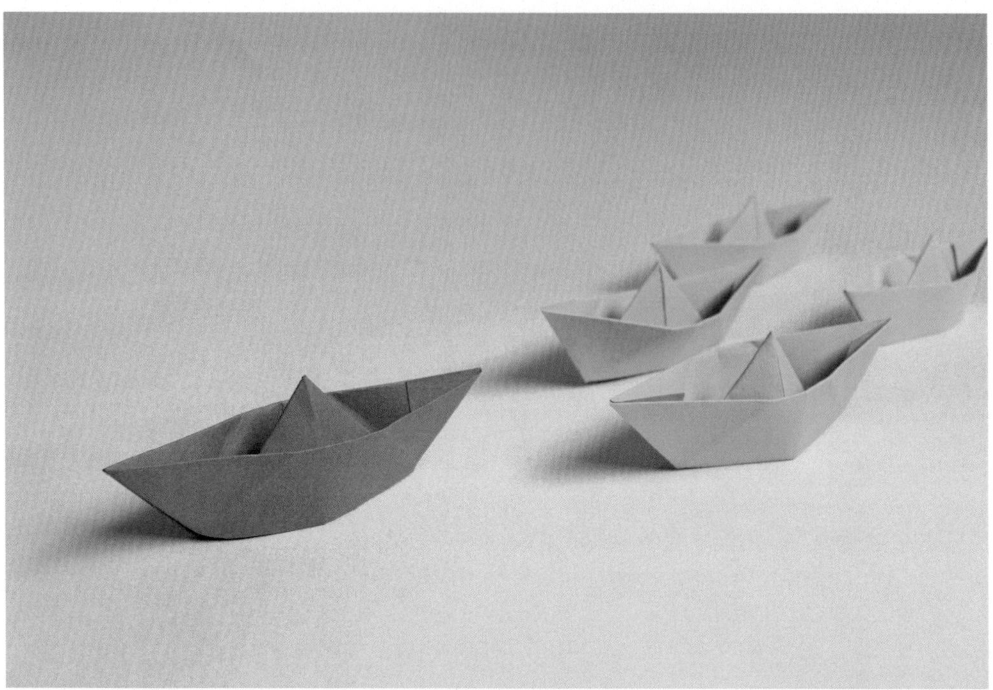

Every team, even a small team, will present a variety of skills and personalities. It will also provide a variety of abilities and working styles. Your challenge is to bring out the best in them all. It is worth the trouble. A team member who feels happy and productive and rewarded will go the extra mile. That team member will work hard for you if you are worthy of respect and demonstrate respect for others. This chapter points out ways to set expectations, provide growth opportunities, and discusses aspects of "hands-on" management of your team. While there are aspects of research leadership discussed, Chapter 5.3 following will address bigger picture leadership practices.

Research Leadership

It is most likely that you will begin your research career as a project leader with a small project. Small or not, the same principles which apply to leading a small group will still apply as you graduate to larger research projects.

In the research environment, a leader has to manage, or at least oversee, the activities of all team members. This requires the leader to understand the core activities that they are responsible for directing. Beyond a basic knowledge of the scientific tools and processes being used by the team, the leader must also be able to do the following:

- Carefully design projects and determine time frames
- Define and explain the work plan clearly to the members of the team
- Create order
- Ensure that project deliverables are met in a timely manner
- Create, and then adhere to, project budgets
- Analyze and think about the project as a whole before making decisions
- Ensure that the roles and responsibilities of all are well defined, and that reporting lines are clear
- Develop effective decision-making processes
- Insist that everyone follows the rules and procedures
- Plan for and write grants
- Juggle many different demands at once

When your project is small and there are very few staff, you, as team leader, will be responsible for many of these diverse aspects of the project. You will probably have a steep learning curve at the beginning as you come to grips with agreements and contracts, requirements of human resources departments, and reporting obligations.

There is nothing easy about leadership—except when everything is going right! Sometimes you will struggle. By definition, the leader is there to manage unexpected crises and issues. There will probably be areas of leadership that you find more difficult than others, such as public speaking or resolving conflict. Once you are a team leader, there is no escape from the aspects you don't feel comfortable with; you have to find a way. In this case, you might seek input from a mentor. If you don't currently have an appropriate leadership mentor, look about you and identify a colleague who appears to fulfill that particular role well. Try to follow your mentor's example, or, probably better, have a conversation about your concerns and request assistance.

Leading and managing in a research context is extra challenging. The very nature of research means that at the outset it is often not quite clear how you will achieve the research goals—which makes leading, planning, and managing difficult. Throughout the life of the project, people are likely to need to learn new skills and use new processes, which may either confuse or stimulate them. All this must be managed by the leader.

> The overall message is that we are all human. Everyone needs positive reinforcement—from the lowliest staff member to *your* supervisors. A little bit of encouragement can work wonders in almost every situation.

Set Expectations

It is important to set expectations for your team. These don't have to be hard and fast rules; it is more of setting up "ways of working." Just as your parents laid down rules at home when you were growing up, you need to make sure that your people know what the general expectations are so they can do their best to comply. Some things you might consider setting expectations around, so as to avoid conflict, are as follows:

- Start and finish timings
- Use of a mobile phone in the shared workplace
- Time off in lieu
- Lunch hours

Many people produce a standard "welcome pack" for new starters that explains the basics. These "rules" are not to create an environment like the one at school, but more to define the norm. Many of these rules could be covered in orientation—see Chapter 2.3.

Manage Staff

You must ensure that each staff member has their own allocated time to talk to you (or their manager). The best practice is to set regular one-on-one meetings between each staff member and their manager, say fortnightly. There should be an agenda, and the more junior team member should minute those meetings, recording decisions.

The agenda and minutes should be stored electronically in a specific place accessible only to the meeting participants.

Performance Review

As team leader you are responsible for the performance of your team members and for ensuring all staff are making the most of their time and resources. It is good practice to set performance goals for all team members. These performance objectives should be determined collaboratively, and like project goals should be SMART: Specific, Measurable, Achievable, Relevant, and Time-bound.

It is good practice to hold an annual or semi-annual performance review, with each staff member, against those objectives usually known as key performance indicators (KPIs). When the performance indicators are precise and measurable it is easy to be objective when assessing whether or not they have been achieved or exceeded.

This performance review process should not be treated as interference or torture, but an opportunity to discuss openly what has gone right, and what could be better—from both sides.

It is usual to offer self-rating for the staff member, and this is reviewed by the manager prior to the meeting. The manager adds their views, and together this provides a basis for discussion. This meeting should be treated as an opportunity to step back from everyday issues and for you to give feedback on the individual's work. Your recognition of good work and effective contributions, especially of the work of other people, will generate enthusiasm and encourage them to continue to try harder. It is also an opportunity to understand roadblocks and revise priorities. Take a positive, collaborative, and problem-solving approach to address any shortfalls.

During the meeting, set the new goals for the coming six months, for both performance (update KPIs) and personal development. This is the time for the conversations about where the person wants to be in 12 months or three years.

Goal setting is often difficult and you may have to push to make your team member nominate a goal. On other occasions they might have a goal which doesn't quite fit your needs. During the goals conversation, remember the vision and mission. If your team member's goals are drifting out of alignment, either bring them back in, or make plans for them to move on. When it comes to the learning goals, remember everyone will be happier and more productive if they feel well looked after, so be as generous as you can. You will both benefit from the professional development of your team.

At this time the position description should be reviewed. It is extraordinary how an individual's job can change over six months. Take a fresh look at the position description to make sure it still captures the essence of the job.

If the goals haven't been achieved, ask yourself why. Is it entirely the fault of the employee, or are some circumstances that have been dictated by you part of the problem? Think about whether a particular project is taking too long. Has it reached "enough," or is the goal important enough for everyone to keep battling on? Could your resources be better allocated?

Underperformance can have a number of reasons, including the following:

- Inadequate skills to do the job
- Poor work organization skills

- Unrealistic expectations
- Personal problems
- Lack of relationship skills

Constructive, thoughtful conversations can usually identify the main reasons for the perceived poor performance, and together you can put plans in place to address them.

Performance Management

As mentioned previously, the smart thing to do, having recruited wisely, is to ensure that you have a probation period, and that you properly assess the new employee before that probation period runs out. Keep an eye on the new employee and if there is any doubt about their ability, move them on while they are still on probation. Resist giving the benefit of the doubt too often: it is not going to be worth the effort in the long run.

Sometimes, though, a poor performer slips through the net and having one on the team tends to take up a lot of time. It is natural for a team leader to focus their efforts on the poor performer in a team. It is all too easy to spend your time and effort on managing this poor performer while you leave your shining stars alone to fend for themselves. Those stars would almost certainly bring much more reward to the team if they were receiving an equal amount of your attention.

Giving Constructive Feedback

There are times when you just have to do it. When you do, get it right. You must design your feedback as a vehicle for improvement, not as an opportunity to get a litany of complaints off your chest.

- Time it well. Don't catch the person on Friday night when they are on the way out the door for the weekend.
- Don't do it when the person is upset and angry and won't be able to take it in. Instead, make an appointment for later, giving them an opportunity to settle down first.
- Be specific and objective. "I am disappointed that although we agreed you would do x by yesterday, it is still not on my desk. Could you please tell me why you haven't done it?"
- Don't rely on second-hand information, dropping the names of others into the problem. "Flossie said that you…"

- If you are discussing a person's failure to achieve a goal(s), refer to the goals you set together in your review meetings or in the KPIs. As these goals, by definition, have been agreed upon, they give you a justification for your concerns.
- Put the issue you want to talk about into context by identifying the research or team needs and explaining the impact or consequences of the behavior or performance from those perspectives.
- Make positive suggestions, or, better, work out ways together for overcoming the problem.
- Focus on behaviors or skills that can change.
- Avoid trying to make yourself feel better by hiding negative feedback in between two pieces of reinforcing feedback. You will only dilute your message.
- Provide your team member with a deadline for review of progress by immediately arranging a next meeting.
- Avoid covering too many topics in one meeting. Realistically they won't be able to take it in.
- Probably the most important of all, don't wait too long to do something about any staffing problem. If your feedback is about one specific incident, give the feedback as soon as possible after the behavior occurred. Even if it is a result of a series of more minor incidents; remember that a bad apple in the team will be affecting everyone. Put yourself in the shoes of the person on the next bench or desk who is wondering "why is she getting away with this? It's not fair."

Although I know it's important, it is hard for me to let people know when their behavior does not meet my expectations. When I first opened the lab, I was more uncomfortable with this than I am now. Basically, I'm quicker to call people on it now. If things are not working and the quality of their work is somehow slipping, or the effort that they are putting in is somewhat dropping, I have an easier time saying, "This isn't right, you have to change it now."

Charles Murry [1]

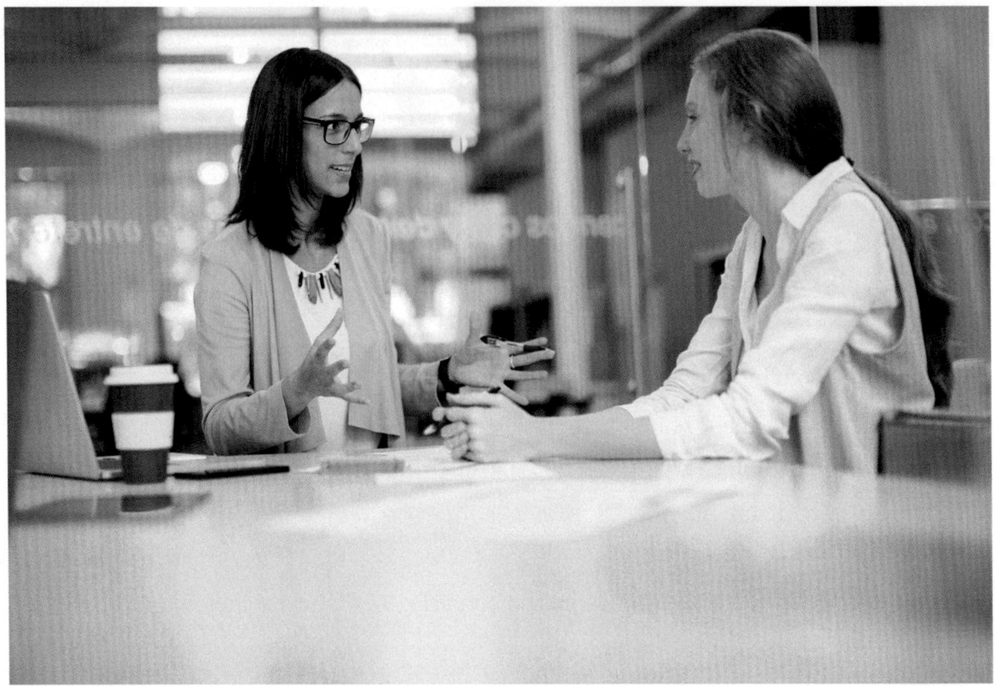

Image Credit: Coaching and advise by Tempura/iStock

Addressing poor performance is easier if you and the staff member have followed the initial advice to set SMART performance indicators, and if you are in the habit of regularly sharing feedback on their progress. The gap between defined expectations and outcomes will provide a clear basis for assessment.

Always document and date your performance review discussions and the planned outcomes. If, in the end, you find that the performance cannot be improved to the extent necessary, your records will be important as background for the subsequent processes. Although rare, persistent unsatisfactory performance needs to be addressed in a formal manner. If the informal methods have not led to improvements, you need to contact your human resources department for advice on how to manage the exit of such a staff member. Leaving situations like this to fester increases the workload for everyone else, while the person causing the trouble is still costing the same salary as an effective staff member.

Conflict in Your Team

On a similar note, watch out for the "bad penny" in your team. This is the person who is too assertive, who doesn't listen, who talks over the top of the others, and who resists and probably resents management. It is also likely to be the person who delegates all their responsibilities while giving the appearance of being busy, who airily allows you to believe everything is done, but who doesn't show the evidence. This is also the person who creates trouble with the others, who complains on the quiet about "management," and who is full of what they believe to be their own good ideas, while at the same time being unwilling to carry out yours.

Don't put up with it. Burying your head in the sand and hoping the problem will go away is not the way to deal with it. Have the difficult conversation and, if the problems continue, have it again. Remember that this troublesome person won't just be upsetting you, they will also be undermining the comfort of other members of the team. Is it worth it?

See more about managing conflict in Chapter 5.4.

Annual Review of the Team's Progress

It is a good idea to plan an annual team meeting to both review the year past and plan the year ahead. While you may want to prepare for this meeting with only your senior team, be sure to include the whole team in the actual meeting. Aim to make it a celebration of achievements rather than a litany of failures. Offer the opportunity to all to provide views on what went wrong and what could have been done better, what were the good things that were learnt, and then plan together for the next year. Seek input on the hopes and dreams and aspirations of the entire team.

Keep an eye on the vision and mission during these sessions. Does it stand, or does it need updating? Has there been "mission creep?"

These meetings can help you avoid potential conflicts within your team and with competitors.

Provide an Equitable Environment

As team leader you should aim to create a culture of behaviors that enable staff to work at their best. Encourage your team to have the freedom to challenge the status quo and exchange ideas. Insist on respectful listening where people can feel confident of being well treated even when exploring creative and unusual ideas.

Likewise, equal employment opportunity initiatives ensure that all employees are treated with fairness and respect. These protect staff from discrimination or harassment in the workplace and require that everyone be given an equal chance to use his or her skills and capabilities.

Equal opportunity in the workplace matters because staff who feel appreciated will contribute to the best of their ability. Where everyone is treated well and impartially, the following effectiveness increases:

- Workplace relationships improve
- Staff are productive, innovative, and creative
- Absenteeism and staff turnover drops

5 PEOPLE MANAGEMENT: FOR YOURSELF AND YOUR TEAM

As leader of your team, you are responsible for ensuring that your staff make decisions and allocate tasks and resources that enable individual members to reach their potential. You must also ensure that they are not discriminated against on the basis of irrelevant characteristics such as race, sex, age, or religious belief.

The social norms and processes you develop should be

- Open
- Transparent
- Inclusive
- Free from discrimination or bias

A respectful culture can be established by discussing with the team the kind of workplace relationships that enable them all to be most productive; one where people will show respect for others' opinions, have open communication, accept diverse backgrounds, and demonstrate supportiveness. When the team is under pressure of deadlines and heavy workloads, reminders of the agreed standards of behavior can help stop destructive interactions at an early stage.

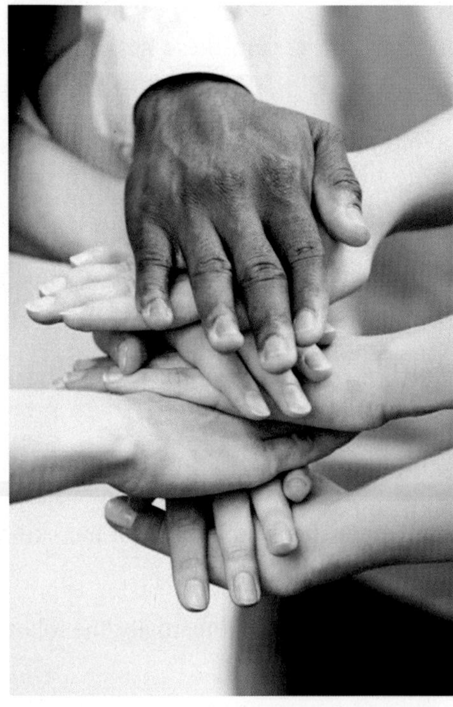

Image Credit: Hands holding together by Africa Studio/Shutterstock

Communicate With Your Team

The best leader is an approachable leader. To be approachable you need to be there, and when there, you need to have your door open. By all means close the door when you are working to a deadline, or for a confidential conversation, but you should aim to be accessible to your team as much as possible.

One way to limit the interruptions is to proactively walk around to visit the team every day. Make it understood that this is the ideal time for the quick chat. Back this up by holding weekly or, at the outside, fortnightly one-on-one meetings with your direct reports.

It is good to also provide opportunities for the whole team to get together in a relaxed environment. Cheap and cheerful Friday lunches with the entire team invited, or weekly afternoon teas where there is time for a chat are simple and effective ways to build relationships. Try instigating a routine where the person "on" for the afternoon tea roster tells everyone something about their life outside work. This little trick can help everyone learn unexpected things about their colleagues. A drink after work on Friday afternoon is always good. Lee [2] suggests a variety of gatherings from wine tastings to dinners with visiting scientists and celebration of every birthday at morning tea to help bring the team together. He recommends the power of chocolate biscuits for doing good and spreading a feeling of well-being.

More formal team meetings are also beneficial. A weekly or monthly whole team meeting with a fixed agenda is good practice.

You can build in an opportunity for a presentation from a junior team member which provides good informal practice in a safe environment for a more formal presentation down the track. Similarly, require a brief presentation from any team member who has attended a conference. They will get the benefit from the need to distill their thoughts about what they have learnt; the rest of the team will share the experience. Use these meetings to formally celebrate the successes of team members—and back up those celebrations by mentioning the successes again at your social gatherings. A little praise goes a long way in the often dispiriting world of research where, by definition, so many hopes don't work out as you wished.

Some other good practices for leaders to promote in a research environment for the benefit of the whole team include a journal club, skill sharing, cross-disciplinary meetings, and annual reviews.

Journal Club

Regular journal club meetings get everyone together and help to reinforce the culture of the team. Discussing a paper relevant to your team provides a great way to review how the writers went about constructing and testing a hypothesis, how they analyzed the results and drew a conclusion. An even more effective meeting can review two papers with opposing views on the same topic.

Another approach is to each independently review a particular paper, completing the referee's report form. Meet with your fellow reviewers as an "editorial board" and decide whether you accept or reject the paper. You can take this to the next step and work independently or together on the rebuttal.

Take the opportunity to reinforce your values while you are discussing other people's work in the journal club.

You can select the journal club papers to further educate your team about your own field, but you don't have to all the time. Try an entirely different field occasionally, and see how they go about presenting research.

Of course the discussion can be helpful background for writing your own papers.

> *[At journal club meetings] we discuss papers and talk about any weaknesses, and it makes it clear that we don't want our papers to have those kinds of weaknesses. I think the scientific rigor issues come up as we go along.*
>
> Tamara Doering, Washington University School of Medicine [1]

A variation on the journal club that can help with scientific writing is to provide the group with a paper which has the abstract removed. Invite your team to carefully read the paper, then prepare what they think would be a good abstract. Later, compare their abstracts with the real one.

Encourage Skill Sharing

A regular skill-sharing meeting for the team is a great way to initiate or confirm collaboration between peers. This meeting gives the opportunity for any team member to present on a special area of expertise, and lets them teach others who have less experience in that area. It is a great way to allow even junior members of the team to shine.

Duplicate the Knowledge Within the Team

You must run your team on the assumption that any one person might leave today. You hope they won't, but things happen. Always, always, always make sure someone else knows how to operate the equipment, create the reagent, open the padlock, use the software, contact the serviceman, and order the supplies.

The sharing of the information across your team is useful in itself, as it can create team bonding and develops in-house training and mentoring skills. It is absolutely not duplication of effort.

The absolutely best practice is having details of these skills written up in a laboratory or project manual.

In a laboratory, aim to share the laboratory management responsibilities through the team, thus teaching them how to manage a laboratory themselves. Whether it is for routine equipment maintenance, sharing being on emergency call, or managing the inventory, have someone in the team take charge of writing up the process and allocating tasks for managing these jobs.

Cross-Disciplinary Meetings

You should encourage cross-disciplinary meeting within your institution. There are many examples of great benefit resulting from bringing disparate groups together. A highly successful example of this has been the Translational Research Institute in QLD, Australia where four medical research organizations, the University of Queensland, Queensland University of Technology, Mater Medical Research Institute, and Queensland Health, have brought their laboratories together into one building. Not only do they meet in the lift and the cafeteria but they also share equipment and, most importantly, ideas. It is extraordinary what someone researching x can teach someone investigating y. At the Translational Research Institute, the work is driven by the needs of patients, a question formed by a clinician, and a solution sought by a scientist. Traditionally, clinicians and researchers worked separately, but this improved method ensures that patient needs are a priority and that teams share knowledge which multiplies with every collaboration. These multi-disciplinary teams create a feedback loop which becomes the translational pathway. With the clinician and scientist working side by side with the patient, results are immediately obvious; much better than waiting for long reports to be read and interpreted.

Provide Networking Opportunities

One of the most important things you can do for your team is to introduce them into the wider world. From the day they arrive with you, you should be helping them to find their feet so they can go elsewhere. It might never come to that, they mightn't want to leave and you might want to keep them, but a really good leader is one who grooms their team members for independence.

Your track record and network of collaborators can open doors for those associated with you and for the mutual benefit of all. Encourage the expansion of their network by doing the following:

- Providing opportunities to meet your collaborators when they visit your institute
- Taking your team to meetings and introducing them to your contacts
- Creating short-term exchanges between institutions
- Encouraging your staff to approach your network using your name (with your approval)
- Encouraging your staff to present at external meetings or institutional meetings with external guests

Encourage Work Life Balance

Life is not all about work. Try not to have unreasonable expectations of your staff. You might well be desperate to get your results sorted, or your paper written by next week, but the need is not necessarily so urgent for your team. Make it clear, up front, what is expected. If work is going to involve the weekend or late nights, say so—and let them decide if they want to be part of the team. If it is not part of the job description, don't let yourself be resentful when the team members don't place the same importance on the tasks that you do, especially on a weekend. Everyone is entitled to work life balance.

Work life balance applies to you too. You will be a much more effective researcher and manager if you can have time elsewhere, thinking about other things.

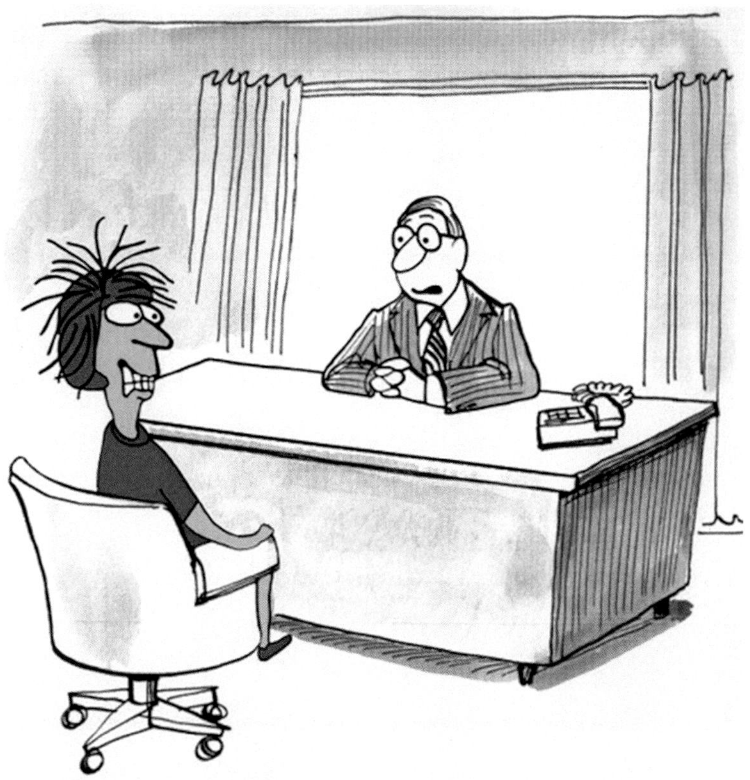

"I'd like you to work more than just 24/7."

Image Credit: Excessive expectations by Cartoon Resource/Shutterstock

Handling Stress

We all know that being a researcher can be very satisfying, but it often comes at a price of high levels of stress and anxiety. Stress could be caused by the pressure of deadlines, writer's block, or sorting out staff matters; perhaps it could be the anxiety of not knowing where your next steps will take you. Research can also be isolating and constant failures are hard on your self-confidence and motivation. Good mental health and well-being can help you deal with the stresses of life in academia, help you and your team make the most of the opportunities around you, and help you deal with the regular knocks that are part of research.

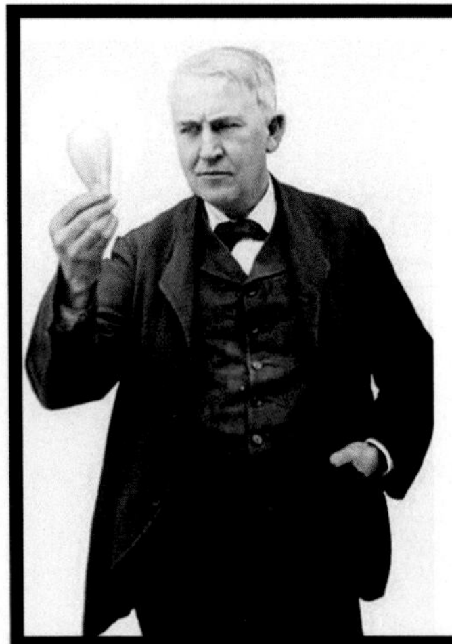

> I HAVE NOT FAILED 10,000 times. I have not failed once. I have succeeded in proving that those 10,000 ways will not work.
>
> When I have eliminated the ways that will not work, I will find the way that will work.
>
> *Thomas Alva Edison*

When you don't have work life balance, you are almost certainly stressed. Stress is the body's response to threatening events. If it's allowed to get out of hand, it leads to a state of mental and physical exhaustion.

Be aware of how stress affects you, your team members, and your or their relationship with your team. Stressed people tend to become irritable and short-tempered, and their judgment is affected.

You can try to manage stress in your workplace by doing the following:

- Shortening working hours
- Granting (or taking) special leave
- Offering exercise programs or yoga or other relaxation

Individuals themselves can contribute to managing their own stress by doing the following:

- Prioritizing their tasks and completing them in order of importance
- Discussing problems with others
- Not creating artificial deadlines or seeking to rearrange pressing deadlines if they can't be met
- Not personalizing issues
- Adding outside interests, such as regular entertainment or sport

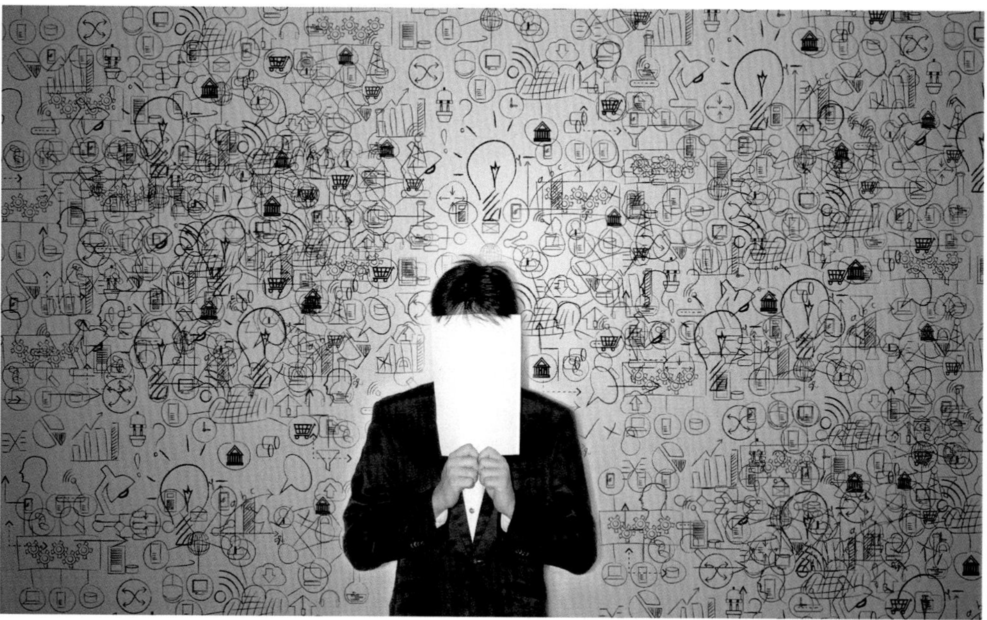

Image Credit: Man covering his face by Technovectors/Shutterstock

Provide a Safe Workplace

A research team leader has a duty to follow safety rules and instructions, use appropriate safety equipment provided, not endanger themselves and others, not be affected by drugs or alcohol, and report hazards/issues to their supervisor.

As a supervisor, you are responsible for ensuring that your staff and students comply with the local Work Health and Safety Regulations and institutional policies. In particular, you are directly responsible for providing a safe working environment, safe systems of work (i.e., safe ways to perform specific tasks), and safe plant such as machinery and electrical equipment for your team. You are also responsible for making sure that your research consumables are in a safe condition (e.g., chemicals are stored safely) and that information, training, instruction, and supervision (e.g., about hazards, procedures, policies) are available for your staff and students. This is one of the biggest challenges in your working environment when you step up to being a project leader—the responsibilities are now yours.

Following best practice for work, health, and safety is good (and cost-effective) insurance against the cost of injury on your research team and its work.

Measure Yourself as Leader

It is worthwhile to reflect on your skills as a team leader. How good are you? Are you providing mentorship as well as supervision to build a world-class research environment?

Lee [2] has provided some of the following exercises that can help you evaluate your success as a leader:

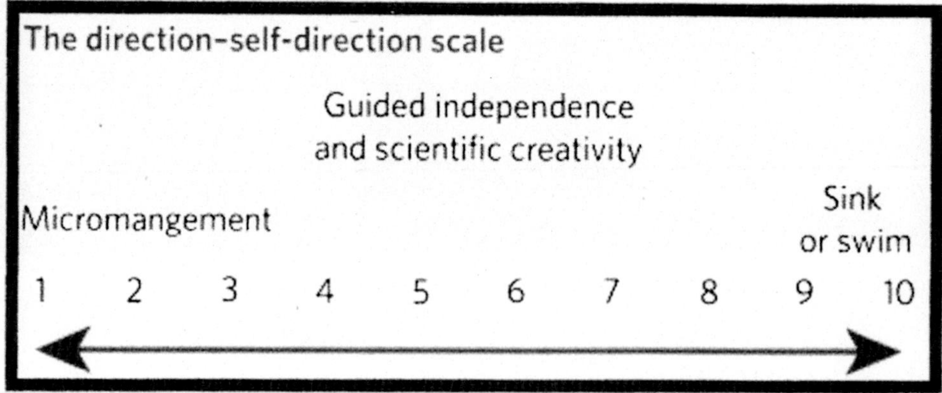

- What strategies do you use to make yourself available to graduate students/early-career researchers?
- When did you last celebrate a student/staff member's achievement? How did you celebrate?

- Where do you place yourself on the "direction–self-direction" scale?
- Describe a deliberate strategy you use to build your group as a social community.
- Describe the steps you take to develop the critical, writing, and presentation skills of your students/staff.

References—Looking After Your Team

[1] Howard Hughes Medical Institute, Burroughs Wellcome Fund, 2006. Making the Right Moves: A Practical Guide to Scientific Management.
[2] A. Lee, Professor Emeritus, University of New South Wales, in conversation.

5.3 Leadership

If I had one piece of advice to give it's that although you've been hired for your scientific skills and research potential, your eventual success will depend heavily on your ability to guide, lead, and empower others to do their best work.

Thomas Cech [1]

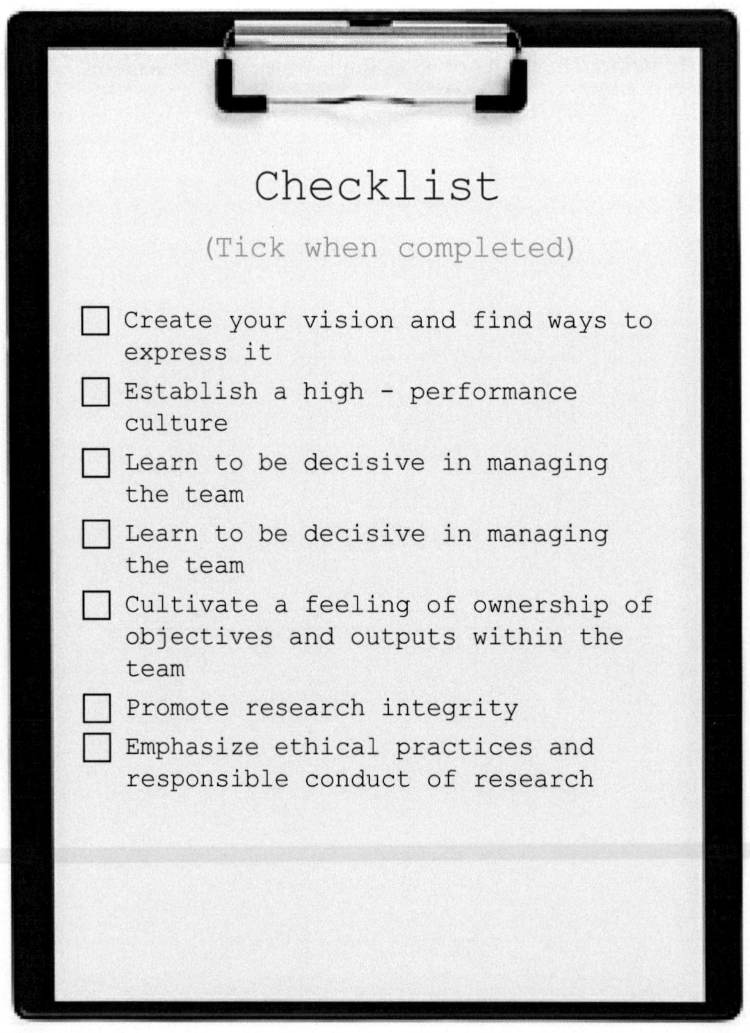

What Is Leadership?

> *A friend of mine, the founder of a company that grew to a billion dollars in annual revenue, best expressed the power of teamwork when he once told me, "If you could get all the people in an organization rowing in the same direction, you could dominate any industry, in any market, against any competition, at any time."*
>
> Lencioni [2]

If you think about it, you will realize that the cost of your team—salaries, staff add-on costs, recruitment, and development costs—is likely to represent at least 60% of your project costs. It is worthwhile looking after that investment of funds as well as possibly making yourself into a good leader of a team that pulls together.

As mentioned in the previous chapter, the leader has to create a vision and set the direction for the group. As leader, you will need to set a specific research vision, leading the research team and creating a culture that encourages high performance even when, as is usually the case in research, the outcomes are uncertain.

You must be able to express your vision (both in terms of research direction and project management) for your research team and your stakeholders (which could include funding agencies, industry partners, and other research collaborators).

In a strong culture the people will work with each other and for each other; where it is weak, they work against each other and for themselves. A good leader enables others in the team to do the work in a unified manner, and together everyone achieves more, demonstrating the qualities listed in Table 5.3.1.

Set Your Team Vision

It is very valuable to define your group's objectives, your vision, and mission. Yes, these sound like marketing words, and to an extent they are. On the other hand, they are very useful in a scientific environment too. Setting your objectives will help you and your team keep on track and stick to the goals.

As described in the Future Leaders Research Program [3], as a team leader you are responsible for helping team members perform at their best. You must provide them with the right sort of

TABLE 5.3.1 Leadership Qualities
Be decisive
Inspire people toward a common/agreed goal
Build and manage the team
Create an environment where people are able to confidently give and receive feedback
Motivate and support graduate students, post-docs, and technicians
Display honesty and integrity
Delegate responsibility to others when possible
Make fair decisions
Manage conflicts
Communicate and listen
Be sensitive to diverse populations and needs
Be a mentor to others, as well as those seeking their own mentors
Encourage networking
Remain focused and keep communicating the vision
And again, be decisive!

environment for clarifying and then solving the problem(s) they are investigating. You must also provide them with an appropriate structure for researching and testing their hypotheses.

Mumford [4] explains that your team will achieve the best outcomes when they all have a clear understanding of their goals (your team objectives). You need to demonstrate the standards you require, provide them with regular feedback on their work, and reward them in recognition of their efforts. Of course you must also supply the resources they need, including training and personal development opportunities and processes for addressing problems.

It is very interesting to learn about what motivates people's behavior and performance at work. Herzberg's [5] now classical research showed that motivators such as salary and good working conditions were necessary for staff to come to work, but these rewards had to be substantial to result in a difference in performance outcomes. Other factors, such as an employee's genuine interest in the work or their social interactions with colleagues or clients, were more likely to make a difference to a staff member's performance. Herzberg found that job satisfaction, intellectual curiosity, good co-workers, and job security were all often higher motivators than salary.

You must always remember, though, that there are considerable individual differences between people, and what is motivating to one person is irrelevant to another. Public recognition at a team meeting might be wonderful for one person, but it can feel like the worst torture to someone else.

Don't under-estimate the power of more informal rewards. If you can do something as simple as show interest in an unexpected result or giving a brief but heartfelt "thank you," you will have a significant impact on a staff member's engagement and motivation at work.

Researchers are always searching for outcomes, so it is important to acknowledge the achievement of outcomes for your team. When you make the milestones in your project plan, make sure you celebrate them with the team, and acknowledge them in performance review records.

Of course your project outcomes will ultimately be acknowledged through authorship of papers, so when that time comes, remember that if it is appropriate for them to be named as first author, doing so could make a big difference to the track record of your PhD students or early post-docs. It is quite common practice to name the junior staff member who has contributed significantly to the project as first author, while the chief investigator is listed as last author. This practice does more than benefit the early-career researcher. It also contributes to building the success of the growing team, as your team will be *recognized* by the funding bodies as one with an interest in developing future research leaders.

The creation of an idea can feel very personal, and it can sometimes be scary to share it. If you as leader can show that you are open to new ideas from the team, acknowledging that they might have possibilities before you start analyzing them critically, you will be helping to create an environment where your young researchers are willing to float new ideas and approaches.

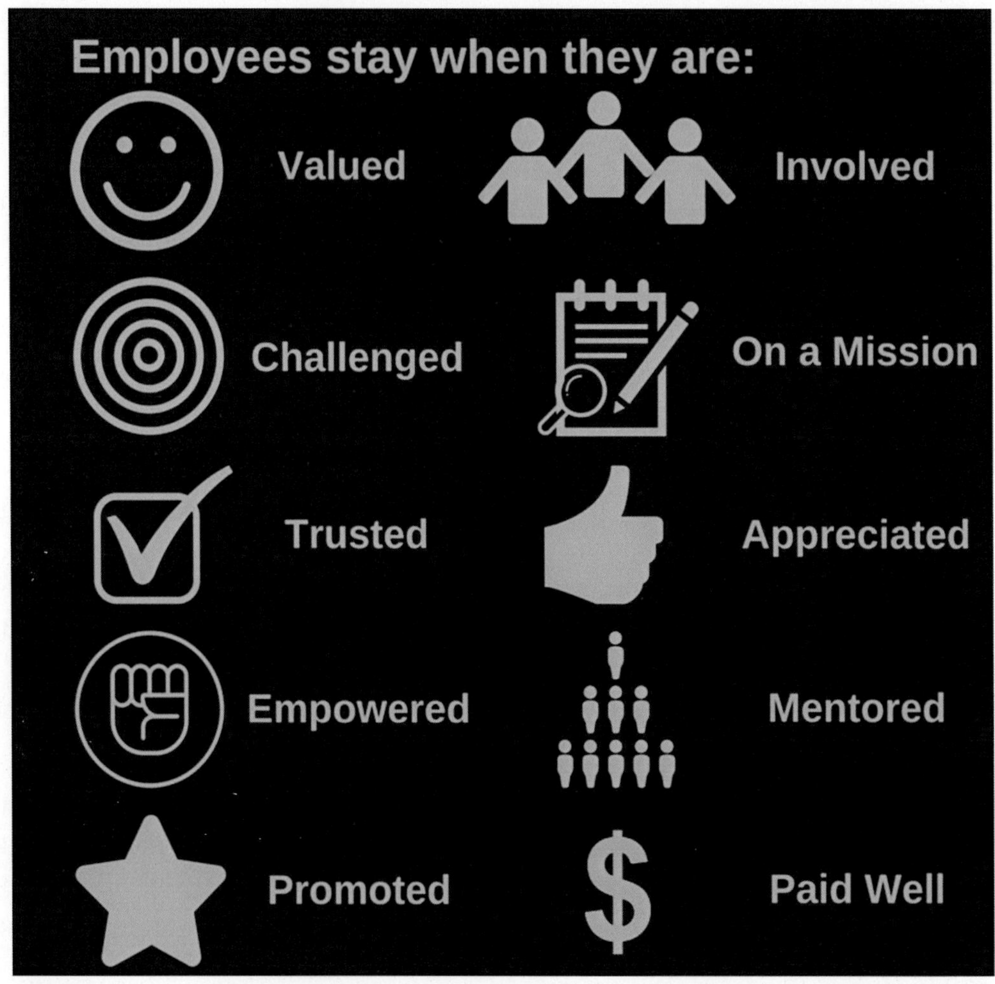
Employees stay when they are:
Valued
Involved
Challenged
On a Mission
Trusted
Appreciated
Empowered
Mentored
Promoted
Paid Well

Image Credit: Corecom Consulting

Establish a High-Performance Culture

The culture of a research team is defined by the character of its internal work climate and personality. This is shaped by its core values and entrenched behaviors, the "normal" way things are done, and its work practices and styles.

A high-performance culture is one in which the following occur:

- Research goals are achieved
- Developments exceed the original expectations

High-performing cultures will normally achieve this when the following conditions are present:

- A strong focus on key outcomes
- Research team members are highly motivated and supportive
- Research team members feel respected and valued by the team leader
- There is an environment where internal communication is encouraged, and everyone is invited to participate
- There is a tolerance of failure and willingness to take risks
- Fostering of collaborative efforts
- Respect for confidences within the team

To achieve this, the research leader will have to do the following:

- Involve others in decision-making
- Provide clear direction
- Encourage a focus on achieving results
- Provide constructive feedback
- Provide particular help to less-experienced team members
- Defuse crises
- Collaborate with other research teams

The resultant behaviors should be a culture where the following occur:

- Team members are focused on the task
- People discuss goals, methods, and activities socially
- Team members are willing to accept constructive criticism of their work
- Team members will offer to assist their colleagues with their work
- The team recognizes and compliments good performance
- Members accept responsibility for project outcomes, positive or negative

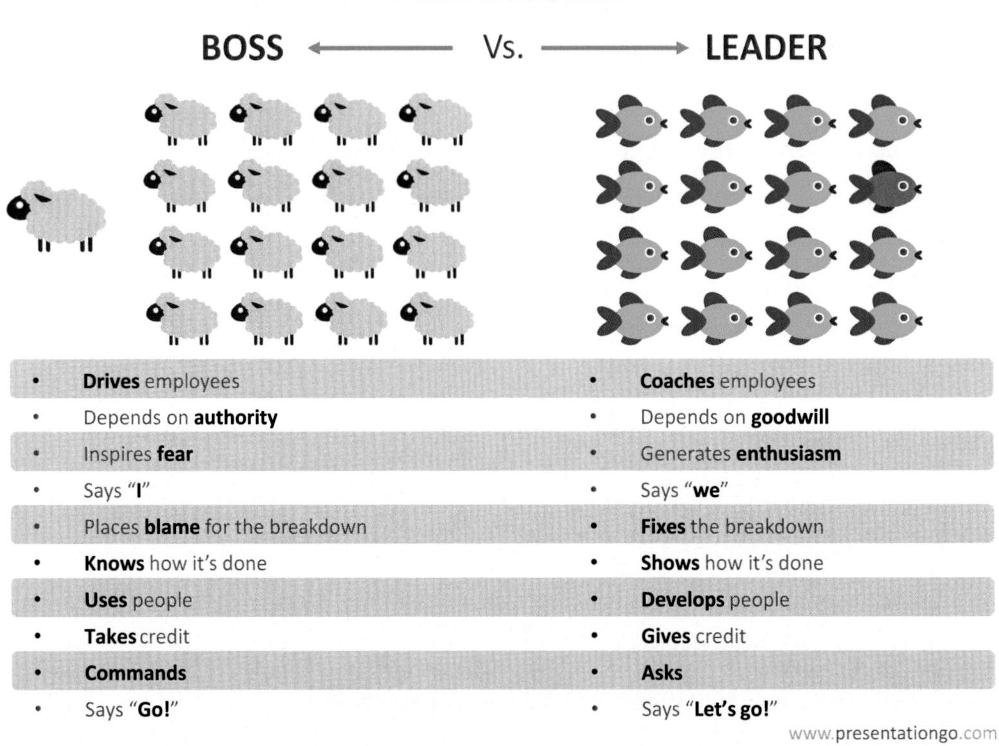

Image Credit: Differences Boss Leader for PowerPoint © Copyright PresentationGo.com

Encourage Collaborative Practices and "Ownership" of Outputs

There is much to be gained by allowing the members of any team to feel a sense of pride for, and ownership of, any outputs they have helped create. You, as leader, might well dream up an objective for the group, but as the idea and the work take shape, you should encourage the team members to feel that this is *their* idea, not yours. Whenever you can, commend them for *their* work as you guide them toward the desired outcomes.

A research team is strengthened by its grant and publication record, so it is good to involve everyone in the team, collaboratively, in the scientific publishing and grant-writing process.

Part of your job as manager is to teach your less-experienced staff how to write publishable scientific papers and successful grant proposals. As mentioned in Chapter 7.2 on publication, it is best practice to have the first author write the first draft, then send the paper around the team for further additions, review, and comment. Later, hold team meetings to discuss the strengths and weaknesses.

You can take a slightly different approach for grant proposals by asking each team member to write a section of the proposal, then put it all together before everyone reviews successive drafts of the whole package. This allows everyone to see the big picture of the team's activities while they also feel a sense of belonging. You might be surprised at the insights of even the least experienced team members.

If you have a post-doc in your team, that post-doc is dependent on you to provide further training and assist her build a track record. A typical post-doc is useful, but by definition she needs experience and needs to be extended. Suggest that the post-doc finds a mentor (in addition to you) to help her with advice and career development. (See Chapter 5.1). You must also ensure that your post-doc contributes to publications. Involve her too in elements of laboratory management or give her responsibility for sections of your project. Many a post-doc has no exposure to management, or to managing a budget, until they suddenly have a big one, and it is terrifying. It is very good for their training to have them assist with your project management.

Promote Research Integrity

It is far more preferable to have an environment where research integrity flourishes than a culture of concern about research misconduct. If you can treat research integrity, ethics, and compliance as central components of research education and training, and indeed of your own research, then the standards will fall into place and everyone in your team will benefit.

To this end, you are encouraged to do the following:

- Be a "role model"
- Encourage discussion of research ethics within the team
- Foster an intellectual climate in which discovery, the pursuit of truth, ethical conduct, and professionalism are highly valued
- Anticipate, negotiate, and discuss issues and problems
- Promote "best practice" in the management of research records and data
- Agree "up front" on publication strategies and recognizing contributions
- Respect people with concerns and respond appropriately

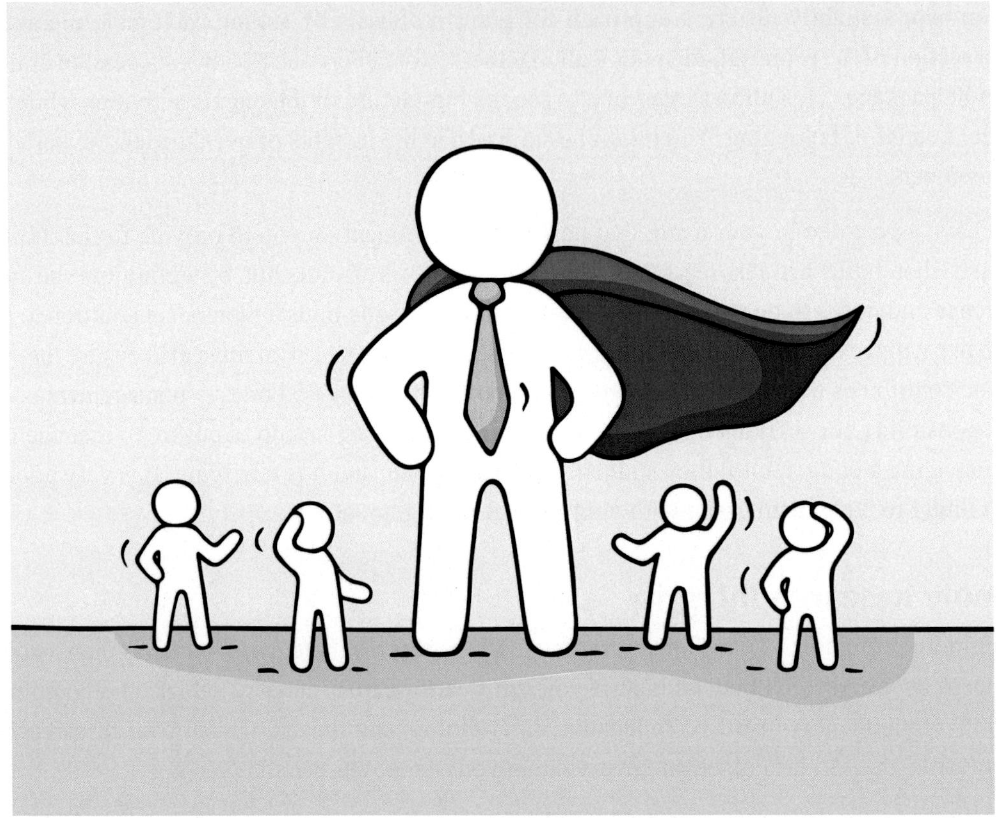

Image Credit: Working little people and big superhero by Sapunkele/Shutterstock

Important Leadership Practices

Good leadership will drive higher performance of the research team. You will need to create the right environment for your team to perform at a higher level. Values that build a culture of creative research include the following:

- Truthfulness, trustworthiness, and integrity
- Ethical business principles
- Respectfulness
- Expectation of high standards for behaviors of your staff
- Taking responsibility and being accountable for your actions
- Open-mindedness and approachability
- A focus on high-quality work

Your laboratory will be an employer of choice if it is known that you adhere to a Code for Responsible Conduct of Research. The best way to communicate responsible conduct in research to your laboratory is to live by its values.

Ensure that there is an emphasis in team meetings on ethical research practices, particularly scientific rigor and avoidance of plagiarism, and conduct audits to ensure there is appropriate regard for privacy and confidentiality. Allow your team to see ethical behavior in practice. Your institution is likely to have a code of practice. Keep a copy in a prominent place and refer to it in team meetings. Include a reference to it in the welcome pack.

A good way to keep an eye on good practice is to regularly (but randomly) ask to view laboratory notebooks. Check to see that detailed, accurate records are being kept by the whole team. This not only benefits all of you when it is time to write up your work but also ensures regulatory compliance and limits falsification of results.

One introduction to the ethical conduct of research is the 2002 report from the Institute of Medicine, "Integrity in Scientific Research: Creating an Environment That Promotes Responsible Conduct" [6]. See Chapters 8.1 and 8.2 for further discussion about ethics in research and responsible conduct of research.

You should also ensure that your research staff may discuss any concerns with you in a confidential manner.

References—Leadership

[1] Howard Hughes Medical Institute, Burroughs Wellcome Fund, 2006. Making the Right Moves: A Practical Guide to Scientific Management.
[2] Lencioni, P., 2002. The Five Dysfunctions of a Team, first ed. Jossey-Bass.
[3] Future Research Leaders Program. http://www.frlp.edu.au/.
[4] Mumford, M.D., Scott, G.M., Gaddis, B., Strange, J.M., 2002. Leading creative people: orchestrating expertise and relationships. Leadership Quarterly 13, 705–750.
[5] Herzberg, F.I., 1987. One more time: how do you motivate employees? Harvard Business Review 65 (5), 109–120.
[6] Institute of Medicine, 2002. Integrity in Scientific Research: Creating an Environment that Promotes Responsible Conduct. National Academies Press. http://www.nap.edu.

5.4 More About Managing Conflict

Lindy was a meticulous record keeper, painfully slow with her work, but an excellent administrator. She worked on a project that collected extensive personal information and she managed its privacy and confidentiality to the very best standards. Her much younger co-worker Jessie displayed the opposite personality characteristics. She was hasty about everything, and Lindy suspected her of "near enough is good enough" practices. Needless to say, they didn't get along. Jessie could have learnt much from her more experienced teammate. Early feedback from their manager and/or a team re-structure could have prevented their problems from getting out of hand, but unfortunately, they were left to sort themselves out. Lindy left, and the team lost the benefit of valuable experience unnecessarily.

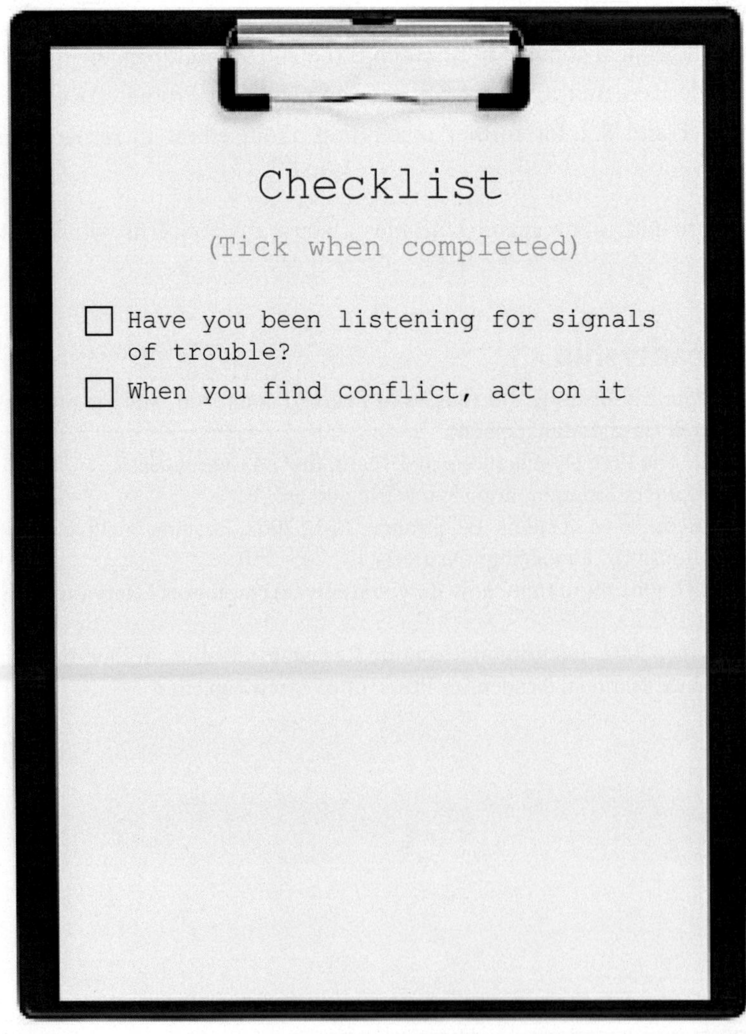

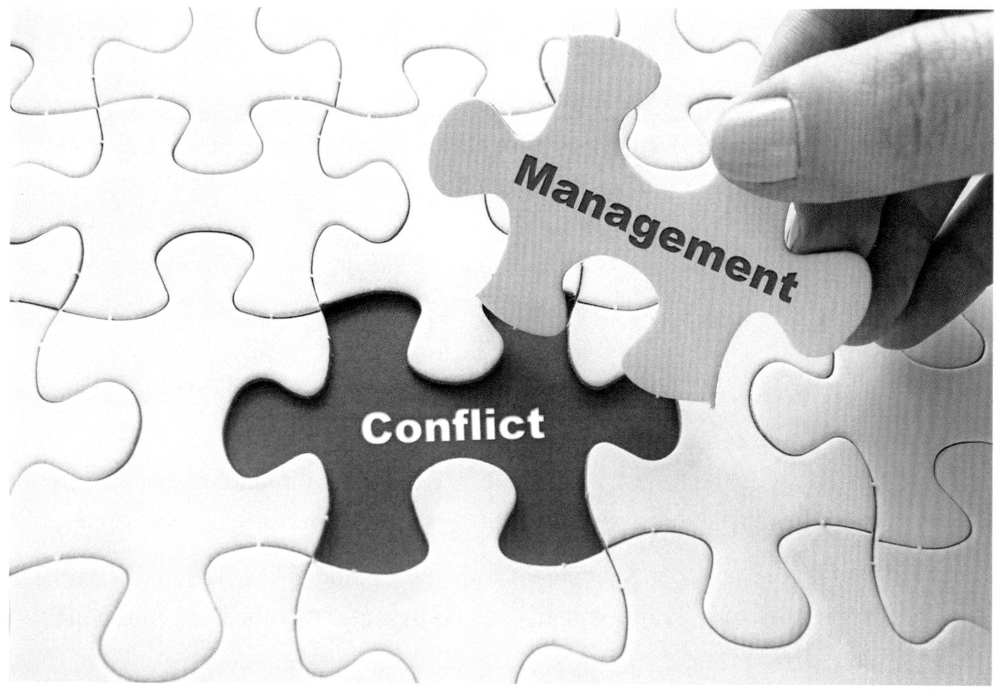

Image Credit: Jigsaw puzzle piece with word Conflict Management by Rei and Motion Studio/Shutterstock

Conflict is any situation where one person's concerns or desires differ from those of another person. In a research team, and particularly a laboratory, conflicts often arise over "turf wars," when two individuals are interested in the same project. By staying on top of what each member of your team is doing, you can often spot potential problems and deal with them before they get out of hand.

Most people try to avoid conflict; however, it does still raise itself from time to time. Depending on how it is managed, conflict can be constructive or destructive, be stimulating or unnerving, lead to original thinking or cause destructive power struggles.

Resolving Conflict Between Team Members

When conflict occurs between two or more members of the team, you need to decide whether it is necessary for you to step in and facilitate a resolution. Usually, most people will be able to resolve their own conflicts, but make sure that a conflict does not fester to the point where it affects morale and the atmosphere for everyone.

Do your best to

- Foster an environment that accepts conflict, as long as the difficulties are faced openly and honestly by the people involved.
- Help the individuals involved in a conflict synchronize the timing, focus, and extent of their overtures and responses. You could, for example, invite the people involved in a conflict to your office at a designated time to discuss the problems openly and honestly and come to a resolution. Encourage each person to try to understand the other's point of view. You can help by summarizing, clarifying, focusing questions, and encouraging each person to listen.

Resolving Conflicts Between You and Others in the Team

There might sometimes be conflicts between you and members of your team. Such conflicts can be influential in mapping out the future direction of the team. It is important that you are seen to be willing to listen, to understand negative feedback—and to learn from it, where appropriate.

It is also important for you, as leader, to avoid the trap of dropping your leadership responsibilities and responding to the challenge by becoming "just another team member."

In other words, as leader, you never have just your interests at hand, but have to keep in mind those of the team as a whole.

When faced with conflict, do the following:

Assess the problem.

Assess the other person's interests.

Acknowledge the constraints.

Select a strategy that balances the importance of the problem, time constraints, power differences, and the relationships.

If you are interested to read more about managing conflict, Thomas and Kilmann [1] provide a useful model for evaluating an individual's behavior in conflict situations along two basic dimensions: "assertiveness"—the extent to which an individual attempts to satisfy his or her own concerns—and "cooperativeness"—the extent to which an individual attempts to satisfy the concerns of the other person.

In the model, illustrated on the following page, these two basic dimensions of behavior define five different modes for responding to conflict situations.

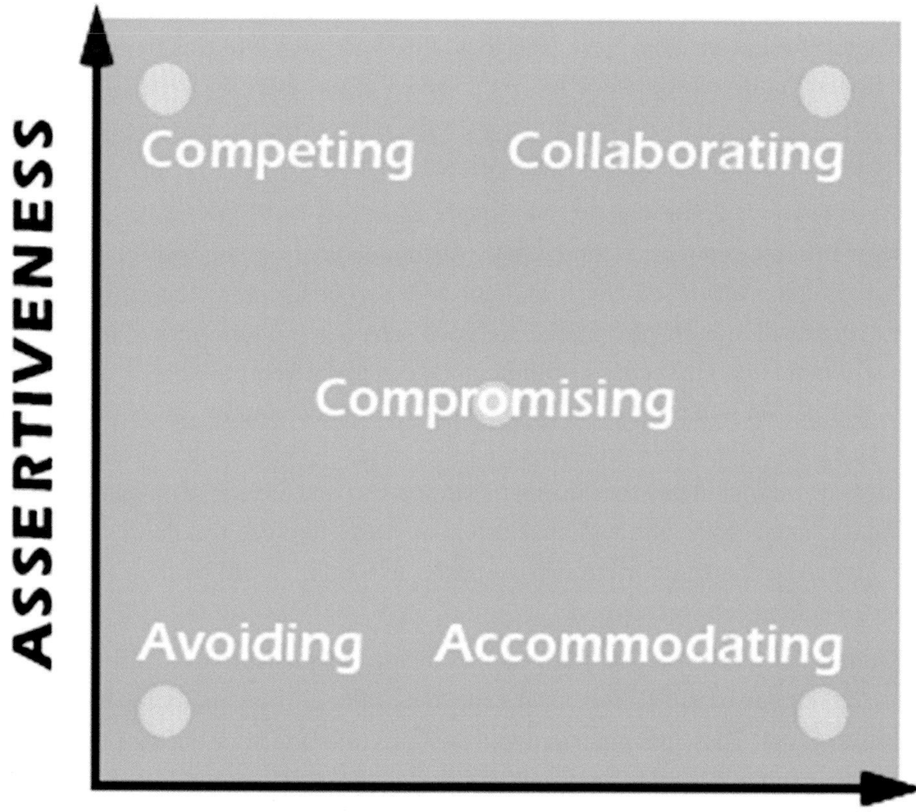

Image Credit: Copyright © 2009–2017 by Kilmann Diagnostics. All rights reserved. Original figure is available at: http://www.kilmanndiagnostics.com/overview-thomas-kilmann-conflict-mode-instrument-tki

An explanation of the behaviors and good examples of each behavior in a scientific environment are given in "Making the Right Moves" [2]. Here they describe the four behaviors from the Thomas–Kilmann model.

- *Competing*: People who demonstrate this conflict-handling mode are assertive and uncooperative. "Competitors" look after their own concerns at the other person's expense. They use whatever methods seem appropriate to achieve their aims, including their superior arguing skills or making use of their rank. This conflict mode works when you are dealing with an issue of great importance, a decision that will be unpopular, or one that needs quick resolution. It is important not to adopt this competitive mode for all situations! An example of being a "competitor" is if the head of another laboratory asks you for a reagent that you have not yet cited in a publication, and one of your post-docs is using it for his or her project. You look after your own interests by refusing to share the reagent until your post-doc has published a paper referring to it. The decision will almost certainly make you unpopular with the other principal investigator, but you are quite fairly putting the needs of your post-doc first.

- *Accommodating*: These unassertive people go out of their way to be cooperative—in other words, the opposite of competing. "Accommodators" often neglect their own needs to satisfy the needs of others. It is a good idea to be accommodating when you want create goodwill or build up "points" for good behavior and for issues of low importance. Keep in mind that the accommodating mode can cause you problems if you expect that the other person will pay you back by being accommodating to you next time. Imagine you and your collaborator are sharing a piece of equipment that has broken down. They insist that you should pay for the repairs since it was one of your team members who was using it when it broke, although their laboratory uses it more. You don't agree really, but you give in on this one for the sake of peace, expecting it will be their turn next time a piece of equipment needs repair.
- *Avoiding*: "Avoiders" evade the issue by being both unassertive and uncooperative. They do not pursue either their own concerns or those of others, but leave them to sort themselves out. These people will avoid conflicts out of fear, or because they don't have confidence in their conflict management skills. Avoiding can work well in cases when the person you are in conflict with is in a higher position or when issues are not very important. Avoiding is also a good strategy when you need to buy time. An example of how to be a successful avoider is to say "These are significant changes. I will need to think about it for a while."
- *Collaborating*: This conflict-handling mode is the opposite of avoiding by being both assertive and cooperative. "Collaborators" attempt to work with others to find a solution that fully satisfies all parties. They thoroughly investigate the concerns of the two conflicting individuals and try to find a solution that addresses both sets of concerns. Some people believe that the collaboration mode is always the best conflict mode to use, but collaboration takes a great deal of time and energy. You should only use this method when the conflict is worth all that time and energy. For example, if two post-docs are arguing over "their space," you might want to spend the necessary time to carefully provide different projects in a way that will satisfy each of them. On the other hand, if your post-docs are in conflict about something as simple as which day to hold a laboratory meeting, the time and energy necessary to resolve the conflict to everyone's satisfaction is probably not worth the effort.

- *Compromising*: The goal of the "compromiser" is as it sounds—to find a mutually acceptable solution that is good enough for both parties. The "compromiser" will give way more than the "competitor," but less than the "accommodator." The "compromiser" confronts the issue more than the "avoider," but does not take as much trouble as the "collaborator." This middle-ground mode of conflict resolution is useful for decisions of moderate importance, when the two people have equal status, or when you are faced with an issue that needs to be resolved quickly.

Thomas and Kilmann show that each of these conflict-handling modes has value; none is intended to be good, bad, or preferable in all situations. A worthwhile goal for you as a research leader is to have a number of different styles of response to conflict situations, giving you flexibility to use the most appropriate for each situation.

You will notice that the people in your team will tend to adopt one style of handling a conflict over another. You will have a mix of "competitors," "accommodators," and "avoiders." Show them by example that there are different ways of handling conflict depending on the situation.

References—More About Managing Conflict

[1] K.W. Thomas, R.H. Kilmann, An Overview of the Thomas-Kilmann Conflict Mode Instrument (TKI). http://www.kilmanndiagnostics.com/overview-thomas-kilmann-conflict-mode-instrument-tki.

[2] Howard Hughes Medical Institute and Burroughs Wellcome Fund. 2006. Making the Right Moves: A Practical Guide to Scientific Management. https://www.hhmi.org/developing-scientists/making-right-moves.

5.5 Mentoring the Next Generation

I believe that mentoring is about the wellbeing of the mentee. Over the years I have observed leaders of some big and important groups who are more concerned with using group members to promote their own scientific standing

Lee [1]

+++ is generous with her ideas, firmly believing that one should give away one's best ideas

Lee [1]

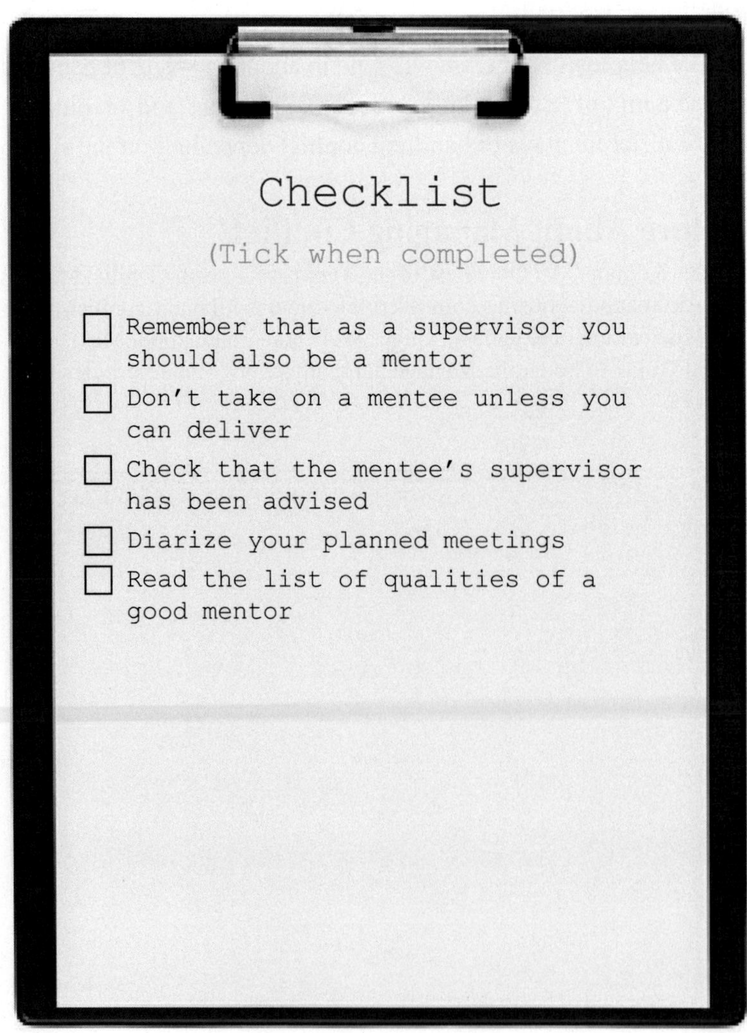

As supervisor of an early-career researcher, it is important to regard yourself as a mentor as well as supervisor. Whether you are a supervisor of a PhD student or leader of a whole team, you have an opportunity to provide a lasting and broad influence on your mentees, and, by setting a good example, their mentees in the years to come. Lee [1] remarks that the distinction between a great mentor and a great supervisor is the mentor's special focus on helping the mentee to build her career, and indeed to help her focus on planning that career.

Good supervision with a focus on mentoring allows you to build a world-class research environment. Take the time to consider some of Lee's exercises in Chapter 5.2, to evaluate your mentoring practices.

It is a privilege to be asked to be a mentor for someone outside your team. The fact that you have been chosen is a sign of respect. While it is your responsibility as a more senior person to take on guiding roles for those who are less experienced, don't treat it as a chore. This is a two-way street: you may be surprised how beneficial it can be for you.

Before you accept, though, it is important to establish a few boundaries and make some investigations. Insist that the mentee informs their supervisor and then touch base with that supervisor to check that all is well. You don't want to open yourself to criticism for doing anything behind the other's back. There is a possibility that the mentee is having problems that you should be aware of—or which you should avoid.

Make sure too that you do have enough time. Once you make a commitment to be a mentor you must be available to do it properly. Establish whether this mentoring role is to be formal or informal, long term or just occasional advice. Set your ground rules early, perhaps by making a commitment to a regular appointment and/or by setting a definite time period for the mentorship. If this mentorship is a success you can always extend it. If it is too burdensome, the time frame gives you an out without a difficult conversation.

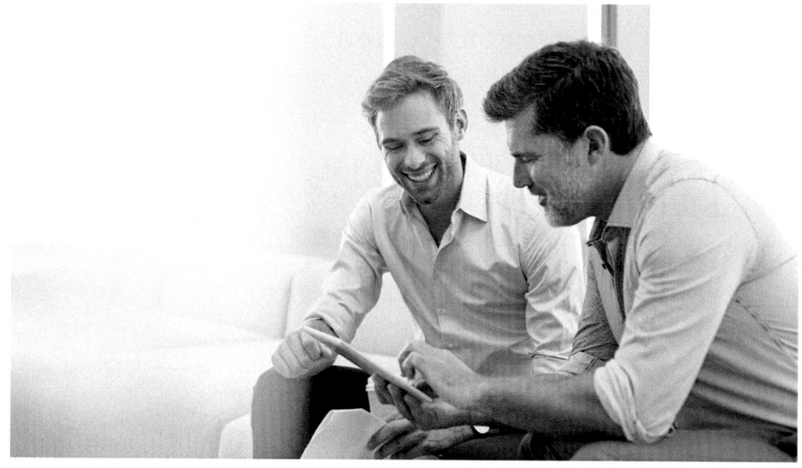

Image Credit: Young man discussing something positive with his mature colleague by marvent/Shutterstock

A good mentor will be

- Kind
- A good listener
- Truthful
- Available
- Open-minded
- Patient

You can assist with the following:

- Future opportunities
- Building a network
- Technical guidance
- Setting goals
- Job hunting
- Publishing
- Skills
- Solutions to problems
- Reviewing research progress

Be aware, always, that the mentees have not come to you because they are going to replicate your career path. They want to gain from your experience and your greater knowledge of the research environment. Always try to be objective with your advice. Listen well, offer possible solutions, and help them set challenging goals.

Be aware that the selection of a mentor for people from underrepresented populations could provide them with difficulty. Women, underrepresented minorities, and international students in the sciences and engineering often prefer mentors who are their same race, nationality, and/or gender. They frequently experience difficulty finding such a mentor because of the dearth of minority, international, or appropriate women in their area of research. You may have been asked to be a mentor because you meet this need.

In "Nature's guide for mentors," Lee [1] lists a number of personal characteristics found in successful mentors. These include enthusiasm, sensitivity, appreciating individual differences, respect, unselfishness, and fostering many researchers. Strategies for good mentorship noted in the same article include good communication, operating an open door policy to ensure ready availability, generating optimism and inspiration, encouraging self-direction while also offering direction, applying effective questioning and listening skills, and celebrating each success. The authors also note the importance of building communities—of researchers and social groups. This overview—which applies just as well to the qualities required for good leadership—is most useful in highlighting the need for generosity, positive and passionate advocacy of research, and realistic consideration of the research environment.

Your mentees should aim to come prepared to your meetings. Allow them the same courtesy, and do your homework ahead of time. Be ready with your comments and advice.

Mentoring can help you because your guidance of the mentee may allow you to identify the same sort of problems within your own team. It will alert you to the needs of your staff. While you are helping your mentee build a collaborative network, your own network will be extending, and new opportunities might come your way.

It may help you too because it will cause you to reflect on why you do what you do, and on the benefits that come with your processes. It may bring you in touch with new methodologies with which you haven't yet had experience with. It opens opportunities for new networks and collaborations. It may even lead to joint publications with your mentee.

As mentor, it is likely that many confidences will be shared. You will become aware of the difficulties your mentee is having at work or at home, of failures in the laboratory, or of personal problems. You must treat these with the utmost confidence.

Remember too that the mentee has come to you as a mentor, not as a friend. While a friendship may arise, you are advised to keep this relationship at arm's length. You will be of more use if you can step aside from personal involvement.

Mentor Versus Adviser

In theory, mentors have multiple responsibilities—being an adviser is only one of these. Many references cite Zelditch [2] who suggests that mentors are the following:

- Advisers: People with career experience willing to share their knowledge
- Supporters: People who give emotional and moral encouragement
- Tutors: People who give specific feedback on one's performance
- Masters: Employers to whom one is apprenticed
- Sponsors: Sources of information about opportunities and aid in obtaining them
- Models of identity: The kind of person one should be to be an academic or a professional scientist

References—Mentoring

[1] Lee, A., Dennis, C., Campbell, P., June 2007. Nature's guide for mentors. Nature 447, 791–797 and Lee in conversation.
[2] Zelditch, M., 1990. Mentor roles. In: Proceedings of the 32nd Annual Meeting of the Western Association of Graduate Schools, 11. Tempe, Ariz., March 1618.

Further Reading

Debowski, S., 2004. Cultivating hidden assets: the developmental needs of university career researchers. Research and Development in Higher Education, 27: 127–135.

Fox, J., 2016. The 7 Dark Elements of Pioneering Leadership. http://www.drjasonfox.com/read/darkpioneering.

National Academies Press, 1997. Adviser, Teacher, Role Model, Friend: On Being a Mentor to Students in Science and Engineering. https://www.nap.edu/read/5789/chapter/8.

Rackham Graduate School University of Michigan, 2015. How to Mentor Graduate Students: A Guide to Faculty. http://www.rackham.umich.edu/downloads/publications/Fmentoring.pdf.

Winter, G., 2017. Think One Team. http://thinkoneteam.com/, quoted by Kate Jones in Sydney Morning Herald 10/05/2015, p. 25.

5.6 Developing Time Management Skills

Annabel was always at work and always overwhelmed. She could never quite get on top of things. Too easily distracted by email and interruptions of others in the team, she could never say no to something new when she sat down to (supposedly) finish off a task.

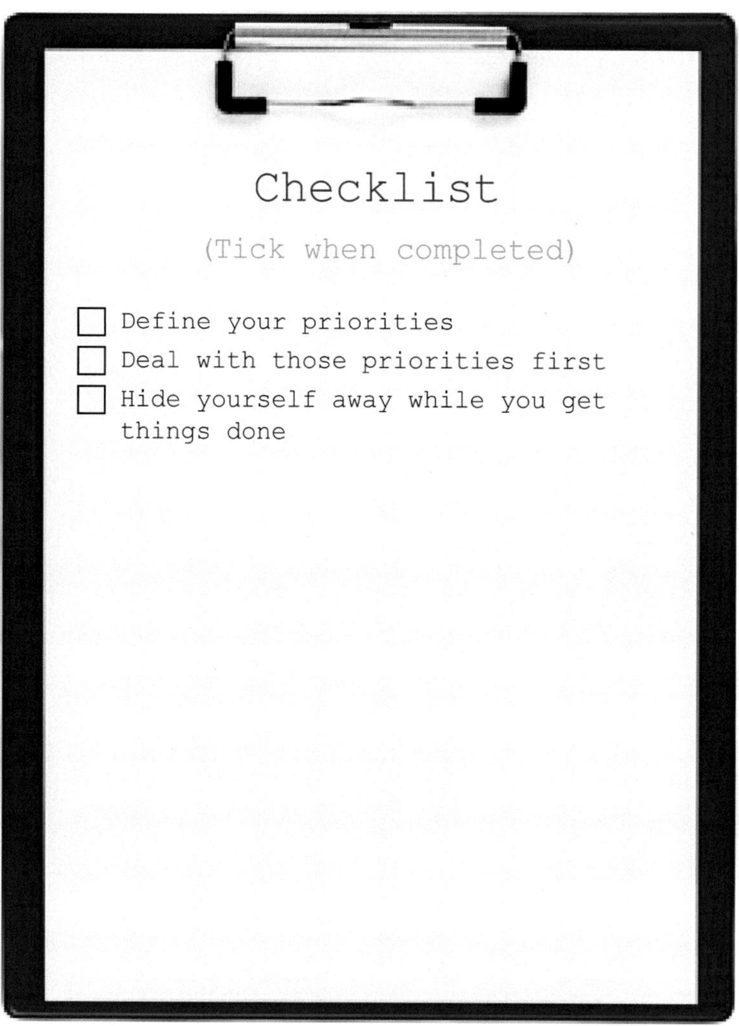

❺ PEOPLE MANAGEMENT: FOR YOURSELF AND YOUR TEAM

While it appears that everyone is busy in this modern life, there would be few environments where people have to juggle more priorities than in research. You must balance the need for outputs with managing and mentoring staff, with applying for further funding, for teaching, and for learning. Somewhere among that, you must find time for keeping up with developments in your field, and find time for thinking and planning. It's tough.

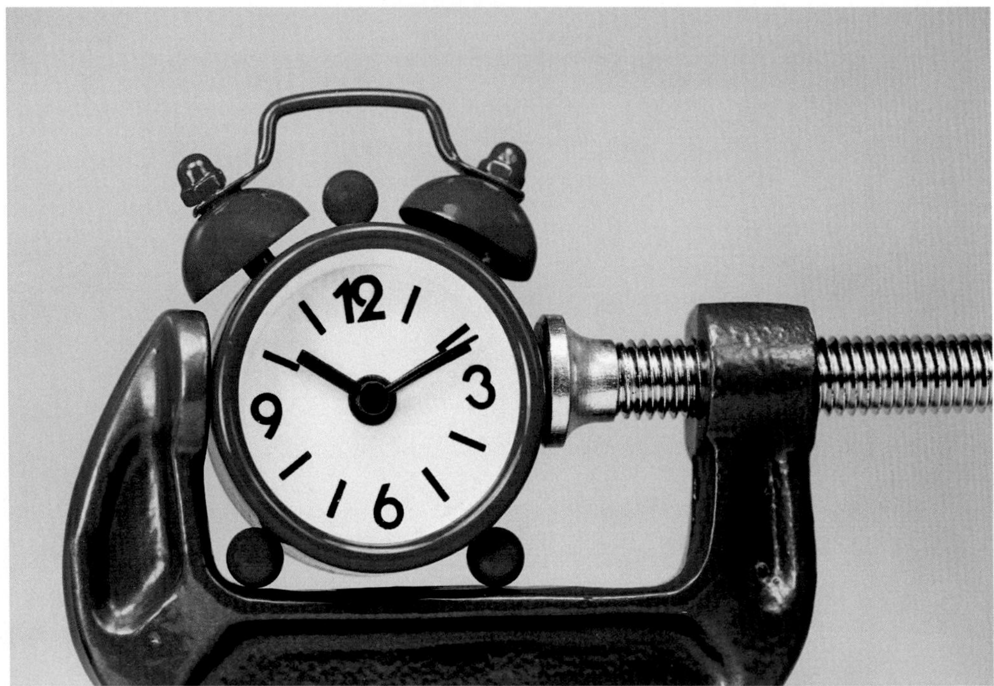

Image Credit: Alarm clock placed in a clamp by Keith A Frith/Shutterstock

The moral of the story is that you must develop excellent time management skills. You can't stint on any of the tasks mentioned above. The old adage of "ask a busy person to be sure you will get something done" applies. It is probably truer in research than anywhere else. Those people who are the ones to get their grant applications in on time, who respond quickly to emails, and who finish their reporting before it is due are nearly always the people who are most productive. It is not that they are super clever. It is usually because they are super organized.

Take the time to reflect on the way you have spent your time in the past week. How much time did you waste; how often were you completely focused?

Start your time management focus by setting yourself a timetable for specific tasks. One of the greatest time wasters and distracters is email. We can't do without it and we can't ignore it, but we *can* manage it. If email is distracting you, try a plan of checking emails in the first hour of the day and then only once or twice through the day, in prescribed time slots. Let your colleagues know that you are not on email all the time. They can always ring, or, even better, come by to talk about whatever it is they want to discuss.

It is very helpful to specifically build some planning or thinking time into your weekly routine. Go somewhere where you won't be disturbed and spend half an hour reviewing progress for the past week and goals for the next. Plan the bigger picture on regular but further spaced intervals.

Effective time management is determined by you defining your goals and priorities. You need to focus on your critical priorities rather than on the less important tasks, however numerous they are. This applies even more for those people who are inclined to be readily distracted and who focus their efforts on the request that just arrived.

At the same time, you must keep an eye out for your work life balance. Not everyone has the freedom or inclination to involve themselves in work, work, work. Your family responsibilities and personal involvement in sport or community activities also have their place, and they must not be neglected if they are important to you.

Kearns and Gardiner [1] explore the time management practices of university staff and students. The authors conclude that having a clear sense of career purpose was most important for perceived effectiveness at work, followed by planning and prioritizing.

Gulli [2], offering a range of suggestions for apps designed to run your life better, lists the following three quick, eminently practical tips for managing your time:

- Make your bed. While a small gesture, it means you have already achieved something within two minutes of waking up.
- Start with your most challenging task. Dreading a particular task? Tick it off your list first to save the easiest for last.
- Prepare for tomorrow today. Writing a "tomorrow list" at the end of your day allows you to leave work prepared for your next workday while reducing dwell time overnight.

References—Developing Time Management Skills

[1] Kearns, H., Gardiner, M., 2007. Is it time well spent? The relationship between time management behaviors, perceived effectiveness and work related morale and distress in a university context. Higher Education Research and Development 26 (2), 235–247.

[2] Gulli, C., Redwire, 2017. 13 Time Management Tools. http://www.vodafone.com.au/red-wire/13-time-management-tools/.

5.7 Change Management

Institution Ajax decided to move part of its team to a different building in another area of town. They just made the announcement one day, right out of the blue, without any prior consultation. The staff were alarmed. There were obviously implications for all of them because there would need to be new travel arrangements, but the rumor mill got going very quickly. The grapevine soon had the institute reducing staff numbers, closing down, being taken over and more. None of this was true, but advanced warning and discussion about the implications would have alleviated many concerns.

Checklist

(Tick when completed)

- ☐ Recognize change may unsettle the team
- ☐ Prepare your communication, pointing out advantages
- ☐ Involve people from all levels
- ☐ Explain every step
- ☐ Provide training
- ☐ Celebrate the change

Change management

An important aspect of managing your staff is change management, which refers to dealing with the impact of change on individuals. That change may be a result of change taking place within the limits of your project, or it might be change in the wider environment. The same principles apply.

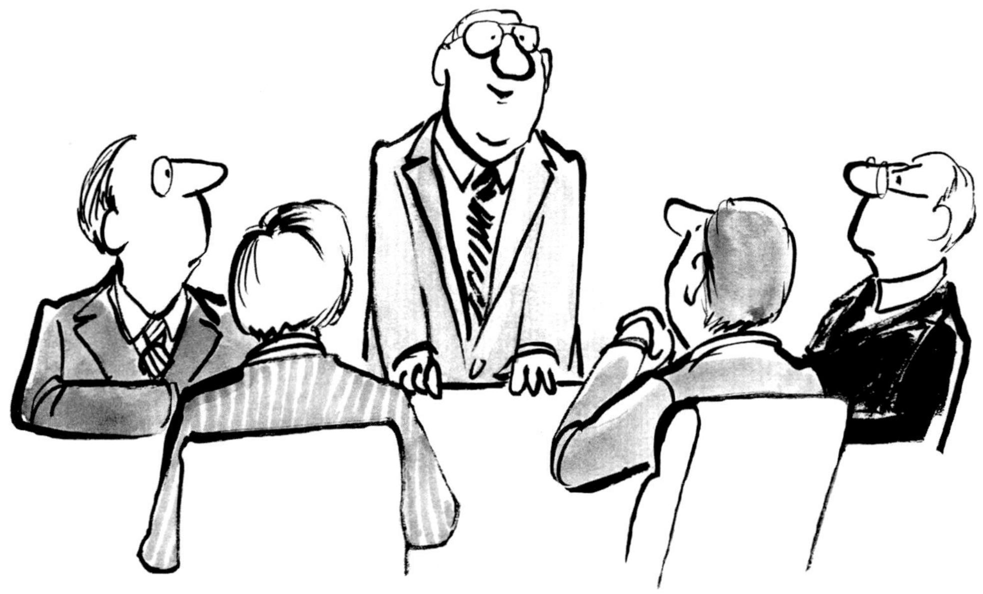

"What if, and I know this sounds kooky, we communicated with the employees."

Image Credit: What if, and I know this sounds kooky, we communicated with the employees by Cartoon Resource/Shutterstock

Applying change management practices should really be just common sense, a reflection of courtesy to your fellow workers.

Often overlooked in a non-commercial environment, *awareness* of the need for change management is half the battle. If you can understand that too much change, too quickly, creates an environment of concern, or even fear, for your staff, then that will help you help them manage change with less resultant stress.

When there is a big change ahead, change management activities should include the following:

- Sponsorship of the change—the support of management
- Planning for change—creating detailed change plans
- Stakeholder engagement—involving everyone
- Implementation—execution of the change plans and ongoing support

The principal tools you will use for change management are communication, training, and thoughtfulness. You will need to regulate and control change to ensure the recipients of change are receiving manageable levels of change.

Managing Organizational Change and Culture

The sorts of change that might affect your research environment, many of which are outside your control, could include the following:

- Change in government
- Re-location of your team
- Change in weather/climate
- Change in competition
- Financial change
- Change in the team
- Change in technology

In the workplace, people often fear change because it might lead to the following:

- Job loss
- Creation of barriers that appear insurmountable
- Damage to friendships and networks
- Negative affect on personal status
- Requirement for development of new skills

People do not like uncertainty.

Dromgold [1] identifies the four key "whats" of change for your team as follows:

- The tools they use
- The way they do their job
- The job they do
- The culture

and recommends that they all need to be approached differently.

Bridges [2] suggests that when change happens, or is proposed, the best things that you can do for your team, as leader, are as follows:

- Communicate, communicate, communicate
- Emphasize the solutions, not the problems
- Empathize and understand their feelings or sense of loss
- Address people's concerns
- Involve the entire team in the change—a shared vision
- Provide training and support
- Set a clear action plan for the change and the transition process
- Set clear goals and objectives
- Compensate and reward

It is a natural human condition to prefer not to change, so don't be surprised if you meet resistance from your team. It is not useful to take the view that "they will just have to get on with it." This does nothing to counter negative responses and nothing to bring people in behind you.

Change fails when it is sprung on the team and they are not involved in planning the next steps. Be sure to take a consultative approach. Take the time to understand concerns and issues, to sell the benefits of the change, and to gain the commitment of your team, and then construct the appropriate change processes and implement them efficiently.

There will usually be some in the team who resist the change more strongly than others. It is a good idea to involve them closely with the process, thus "keeping the enemy inside the tent." If the dissidents are included in the working group administering the change, they will get to have a voice and will thus feel recognized. They will also be exposed to the reasons for the change and will eventually develop a greater understanding.

Bridges [2] explores the following three transitions people must go through:

- Ending, letting go—this is a time when you need to help people deal with their losses
- Neutral zone—the old is going but the new isn't yet fully operational
- New beginning—people are developing a new identify (Table 5.7.1)

TABLE 5.7.1 Transitions of Change

Ending, Letting Go	Neutral Zone	New Beginning
What are people going to lose?	Communicate that it will be an uneasy time	Beginning cannot occur until other transitions have been dealt with and completed
Understand the subjective losses	Training	Clarify and communicate the purpose
Acknowledge losses with sympathy	Policy and procedure change	Everyone must play a part in the process
Let people vent	Rewards	Quick successes
Can I compensate people?	Staged changes—not too many at once	Celebration and recognition of a new beginning
Provide accurate information	Short-range goals	
What is over, and what isn't	Encourage experimentation and innovation	

You need to plan all of the activities involved in your change processes. Consider the following critical factors:

- What actions need to be taken and by whom?
- What resources are required?
- How long should it take for the action to be completed?
- Who is responsible for ensuring that the tasks are completed to an appropriate standard?
- What are the criteria for measuring that your activity is complete?

If your change is complex, you might like to break it into the following phases:

- Initial planning
- Introducing new technology
- Staff restructure
- Monitoring and adjustment

Training is important, as demonstrated by this extreme example:

> *When World War II started, no one had given pilot training much thought. People didn't understand what a gigantic step it was from those little biplanes to the new multiengine monoplanes. Our class was assigned to A-20s. It had over ten times the horsepower of our basic trainers. The landing speeds must have been twice as fast. But there were no "trainer" versions of the aircraft with two sets of controls and instructor seats. The instructors just handed out aircraft manuals and said, "you have one week to make your first flight."*
>
> *Half the class died that week in Mississippi, thousands of miles from the war. After my combat tour was over and I was assigned to the Pentagon, I found more pilots died in training than in combat. The worst was during my training. Six thousand aviation casualties in one month! These numbers were classified then—the American public would have been outraged if they knew the truth.*
>
> Lt. Colonel A.B. Farry, Sr US Army Corps & US Air Force Pilot 1942–68. Adapted from Hooks and Farry [3].

Use Table 5.7.2 as a guide to schedule your change processes.

When the change project is over, check to ensure that your goals have been reached.

Universities are some of the most difficult environments into which to introduce change because of their size and the inherent bureaucracy.

TABLE 5.7.2 Example: Moving Office

Change Process					
Business criteria	Plan what you need	Space	Location	Transport	Price
Activity	Find new premises	Advise new location	Provide assistance	Book removalists	Celebrate new start
People	Advise staff that a move is coming	Form a committee to discuss	Announce results of search criteria	Announce new location and sell advantages	
Resources	Which equipment can move with you	New equipment to be purchased	Revivalists		
Milestones (include start and finish)	June	July	August	September	October
Accountability	CEO	Human Resources	Human Resources	Human Resources	CEO

References—Change Management

[1] Dromgold, D., LinkedIn, 2017. Change Management It's Not that Complicated. https://www.linkedin.com/pulse/change-management-its-complicated-diane-dromgold?trk=hp-feed-article-title-share.

[2] Bridges, W., Mitchell, S., 2009. Managing Transitions: Making the Most of Change. Da Capo Press, Philadelphia.

[3] Hooks, I.F., Farry, K.A., 2001. Customer-centered Products: Creating Successful Products through Smart Requirements Management. AMACOM Div American Mgmt Assn, p. 76.

6 WRAPPING UP YOUR PROJECT

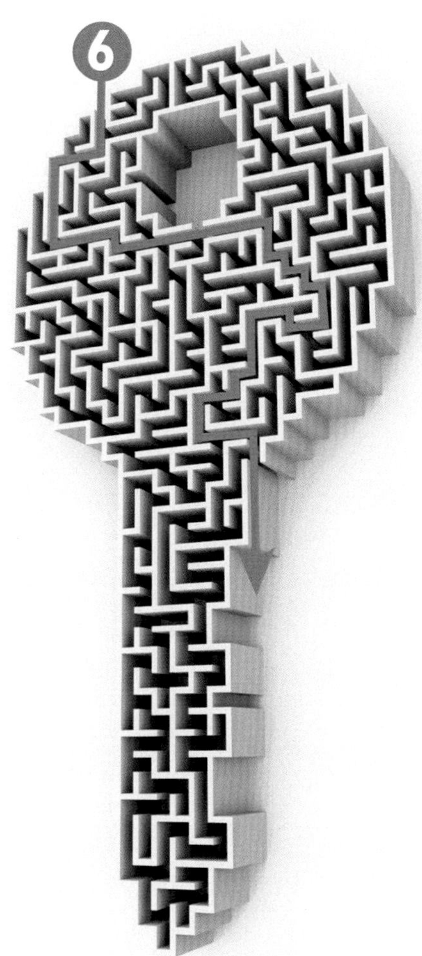

6.1 Considerations in the Last Months of Your Project

Project Jellybean came to the end of its time and budget, then work stopped. There was no more money for a research assistant or project coordinator and Chief Investigator Gus was involved in new adventures. The data were left on the server, and no one quite knew how to access the files. Nothing was written up. Eventually the funding body made a fuss about missing reports and asked difficult questions about project outcomes. Gus focussed his attention and tried to deliver, but his job was difficult. The end result was damage to his reputation, and his institute was less than pleased.

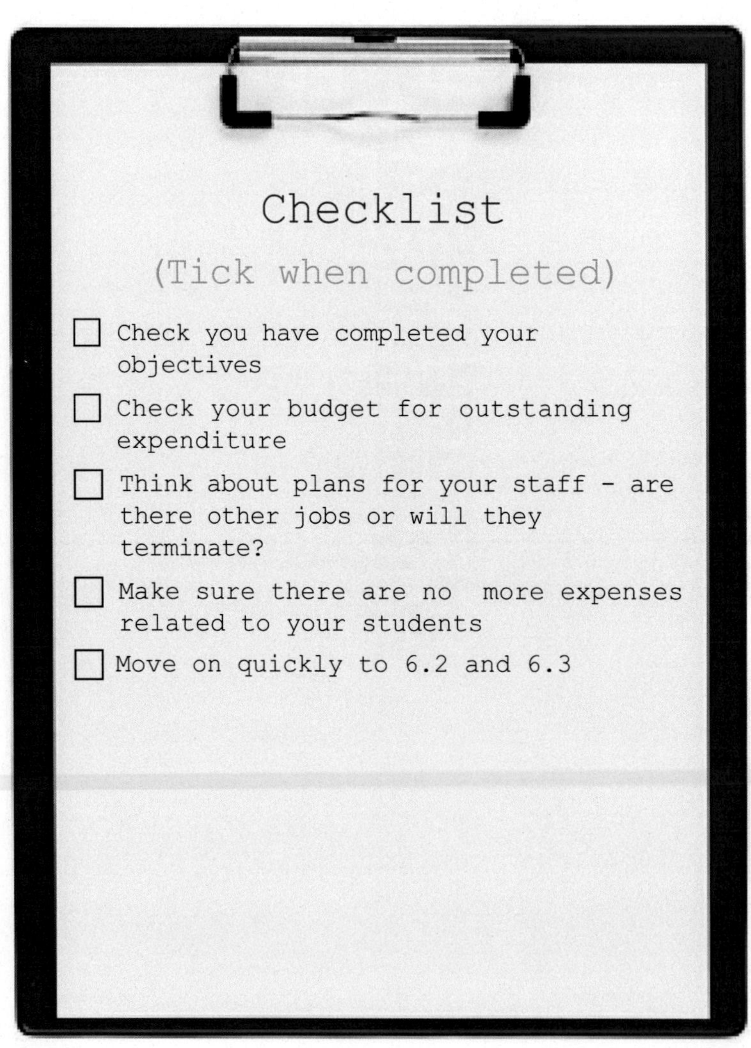

There is more to closing a project than just stopping work and intending to write it up sometime.

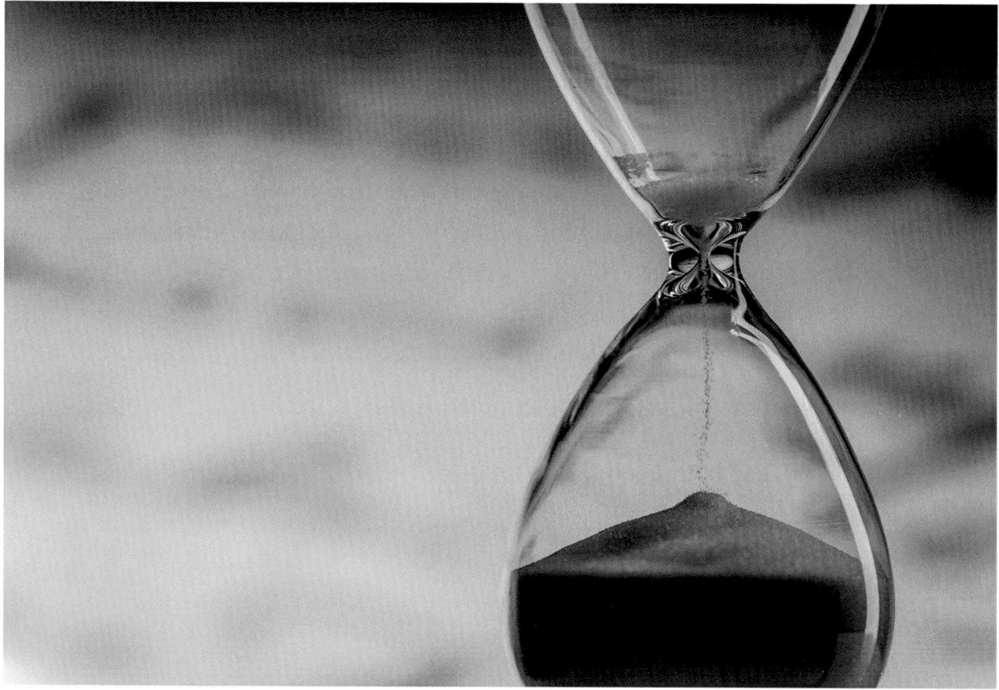

Image Credit: Sand running through an hourglass by sergign/Shutterstock

There is actually a surprising amount of closing detail to be attended to, and some of it absolutely must be done *before* the project finishes completely. That means that toward the end of your project you need to be sure you have met a number of obligations.

- Have you completed all the project objectives?
- Have you finished your project spending and actually paid all outstanding accounts?
- Have you sorted out the future of your staff and their entitlement payments?
- Have you planned who will write the final reports?

In many research institutions, staff are employed for their whole career on short-term contracts. They simply move from one project to another as funding dries up and they are allocated to another. Along the way, these staff learn a range of valuable skills, and with this experience they often become more and more attractive to the next project which is looking to build a team. You may wish to retain them yourself for another project, or you might be able to help them be re-deployed somewhere else within your institution.

6 WRAPPING UP YOUR PROJECT

If you wish to retain them for another project, and have other funding available or potentially available, remember to hold the conversation with them in plenty of time, to avoid them having concerns about their future. They have to worry about themselves first and foremost, and they mightn't be able to guess that their future is secure. Discuss the possibilities and probabilities in good time. There are usually great benefits in keeping your team together.

If you don't have the certainty of more funding, let them know and you can plan their next steps together. There may be other positions available within your institute or your university, or within your network. If your staff member is a good performer, you should be glad to offer assistance wherever you can and provide a good reference. If the staff member is to move to another team nearby, you may be able to assist with a smooth transition by allowing some project crossover time where the person is employed part-time on each project.

You will also need to plan for any students who are impacted by the end of the project.

After work is completed, and before too long, you will need to focus on the following:

- Reporting
- Publication
- Disposal of equipment
- Storage of data
- Communication
- Next steps for the actual work

The end of the project is also an opportunity to review the project as a whole.

- Did you meet your aims?
- Did the hypothesis change? Why?
- Did you reach firm conclusions?
- Is there a natural next step or steps?
- Are you within budget?
- Who should you thank?
- Who should you tell about it?

6.2 Winding Up Your Project Budget

Project Vagabond reached its end. Its Principal Investigator had been unsuccessful in attracting more funding and was now going to move to another institute. The project team had to be broken up. It turned out that between them, the three staff were owed many weeks of accumulated leave, and there was no more money in the project budget to cover the $20,000 required.

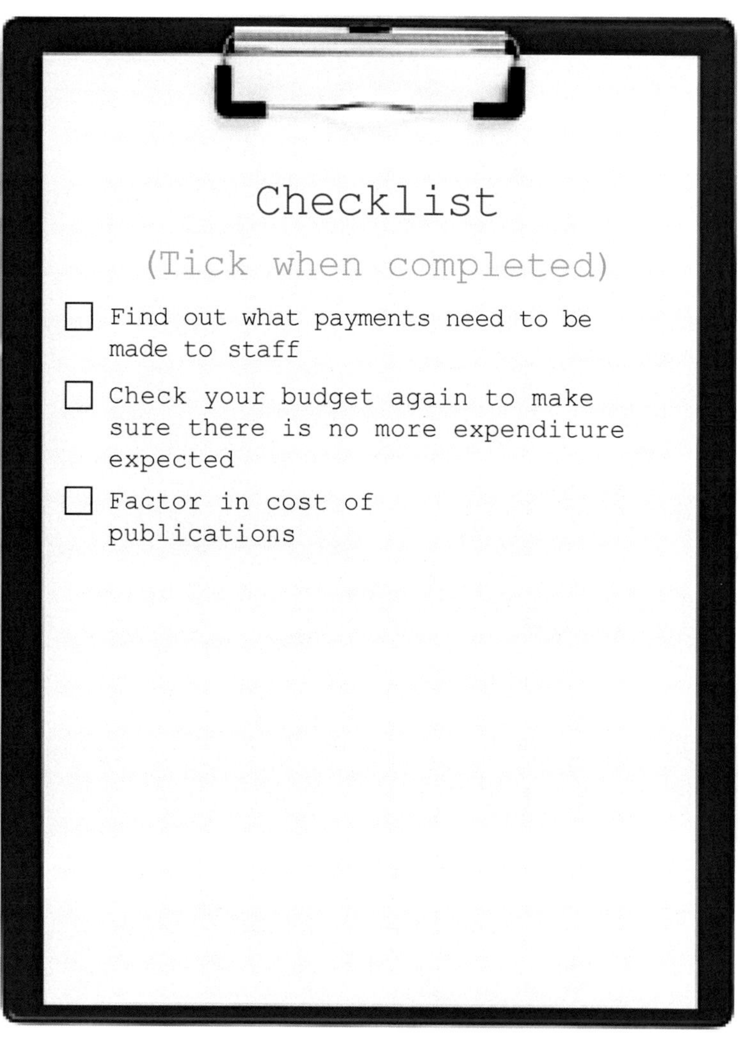

6 WRAPPING UP YOUR PROJECT

Closing your project budget properly is very important. If you don't manage this element of project close-out effectively, you run the risk of having to make up shortfalls in funding from other accounts, or of having to return unallocated monies (even if they have been spent, just not properly accounted for). You can even lose your entitlement to the last project payment. These sorts of financial mistakes aren't just upsetting; they reflect badly on your reputation and that of the team.

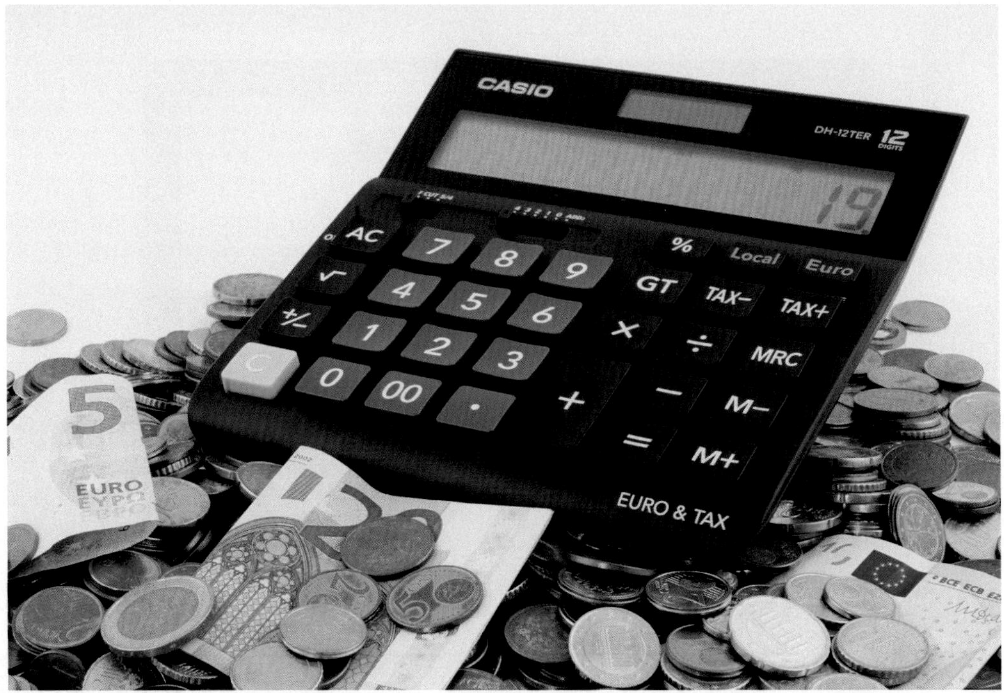

It is important to remember that once a project is officially closed off *there is no more money*. You may not suddenly remember something later and ask for more. Toward the last few months of the project, you should take the time to think about any likely remaining expenditure. This could include payments relating to staff, students, or publications, all of which are discussed in more detail below.

There are non-salary payment considerations for your staff who are leaving altogether and which are often forgotten in the wind up of a project. While these should have been in the project budget at the beginning, these hidden costs can take the investigators by surprise. These include annual leave, long-service leave and termination pay, all of which must come out of the project budget. To avoid this, try to ensure that your staff have taken all their accumulated leave during the life of the project. They will carry forward their long-service leave if they move to another project with the same employer, but termination pay for a long-term employee who is moving elsewhere might be quite significant. If your staff member has been at the university for, say, 15 years, the severance pay accumulation from the whole 15 years will be substantial and may have to be paid by your project's budget. Have the necessary conversations with your human resources team about these liabilities in plenty of time.

Student Payments

Similarly, you must not forget any PhD stipend payments which may remain due to students working on your project, and which should be paid from project funds before they are closed off.

Consider whether there will be any further costs for the student's project that should be met by the project and not come out of the stipend. This might include costs for travel, conference attendance, publication, or data.

Cost of Publications

In these days of open access publications, there is often a significant fee due to the journal on acceptance of your paper. These fees should be paid by the project—or else they may have to be paid by the investigators!

6.3 Other Important Elements to Tidy Up at the End of Your Project

Project Mayhem lurched to the end of the time, then everyone left for greener pastures. The folders of files gathered dust on the bookshelves; benches remained lined with unspecified bottles. Another project took over the computers and deleted the data. Good planning? No way!

Checklist

(Tick when completed)

- ☐ Assist your team with their transition
- ☐ Hold exit interviews
- ☐ Notify the appropriate person about insurance
- ☐ List the intellectual property which has been created
- ☐ Store study records
- ☐ Dispose of equipment and consumables
- ☐ Complete final report(s)to your funding body
- ☐ Complete final ethics report
- ☐ Start your write up

Sorting Out Your Team

Whether they are to be re-deployed or not, you must consider both the welfare of your team and the payments due to them before the project comes to an end (discussed in Chapter 6.2).

Before they leave you, interview project team members together on their project experience and hear their suggestions for any future projects. It is good practice to conduct an individual exit interview for each team member as well to review their contributions, affirm their achievements, and assist with their exiting the project.

Make sure you have contact details for them, and check that they have returned equipment and keys. Particularly remember to ensure you have access to their computer files, and make sure you know where relevant materials are stored. You don't want to be fruitlessly hunting for something you particularly need while they are backpacking though Europe and out of reach.

Insurance

If there is a specific insurance policy or amendment to an insurance policy relating to your project, you will need to advise either the insurance company or the person in your institute who handles the relationship that the project is over. This step is often overlooked, but your institution will be grateful to not be paying unnecessary premiums.

Intellectual Property

At the end of your project you should create a register of the IP outcomes from your project. It is often a requirement that you do so, but it is always good practice to capture and report on all IP generated in a project. Also, if there is to be any commercialization of IP, it will be important to be able to verify in future what IP was generated during this particular project and what stage of development it was at when the project ended. Similarly, if there is to be a follow-on project in a similar area, or involving similar personnel, it is extremely useful to have a record of the status of any IP at the conclusion of the prior project (Table 6.3.1).

TABLE 6.3.1 Intellectual Property Register

IP Description	Owner	Date Created	Related Project	Format	Storage Location
Data set x	Dr. Lightning	1/4/2017	Project Thunderstorm	SAS	H:\Thunderstorm\Data\2017
Data set y	Dr. Lightning	2/6/2016	Project Thunderstorm	Excel	H:\Thunderstorm\Data\2016

Safe Storage of Study Records

Many a project has ended, its records have been stored in a box in the basement; its staff have moved on and all is forgotten—then one day somebody wants to know something about it. What happened to the data? Where are the records? Where did Fred move to?

This can be a terrible waste of years of labor and of institutional IP. You can't prevent the project coming to an end and the staff moving on, but you can leave behind good records and safely stored data. So, you must do the following:

- Back up, label, and store on appropriate media all study records.
- Safely store physical study records, ensuring confidential records are secure.
- Record the physical location of these records and let someone else know where they are.
- Delete all data from equipment used during the project before it moves elsewhere.

These days, once your data have been published you will be likely to upload the project data to an open access repository.

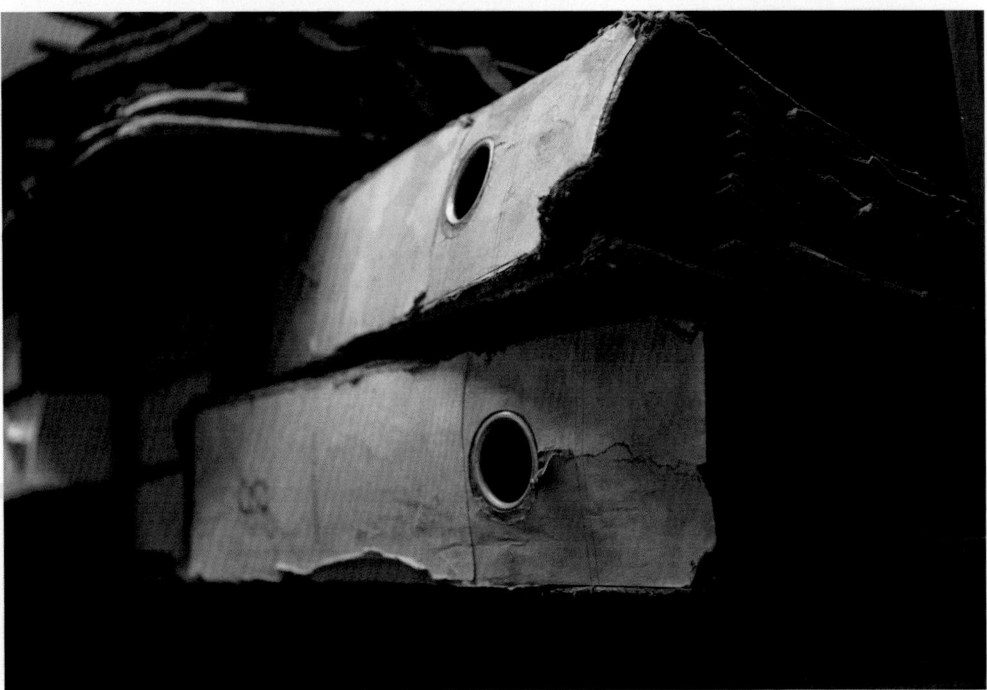

Image Credit: Archive Files by vuralyavas/iStock

Disposal of Equipment and Consumables

Your funding agreement may stipulate what happens to assets purchased with your project funding. Equipment will often be able to stay at the institution, but sometimes it must return to its origin, or sometimes there is a requirement for it to be sold and the funds returned to the funding agency.

Disposal of the equipment is an important part of winding up your project. A record needs to be kept, particularly when the equipment is disposed elsewhere. You should note the name of the person authorizing the sale or transfer of the equipment in your records.

End of Project Reporting

At the end of your project, reporting obligations must be met for both the budget and the research outcomes of the project.

Reporting to Your Funding Body

Your obligations to your funding body will have been spelled out in your funding agreement. They will certainly include financial reporting (See Chapter 4.14) and will probably include reporting on outcomes of your work. Some funding agencies require separate financial and technical final reports.

It is extremely important that all reporting is done on time, both throughout the project and at the end of the project. Sometimes unforeseen circumstances may lead to a deadline not being met. If you are going to be late, it is vital that the funding agency is notified and you have made a request for a later submission of the final report well before the deadline. Note that if an extension of the final report deadline is sought two days prior to the deadline, the extension requested should not be for more than two days. It is not reasonable to ask for a two-month extension two days before the report is due. It would have been obvious to the chief investigator several weeks before the deadline that two months more were needed, so try not to let everyone down with a sign of poor research management.

As mentioned in the Chapter 4.14 on reporting, be sure to bear in mind the focus of the funding body when you write the end of project report to your funders. It is likely that it will be read by laymen, and it is in your interest if they understand what you are saying. If your funding organization is a commercial one, they will be interested to read about translation into product or practice, and other such practical potential outcomes.

Ethics Committee Reporting

There is likely to be a standard format for reporting to your IRB or ethics committee. This report will essentially be advice that the project is complete, and the committee no longer needs to have it on their list of concerns. The report is likely to require that you summarize all ethical issues which arose during the life of the project in one document.

6.4 Further Project Communication

Project Starlight was finished, but no one really noticed. It just petered out. Later, everyone was distracted with new things, and no one quite remembered to pay attention to the outcomes or to think about whether there was a possibility to move on to the next step. Opportunities available while the subject was "fresh" slipped by.

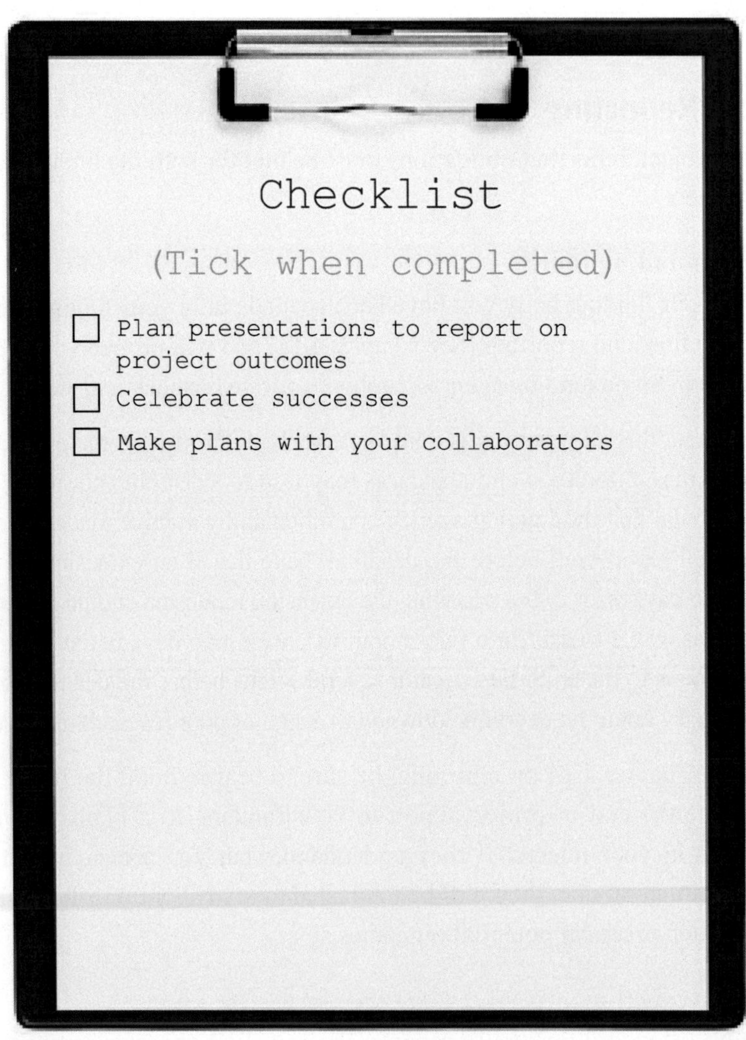

By no means last in the priorities at the end of your project is your obligation to communicate its outcomes. With any luck the project has been a success, but whether a success or failure, it is a research task completed, and you need to mark its end appropriately.

You should celebrate your projects successes with the following people:

- Study staff
- Study participants
- Colleagues

It is useful to canvass stakeholder feedback on the benefits of the project and its potential impact. You should organize a meeting to discuss their collective views.

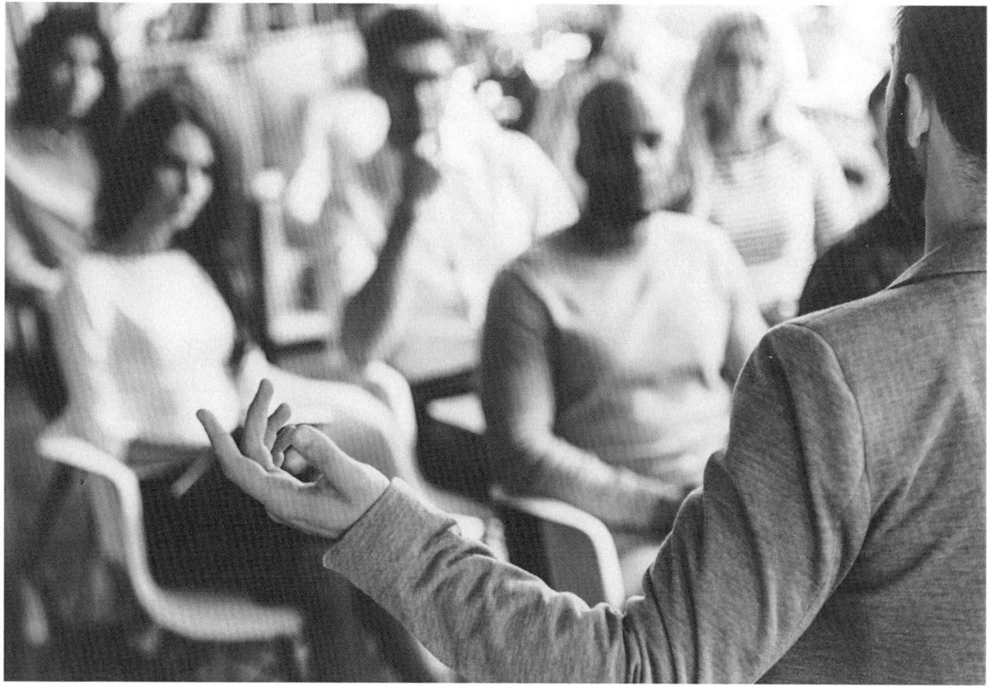

Image Credit: View of man gesturing with hand by g-stockstudio/Shutterstock

It is a good idea to present a seminar on the project and its outcomes within your institution. This applies whether the project has achieved all its objectives or otherwise. This presentation gives you an opportunity to explain what you have all been up to, and what you have learned, or even failed to learn, will be of benefit to your colleagues.

You should also create an opportunity to present your project outcomes at an appropriate external meeting once your research project findings are published, or are otherwise in the public domain.

Last, ensure stakeholders are advised of your publication plans and achievements, and your intentions, if any, to continue with the work.

Remember to update your website with the project's successes and outcomes, and provide copies or abstracts of your publications on the website as they become available. You should also provide a forwarding contact address to all stakeholders.

Talk to Your Collaborators

You are very likely to continue working with your collaborators at the end of your project, particularly if further opportunities have opened up for your work together. In the meantime do the following:

- Continue working on publications from your study, in collaboration with the team
- Consider whether there is an opportunity for further collaboration with your study partners and prepare further funding applications together

6.5 Post-Project Evaluation

Did the project make any difference? Could we have done better?

"I don't know. We never really thought about it." Don't let this person be you.

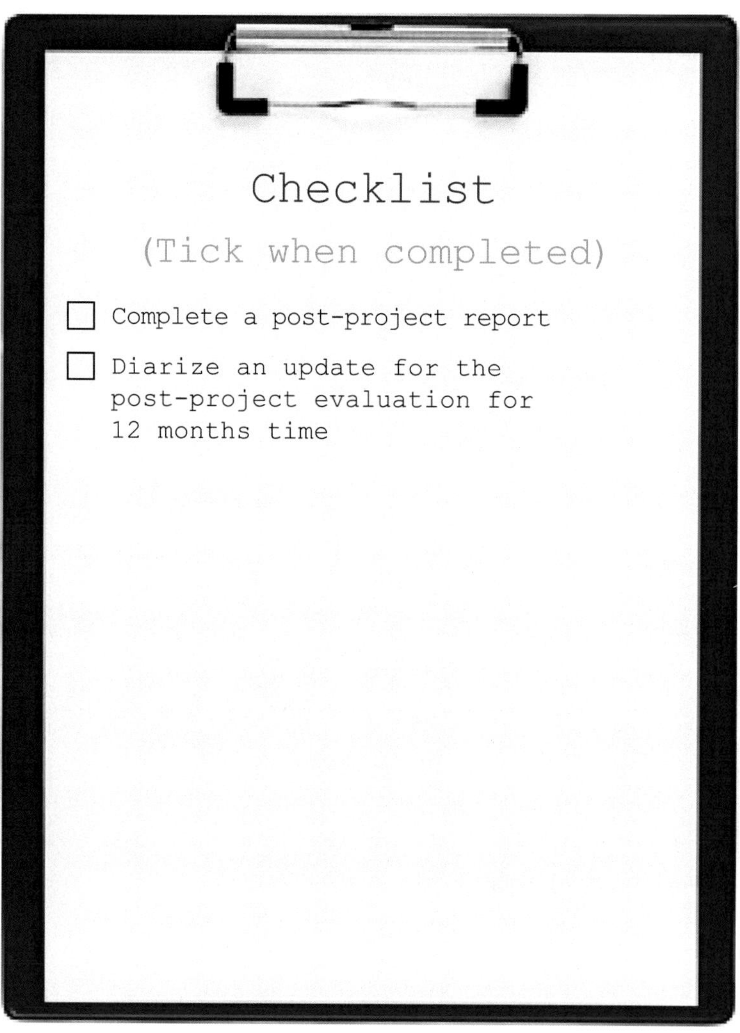

6 WRAPPING UP YOUR PROJECT

The last steps for your project should involve a complete post-project evaluation. This is a standard activity in good project management and applies just as much for research project management as it does for business.

Post-project evaluation will summarize both the outcomes and the lessons learned during your project. It is valuable to share these learnings with your peers. This evaluation can be carried out at the project end and should be updated after about a year, once publications have been written, and there has been an opportunity for the results of your research to be communicated to the outside world.

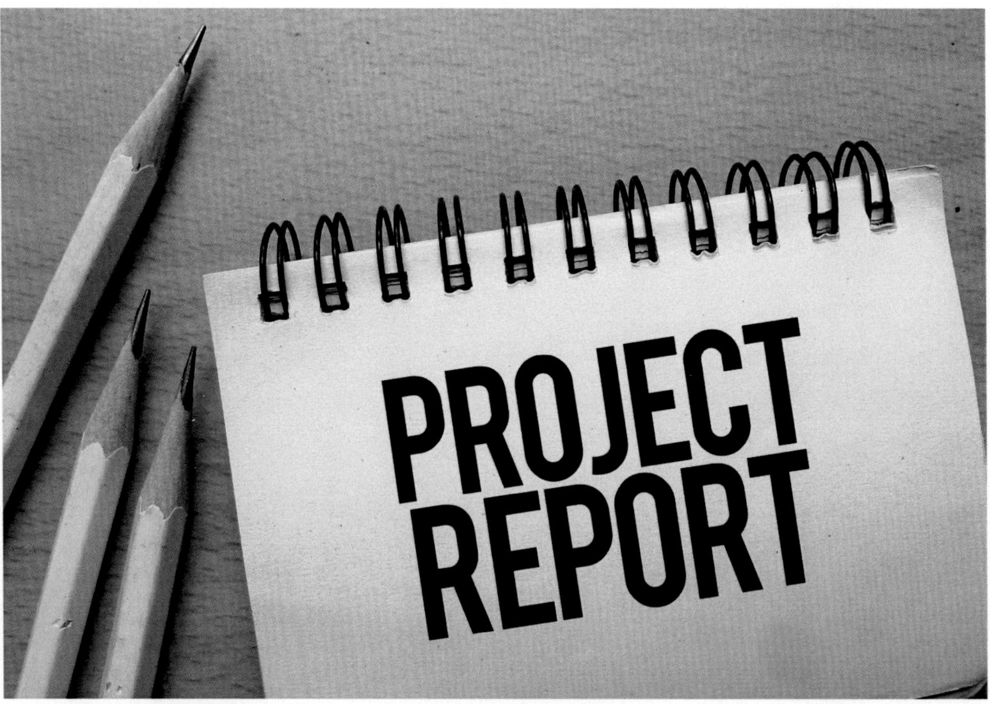

Image Credit: Project report by Zuraihan Md Zain/Shutterstock

This post-project review is a tool for facilitating both continuous improvement and quality management. It will help you identify what went wrong and what could have been done better—as well as what went well. It will also help you prepare for planning and budgeting for future projects.

Your review should cover an assessment of whether the project met its objectives as defined in the project plan. It should also assess whether it was well managed and whether the team was effective.

Before you begin the assessment process you should consider the criteria by which you will measure the project's success. These should be SMART goals:

- Specific
- Measurable
- Achievable/Attainable
- Realistic
- Time-bound

and should be applied to the following:

- The immediate (and possibly commercial) outputs of the project
- The potential outcomes created by the project in the future

The Form 6.5.1 Post Implementation Review Form and Form 6.5.2 Report for a Completed Project Analysis (following) can provide assistance in your report preparations and help you leave an easy to understand trail about your project for people in the future.

Further Reading—Wrapping Up Your Project

Note that these references are pertinent for the whole of Part 6 and for general project management.

National Institutes of Health (NIH) provides a detailed end of study report template which can be found at: https://www.nidcr.nih.gov/research/toolkit/Documents/dsmb_final_study_report_template_v2_21APR2014.dotx.

Payne, J. M., France, K., Henley, N., D'Antoine, H. A., Bartu, A. E., Elliott, E. E. & Bower, C., 2011. Researchers' experience with project management in health and medical research: Results from a post project review. BMC Public Health, 11. https://bmcpublichealth.biomedcentral.com/articles/10.1186/1471-2458-11-424.

Singer, S. L., 2010. Project Management in the Research Environment. https://www.bestthinking.com/articles/science/applied_science/project-management-in-the-research-environment.

The University of Tasmania provides a helpful guide to project closure, plus associated documentation at: http://www.utas.edu.au/project-management-methodology/project/closure-and-review.

Associated Documents—Post-Project Evaluation

6.5.1 Post Implementation Review Form

(for use approximately one year after project completion)

Project Title	Click here to enter text.
Date of Review	Click here to enter text.
Original Project Aims	
Click here to enter text.	
Original Project Timelines	
Click here to enter text.	
Project Outcomes	
Click here to enter text.	
Funding Source and Total Cost	
Click here to enter text.	
Publications Resulting	
Click here to enter text.	
Presentations Resulting	
Click here to enter text.	
Further Funding Sourced	
Click here to enter text.	
Risks and Issues encountered	
Click here to enter text.	
Location of Study Documentation (include electronic and physical location of documents). If physical documents have been sent offsite, please record the box numbers, contents of each box and destruction dates of each box.	
Click here to enter text.	
Sub-studies or Further Projects Associated with this Project	
Click here to enter text.	

6.5.2 Completed Project Analysis Report

Project Title	Click here to enter text.
Report Date	Click here to enter text.
Analyst/Investigators:	
Click here to enter text.	
Name(s) and Location(s) of Key Data Set(s):	
Click here to enter text.	
Statistical (or other) software used:	
Click here to enter text.	
Location of Code/Program(s) Used to Analyze the Data:	
Click here to enter text.	
Types of Analysis(es) Carried Out:	
Click here to enter text.	
Date Completed:	Click here to enter text.
Citation(s) for Associated Publication(s):	
Click here to enter text.	
Any Other General Comments:	
Click here to enter text.	

Paper Submission History

Paper Name	Click here to enter text.
Target Journal	Click here to enter text.
Date Submitted	Click here to enter text.
Response Date	Click here to enter text.
Outcome	Click here to enter text.

7 RESEARCH DISSEMINATION

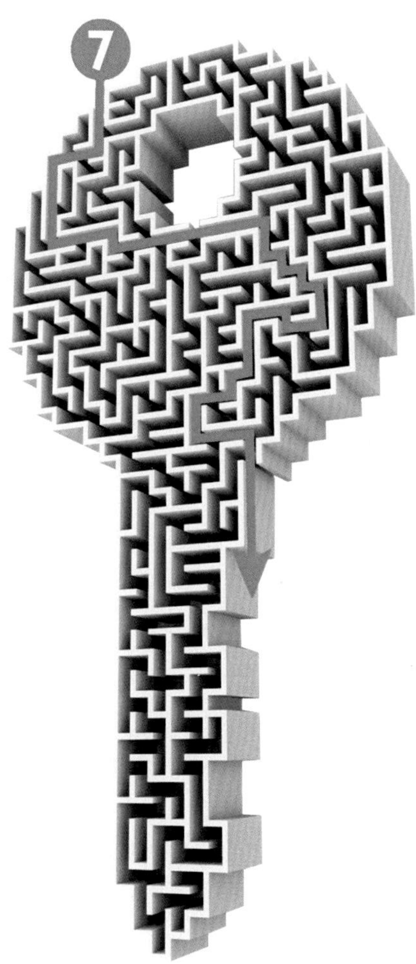

7.1 Posters and Presentations

It's all too familiar: the slide presentation where the presenter stands in front of you and reads every one of the hundreds of words squashed on to each slide. You'd prefer to count the number of tiles on the ceiling. In the same category, the poster so densely covered in minute text (with no images) that you almost have to put your nose onto it to work out the subject matter. You go and have a cup of tea instead.

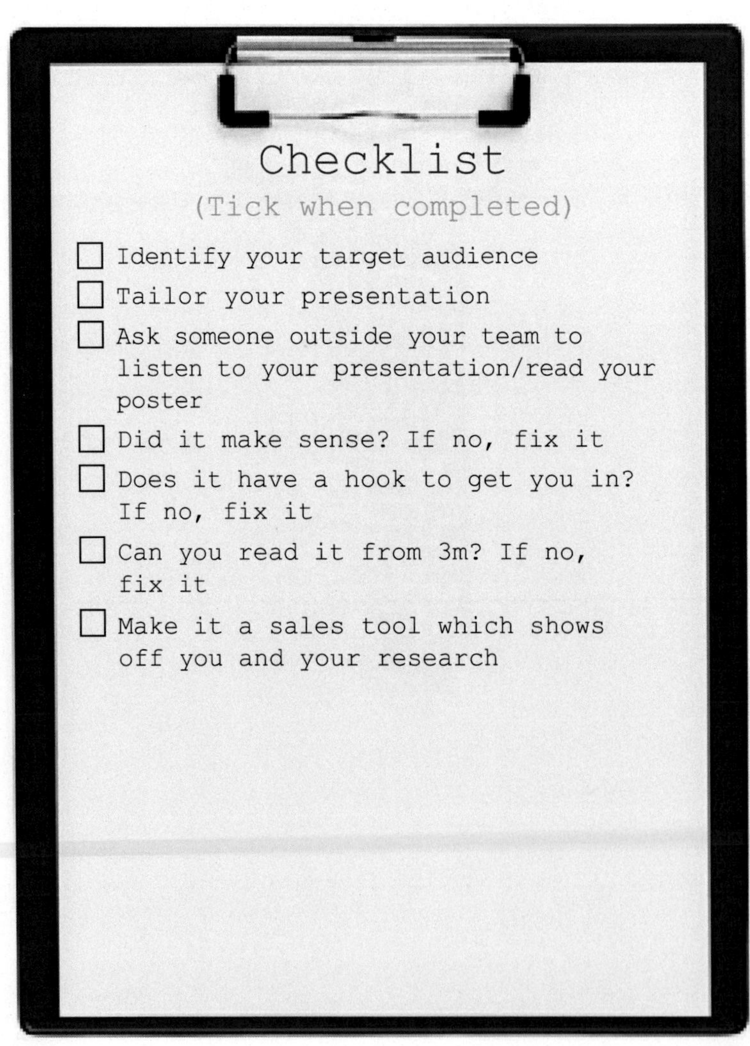

Elements of a Good Presentation

As with any form of publication, the two most important things to keep in mind when you are presenting are that

- these are *people* who will be listening to you at your presentation and
- you are likely to know, and probably care, way more about your topic than they do.

This means that you need to think about the makeup of your audience and tailor your presentation so that it piques their interest and they pay attention.

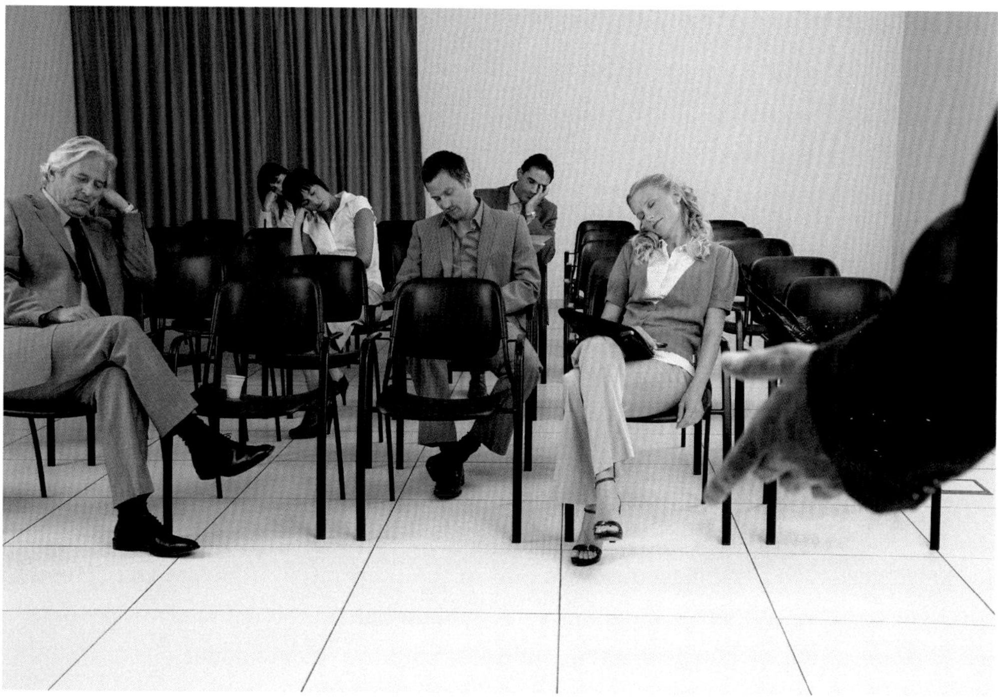

Image Credit: People sleeping during a seminar by sirtravelalot/Shutterstock

We have all suffered from "Death by PowerPoint." PowerPoint certainly has its uses, and in a presentation it can be particularly valuable. What you don't need though, is millions of slides and too many words. What you absolutely don't need, ever, is a presentation where you speak to the words on the slide. Not only is this boring and unimaginative for the audience, but you will find that they are automatically reading the slide, not necessarily taking it in, and almost certainly not listening to you.

If you want them to *really* listen, have images on your slides, and no words. Watching some TED Talks [1] will show you some great examples of people captivating their audiences with very few visual aids.

In her article "How to Prevent Death by PowerPoint" [2] White reminds us that when presenters use PowerPoint as a script, or overload slides with text or data, it becomes a barrier between them and the people with whom they are trying to communicate. She tells us, when preparing our presentation, to do the following:

- Set clear objectives—what is the purpose of this presentation? Passing on knowledge? Looking for a decision? Changing an opinion? The answers should provide an indication for your content.
- Speak their language—avoid jargon if they are not going to understand it.
- Plot it out and set it up. The opening is when you can grab their attention. Preview what you are going to say to let them know what's in it for them and engage their attention.
- Have three key messages and an organized closing. Your audience is likely to remember only three key things. Work out what they are, feature them, and repeat them in closing with a call to action.
- Follow the 6-6-6 rule. If you must use words, no more than 6 words per bullet point, no more than 6 bullet points per slide, no more than 6 minutes on a slide.
- Bring the data to life. If you can work it, speak to some of your points by drawing on a whiteboard. Watching this activity is much more interesting than a slide.

White also suggests you ask for feedback as part of the preparation. Practice your presentation with colleagues and ask if there is anything you could do better. You could also ask someone to film you. Watching yourself can give a good indication of how you are doing.

The Three Minute Thesis

A great way to practice your presentation skills is with the Three Minute Thesis. What an impossible task, you think! How to distill three or four years of work into three minutes? It is a fabulous concept which has helped train researchers all over the world to talk coherently, and succinctly, about their work. When you get this right, you have really nailed it.

Designing a Good Poster

As you will be aware, posters are widely used in the academic community, and most conferences include poster presentations in their program. Research posters should summarize information or research concisely and attractively to help publicize it and generate discussion.

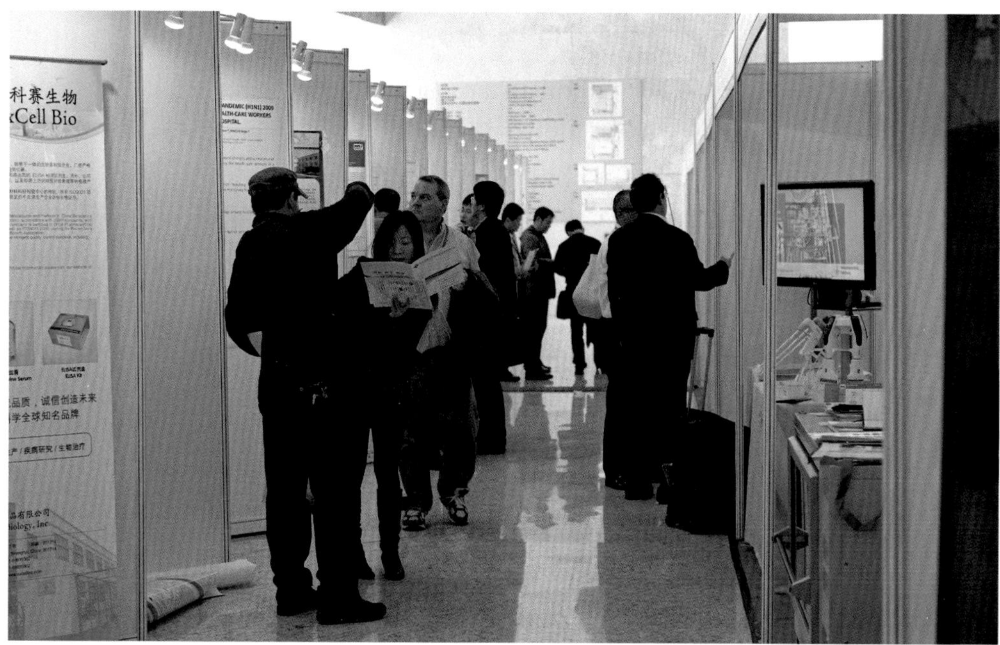

Image Credit: Visitors look at posters by Testing/Shutterstock

The poster is usually a mixture of text mixed with tables, graphs, pictures, and other presentation formats. At a conference, the researcher stands by the poster display while other participants can come and view the presentation and interact with the author.

> Typically, the poster is also visually unappealing, crammed with text, and hard to read. Don't let yours be like this!

In an effort to make scientists make a really big effort to produce great, easy-to-read posters the Royal Society of Chemistry held the world's first Twitter-only conference in 2015. The conference allowed researchers to upload their academic posters as tweets, replacing a physical meeting. Reporting on the success of the conference, Randviir [3] concludes that the conference reached many researchers across the world and created an opportunity for participants to share their work not only with academics but also with other interested parties such as writers, industries, friends and family, and even policy makers. Over 80 posters were tweeted. Whether or not Twitter conferences become a standard format, this emphasizes the fact the posters are for communication about your research, and your focus should be more about the audience reading and understanding your messages than dazzling people with the maximum number of words you can squash on to the page.

So What Makes a Good Poster?

NYU Libraries [4] provide great, clear information about creating better posters.

- Important information should be readable from about 10 feet (3m)
- Title is short and interesting
- Word count of about 300–800 words
- Text is clear and to the point, and not too full of jargon
- Use of bullets, numbering, and headlines make the text easy to read
- Effective use of graphics, color, and fonts
- Consistent and clean layout
- Includes acknowledgments, your name and institutional affiliation (with logo not text), and funding bodies

NYU suggest that when you start planning your poster, you should answer these three questions:

- What is the most important/interesting/astounding finding from my research project?
- How can I visually share my research with conference attendees? Should I use charts, graphs, photos, and/or images?
- What kind of information can I give during my talk that will complement my poster?

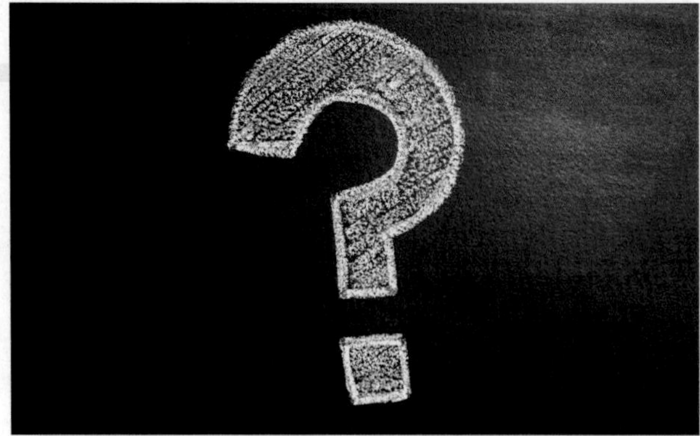

There are great examples of good poster design available on the Better Posters blog [5]. This blog quite correctly notes that academic conference posters are often ugly, with tiny text, confusing layouts, and dubious color schemes. Better Posters is about making posters informative and beautiful, and the comments they provide in their regular critiques are a rich source of design ideas.

See two of their excellent examples in the images following.

The parthenogenetic marbled crayfish, Marmorkrebs, in Texas

Teresa Patricia Feria and Zen Faulkes, Department of Biology and Center for Subtropical Studies, The University of Texas-Pan American

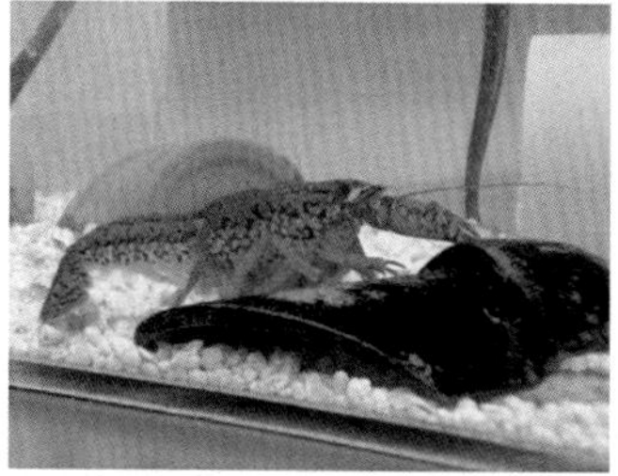

Marmorkrebs (*Procambarus fallax* f. *virginalis*) are parthenogenetic crayfish (Scholtz et al. 2003; Martin et al. 2010) that have been introduced into natural ecosystems in several countries (e.g., Jones et al. 2009; Kawai & Takahata 2010; Chucholl & Pfeiffer 2010), and could become an invasive species. They are sold as pets in North America (Faulkes 2010); for example, www.marbledcrayfish.com is a business in Texas that sells Marmorkrebs, often promoting their use as live bait.

Because many exotic species have been introduced into natural ecosystems by the accidental or deliberate release of pets, we wanted to assess the threat posed by Marmorkrebs should it be released in Texas.

We modeled Marmorkrebs' potential distribution using MaxEnt, with four sets of training data:

1. The distribution of Marmorkrebs in Madagascar (where they are an exotic species) and *P. fallax* in the U.S., plus single European Marmorkrebs in (European *populations* were found after this study; Chucholl & Pfeiffer 2010). This model probably best predicts the potential distribution.
2. The distribution of Marmorkrebs populations in Madagascar.
3. The distribution of *P. fallax* in the U.S.
4. The distribution of Marmorkrebs in Madagascar and *P. fallax* in the U.S.

Texas crayfish distribution from Johnson & Johnson (2008, 2009).

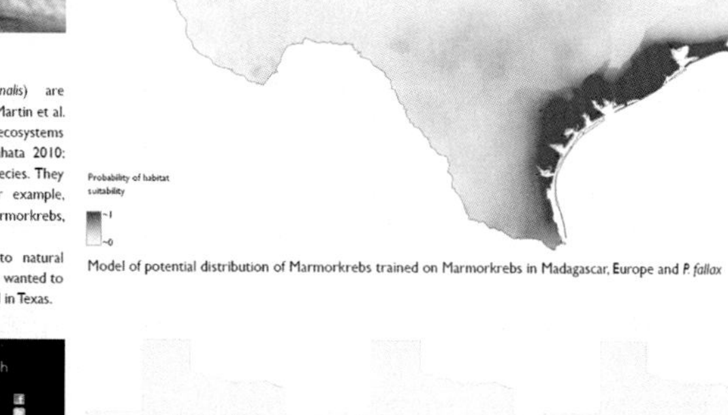

Model of potential distribution of Marmorkrebs trained on Marmorkrebs in Madagascar, Europe and *P. fallax*

Model of potential distribution of Marmorkrebs trained on Marmorkrebs populations in Madagascar

Model of potential distribution of Marmorkrebs trained on *P. fallax*

Model of potential distribution of Marmorkrebs trained on Marmorkrebs in Madagascar and *P. fallax*

The most suitable habitats for Marmorkrebs in Texas are areas with high native crayfish biodiversity and rice production. Marmorkrebs could threaten Texas's 39 native crayfish species through competition, and eat rice meant for harvest, as they do in Madagascar (Jones et al. 2009). Pet owners and sellers need to be aware of the consequences of exotic species introductions.

This work is in press in *Aquatic Invasions*.

References

Chucholl C, Pfeiffer M. 2010. First evidence for an established Marmorkrebs (Decapoda, Astacida, Cambaridae) population in Southwestern Germany, in syntopic occurrence with *Orconectes limosus* (Rafinesque, 1817). *Aquatic Invasions* 5: 405–412.

Faulkes Z. 2010. The spread of the parthenogenetic marbled crayfish, Marmorkrebs (*Procambarus* sp.), in the North American pet trade. *Aquatic Invasions* 5: 447-450.

Johnson SK, Johnson NK. 2008. *Texas Crawdads*. Crawdad Club Designs, College Station, Texas.

Johnson SK, Johnson NK. 2009. Texas Crawdads Supplement. http://texascrawdads.com/yahoo_site_admin/assets/docs/2009_Texas_Crawdads_Supplement.73195937.pdf (accessed 6 January 2011).

Jones JPG, Rasamy JR, Harvey A, Toon A, Oidtmann B, Randrianarison MH, Raminosoa N, Ravoahangimalala OR. 2009. The perfect invader: A parthenogenic crayfish poses a new threat to Madagascar's freshwater biodiversity. *Biological Invasions* 11: 1475-1482.

Kawai T, Takahata M. 2010. *The Biology of Freshwater Crayfish*. Hokkaido University Press, Sapporo.

Martin P, Dorn NJ, Kawai T, van der Heiden C, Scholtz G. 2010. The enigmatic Marmorkrebs (marbled crayfish) is the parthenogenetic form of *Procambarus fallax* (Hagen, 1870). *Contributions to Zoology* 79: 107-118.

Scholtz G, Braband A, Tolley L, Reimann A, Mittmann B, Lukhaup C, Steuerwald F, Vogt G. 2003. Parthenogenesis in an outsider crayfish. *Nature* 421: 806-806.

Visit us online at Marmorkrebs.*org*

Image Credit: Better Posters

7 RESEARCH DISSEMINATION

Note the clear headings, white space, and bright images.

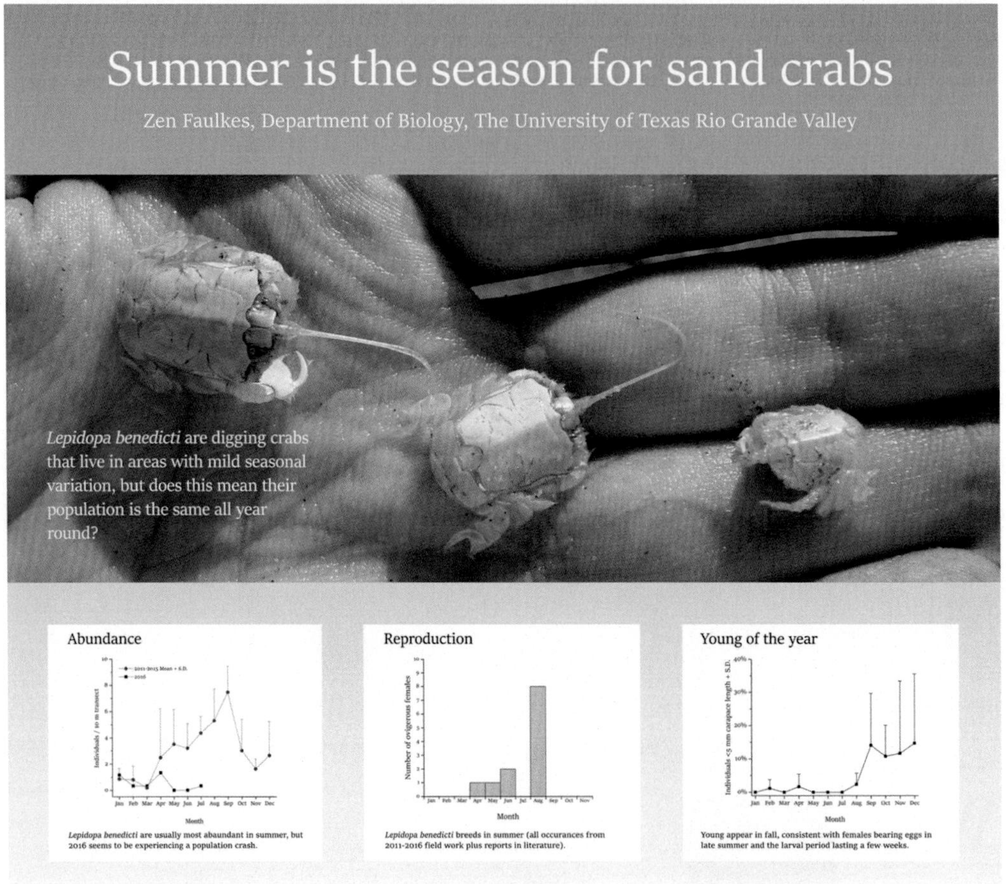

Image Credit: Better Posters

PowerPoint is the popular, easy-to-use option for creating your poster. If you have more sophisticated design software available, such as Adobe Illustrator or InDesign and the ability to use it, they are good for posters which include lots of high-resolution images and help you produce a high-quality product. There are open source alternatives such as Inscape, Gimp, or Lovely Charts.

References—Posters and Presentation

[1] TED Talks. www.ted.com.

[2] White, S., August 2015. How to prevent death by PowerPoint. Journal of Accountancy 220 (2) ProQuest Central p. 20.

[3] Randviir, E.P., Illingworth, S.M., Baker, M.J., Cude, M., Banks, C.E., 2015. Twittering about research: a case study of the World's first Twitter poster competition. F1000Research 4 (798). https://doi.org/10.12688/f1000research.6992.3.
[4] NYU Libraries, How to create a research poster: poster basics. http://guides.nyu.edu/posters.
[5] Better Posters blog. http://betterposters.blogspot.com.au/.

Further Reading

Presentations

Bulska, E., 2006. Good oral presentation of scientific work. Analytical and Bioanalytical Chemistry, 385: 403–405. https://doi.org/10.1007/s00216-006-0441-2.

Fischer, D., 10 Hints for Improving Presentations for the Three Minute Thesis Competition. https://grad.ucsd.edu/_files/student-affairs/grad-slam/3MinThesisHints.pdf.

Illman, J., December 15, 2010. Stand and Deliver. Nursing Standard, 25 (15–17): 62. http://connection.ebscohost.com/c/articles/57289670/stand-deliver.

Mewburn, I. (aka@thesiswhisperer). How to sell your thesis in 3 minutes or less. https://thesiswhisperer.com/2010/07/01/how-to-sell-your-thesis-in-3-minutes-or-less/.

Powell, K., 2012. Presentations: Billboard science. Nature, 483: 113–115. https://doi.org/10.1038/nj7387-113a.

Posters

Duke, S. P., Bancken, F., Crowe, B., Soukup, M., Botsis, T., and Forshee, R., 2015. Seeing is believing: good graphic design principles for medical research. Statistics in Medicine, 34: 3040–3059. https://doi.org/10.1002/sim.6549.

Erren, T. C., Bourne P. E., May 2007. Ten Simple Rules for a Good Poster Presentation. PLoS Computational Biology, 3 (5): e102. http://journals.plos.org/ploscompbiol/article?id=10.1371/journal.pcbi.0030102.

Gopal, A., Redman, M., Cox, D., Foreman, D., Elsey, E. and Fleming, S., 2016. Academic poster design at a national conference: a need for standardized guidance? Clinical Teacher. https://doi.org/10.1111/tct.12584.

Miller, J. E., 2007. Preparing and Presenting Effective Research Posters. Health Services Research, 42 (1 Pt 1): 311–328. PMC. Web. 3 March 2017.

Pedwell, R. K., Hardy, J. A. and Rowland, S. L., 2016. Effective visual design and communication practices for research posters: Exemplars based on the theory and practice of multimedia learning and rhetoric. Biochemistry and Molecular Biology Education. https://doi.org/10.1002/bmb.21034.

7.2 Step-by-Step Guide to the Publication Process

Your reputation is built by publishing and by people knowing about your publications. Do it well; do it often.

Checklist

(Tick when completed)

- ☐ Check if there are any limitations on your publishing
- ☐ Define your audience
- ☐ List the most appropriate journals for your work
- ☐ Select your target journal
- ☐ Involve the whole team in the writing
- ☐ Write a very careful abstract
- ☐ Think very carefully about the authorship list, who should be on it and in what order
- ☐ Remember to acknowledge funding bodies and other assistance
- ☐ Listen to your reviewers - take their advice
- ☐ Try again (and again, and again)
- ☐ Go to the next chapter and read about promoting your accepted paper

Before You Start Writing

There are some questions you need to consider before publication and dissemination of your research findings:

- Are there to be any limitations of access to or dissemination of your results? If so, what are they?
- Are there any restrictions on when and how you publish?
- Are there any outstanding intellectual property (IP) matters to be resolved? If you are hoping for a commercial outcome, you will need to decide who has contributed and agree on IP ownership and licensee rights. Often this will have been spelled out in the funding or collaborator agreements. IP is usually not a problem as long as there are no commercial undertakings for this project, but there could be trouble if you release data prematurely or in a way contrary to agreements.
- Have you worked out a process for consultation between the partners when you are preparing for publication? Who will make the decisions about joint publications? Again, this should have been covered in your collaboration or funding agreements, so check what they say.

Define Your Target Audience

Before you write the first word for your new publication, indeed, before you select the target journal, consider your audience. Who are you writing for? What is the purpose?

Assuming you are not simply targeting the only journal likely to accept your work, or the open access (OA) journal hungriest for your fee, these questions will help you define the journal to aim for, and then the style of writing.

If you are not writing for a journal at all, but for an abstract for a conference or a brief for your media office, you might—should—choose to use different language.

Having considered your audience, remember it is made up of *people*. You are closer to your subject than they are. They need to properly understand the background for your research and what it is about. They need to understand the "why." For conference papers, you must be able immediately to catch the attention of potential readers. If there are hundreds of abstracts or short papers to read, their question will be do I bother to read this one?

Choosing a Journal

Getting your paper published can take much longer than it took to actually do the work. You can expedite the process by doing some thoughtful homework first. Choosing the correct journal to approach can save a lot of wasted time because while you are waiting for a response your hands are tied.

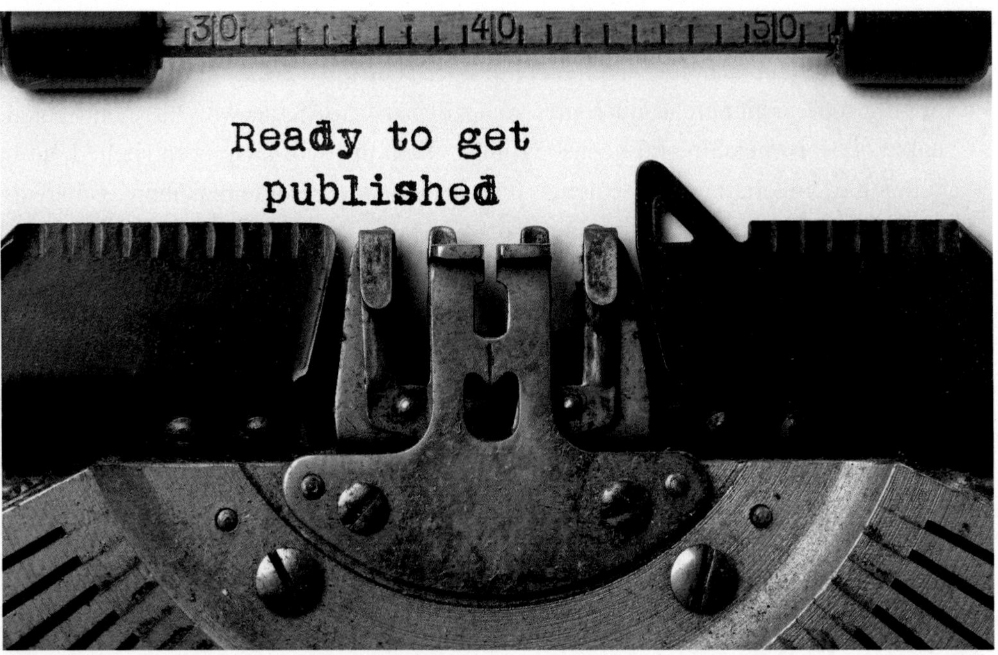

Image Credit: Vintage inscription made by old typewriter by MyImages-Micha/Shutterstock

You are likely to be publishing jointly with a number of others, and you may all have a different view on which journal to approach first. You will be certain to agree that the higher the impact factor the better, but simply because everyone wants exactly that, the competition will be stiffer. Trying to publish in *Nature*, *Science*, or *PNAS* may simply be an exercise in frustration. Conversely many Nobel Prize–winning pieces of work, e.g., Zinkernagel and Doherty [1] were published in relatively obscure technically focused journals. There are views that the emphasis currently placed on impact factor in many institutions is a relatively recent, and possibly passing, fad pushed by university and research institute managers who are encouraged to use relatively crude metrics to attempt to quantify productivity of their staff.

When choosing your target journal(s), (it is a good idea to have more than one as you might well be rejected by the higher ranking publications), consider the following:

- Is your field one of particular interest to that journal? If yes, is there a time of year (and therefore issue) when they publish on your particular topic?
- When you conducted your literature review, was there one journal or group of journals that frequently included related work?
- Is there a journal that champions the work of early-career investigators in your field?
- Is your topic of specialist interest (and therefore should be directed to a specialist journal) or would it be better suited to a broader interest publication?

Publishing articles in high-impact factor journals is a good strategy to have your work recognized, but *a much better strategy is to publish research in journals that target the audience of your paper*.

You may wish to check that you have chosen an appropriate journal by making an initial approach to the editor. If you have checked that your paper appears to meet the guidelines for the journal, send an email to the editor, including an abstract, and ask whether it is of interest. In the covering email you can explain the background to your research question and the reason why your findings matter. You are likely to receive a response fairly promptly. If the paper is not of interest, you can immediately proceed to the next journal on your list. If, on the other hand, there appears to be some interest, you already have a foot in the door and might already be in a position to respond to a comment or two.

Some Further Thoughts Before You Get Started

Journal Impact Factors

Note that "journal impact factors" are calculated on the basis of citations in the two years following publication, to try to track trends in impact factors. This can have problems. A paper that receives very few citations in the first couple of years might go on to receive hundreds of citations. This is one reason for being wary of choosing a journal based on impact factor alone.

Open Access?

Another consideration is whether you want to publish in an OA journal. OA can have great benefits to individual researchers and institutions. It can increase citations to your work, build networks with like-minded researchers, promote research translation and policy change. It means sharing your ideas with everyone—not just to those who can pay. The downside to publishing in an OA journal is that you have to pay to publish with them. The fees for OA journals, known as "article processing charges," can be quite significant, so make sure you have allowed for them in your budget.

A more significant downside is that some of the new OA journals that have popped up since OA became an obligation for many researchers have been found to be unscrupulous.

When selecting your journal, you should beware of the proliferation of predatory, bogus, and ultra-low-impact OA journals interested only in your publication fee. Be warned that the "editors" of these "journals" frequently approach authors soliciting manuscripts and can appear genuine and persuasive.

See Chapter 7.3 for more about OA, via your institutional repository.

Don't Overclaim

Something to be careful about with your results and conclusions—don't overclaim. The journal, or your reviewers, will challenge any unreasonable statements, and this will lead to delays. Don't leap to conclusions and write about what you *wish* your data were showing. Publish what you have and perhaps find a way to allude to results you hope to manage in the future. Being fanciful won't help your reputation or improve the likelihood of your paper being accepted.

Writing Your Papers

Once you have selected your target journal, you can start writing, tailoring your paper to that journal's requirements.

In science, your paper will be a collaborative effort, almost by definition.

The usual practice is for the first author to have a go at the first draft. The next step is to pass it around to the rest of the team for review and comment. Hold team meetings to workshop the paper, discuss the strengths and weaknesses, and plan the next steps. It is invaluable experience for all.

Diedrich [2] encourages more collaboration in the scientific writing process. He notes that the best science is performed by collaboration of researchers with different expertise; asking a collaborator for help with a specific technique is encouraged. At the same time, asking for help with writing can be frowned upon. If you find yourself in this situation, ignore it. It is the responsibility of all investigators who will be named on the paper to take part in the writing. If writing doesn't come easily to you, and one of your colleagues is better at this skill, encourage them to assist. You are all in this together.

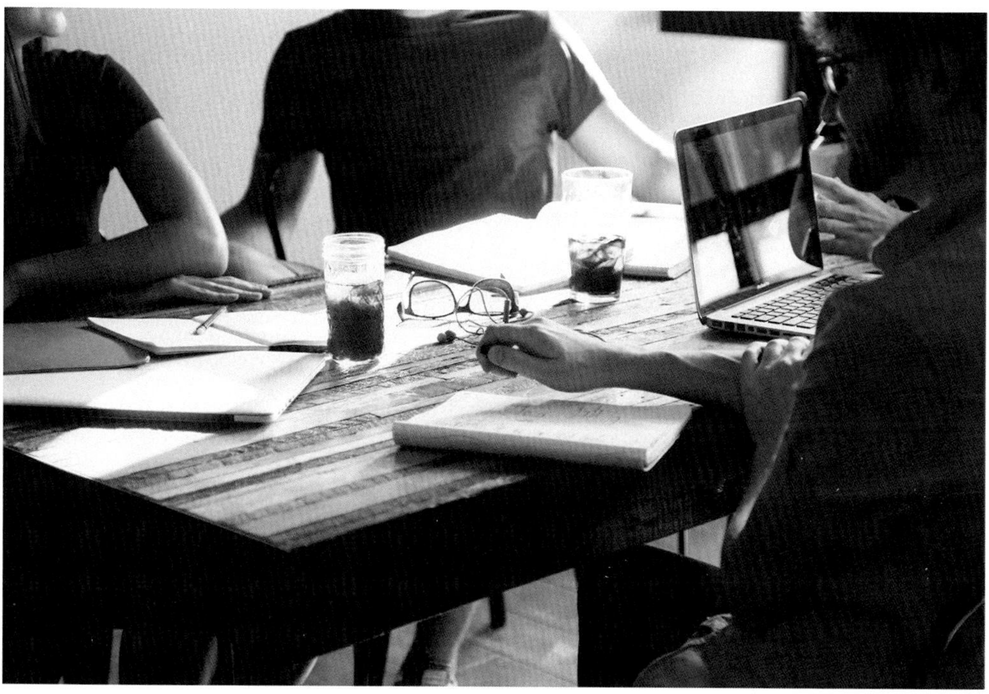

Diedrich hopes the stigma against asking for help with it can change. *"I hope that writing can eventually just be viewed as another technique that is part of the scientific process. When someone needs help with it, they shouldn't be embarrassed; they should ask for help. Remember, it takes a village to make good science happen!"*

The Abstract

By the time you have reached the stage of your career where you are reading this book, you should understand the basics of writing papers; however, special mention must be made about the abstract.

The abstract is not something to be thrown together at the last minute before you submit the paper. The importance of abstracts cannot be understated.

In some cases, the abstract may be the only thing a reader will see to determine if your work is worthy of further attention.

For reviewers, this is the first opportunity to understand what you are about to present. The abstract is your first and possibly only chance to attract the attention of a potential reader.

Your abstract is the "bait" that catches the attention of your reader. You have to include enough information to encourage the reader to go on to peruse the whole paper. You need them to understand any subtleties or qualifications, as well as your detailed interpretations and suggestions for further work.

Each journal has unique requirements regarding how the abstract should appear. Get it right or all your efforts might well be in vain.

Responding to Reviewer's Comments

When the editors select the reviewers for your paper they will have done their best to match the reviewer to your field of expertise. Although they may have chosen not to follow your recommendations, those recommendations will have been the starting point of their selection process, along with their own knowledge of your field. Whoever it is, it is likely that your reviewer will be someone able to offer an independent and entirely reasonable perspective.

One day you will be called upon to be a reviewer yourself. You need to remember that peer reviewers are experts in the field who are voluntarily, and free of charge, giving up a large amount of their time and effort to assess and inevitably improve any publishable manuscript. Rather than feeling resentment or annoyance at reviewers' comments, you as an author should actually feel profound gratitude. Listen to what they have to say, and do your best to take their advice.

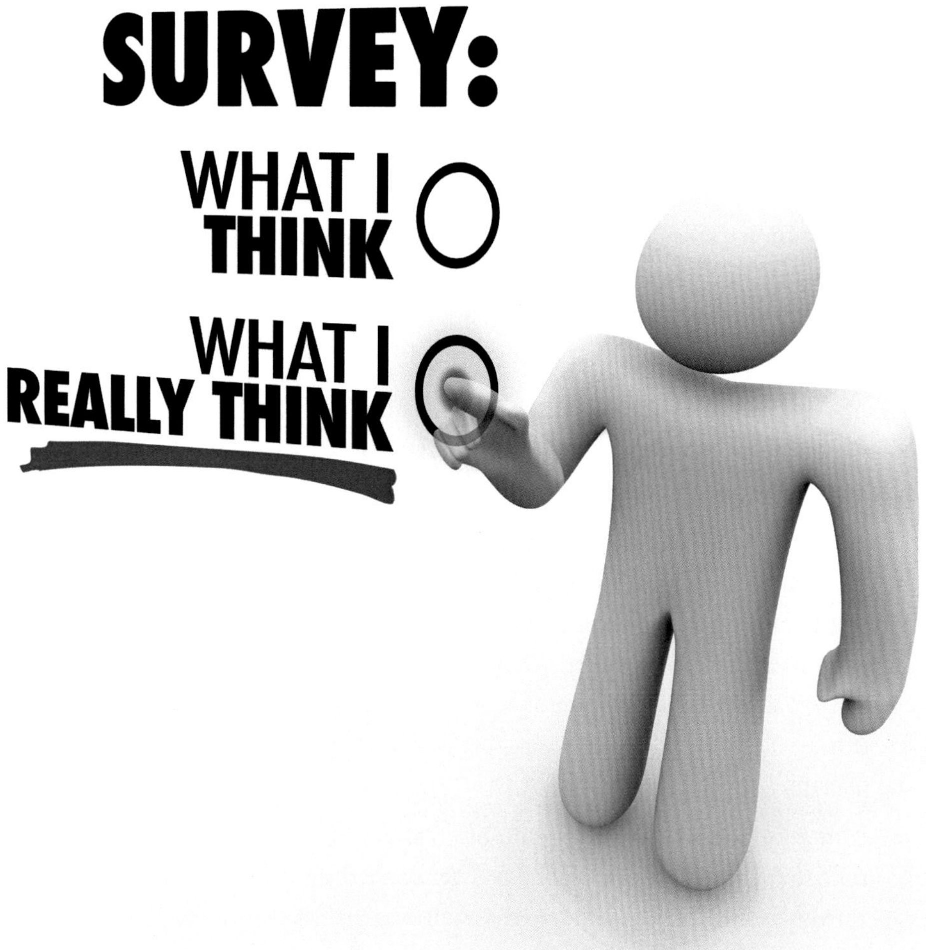

Image Credit: Response button for What I Really Think by Iqoncept/Shutterstock

It is very rare for a paper to be accepted without the need for some changes. Comments will come back from your reviewers, and your immediate response will probably be to feel they are unfair. You are human, after all. Remember that these reviewers are looking at your paper with fresh eyes—and they are experts in your field.

There are a number of possible situations you could be in:

- The paper might be accepted subject to some minor alterations.
- The paper might be rejected as not sufficiently novel or too preliminary.

- The paper might be rejected because it is out of scope for the journal.
- The editor or reviewers might feel that the work is plain wrong (this is particularly the case with papers which challenge the status quo).

Read the reviewers' comments and the editor's response with care, and discuss your strategy with your team before you start your response.

There are rare occasions when opposing groups go to lengths to prevent or delay publication of something new, particularly if it might put their reputation and body of work at risk. This is unethical behavior. If you feel that your paper is not been handled ethically you may be able to seek guidance from the Committee on Publication Ethics (COPE) [3].

It is more likely, where you are trying to change the status quo, that people are having difficulty understanding your point of view. Provide a more detailed explanation of your methodology and results and give clear reasoning for why you are right, and why the accepted dogma is no longer correct.

If you think a referee's comments are completely incorrect or unfair, you should write a rebuttal letter to the editor explaining your concerns. Similarly, if you think a requested additional experiment or other piece of work is unreasonable, write to explain why the experiment cannot/should not be done or why it will not help strengthen the conclusions of your paper. It may be possible to discuss your concerns with the editor before working on a revised manuscript.

The responses to your paper's review should be treated in a similar way to responses to a grant application. Take the reviewer seriously and answer each point thoroughly. The problem may just have stemmed from a lack of understanding that will be clarified by your responses. If a little more work is suggested, do it and supply the results. If there is extra work suggested that you do not have budget for, or that you don't believe merits the trouble, respond accordingly with a thorough explanation for why you will not be doing it.

If you think that the reviewers have entirely missed your point, reflect on whether this could be because you have not made it clearly enough. You are closer to your topic than they are. Have one of your colleagues read your paper, bearing this in mind. If your colleague, too, doesn't understand, then try to re-write some of the paper, altering the focus to clarify the problem. If the general consensus is that you were clear, discuss the matter with the editor. It is possible that your reviewer did not understand the field sufficiently. The editor might decide to approach someone else. Warning: Do not openly criticize your reviewer to the editor.

Submitting to Another Journal

If your paper has been rejected by your target journal because it is not a good fit, or the work is not sufficiently novel, you will need to aim for another. Don't be distressed: this is not uncommon, particularly for high-impact journals. Nature rejects 95% of papers sent to them, so you are in very good company.

Before you try again with an alternative journal, ensure that you address any comments made by the reviewers at the first journal. You must assume that it is likely the same people will be called upon to review your paper at the second journal, and this is in fact an opportunity to make your paper even better. They will see your improvements and be pleased you took their advice. Note that if you are ever tempted to break the rules and submit identical or near-identical papers to two or more journals simultaneously, there is a good chance you will be caught out when the different journal editors choose the same reviewers—there is a limited pool of experts. Don't do it!

If you feel you have had a "near miss" from your original journal, it could be worthwhile mentioning that you have received reviews and positive feedback from "Journal X," have addressed the comments and are now submitting to this more targeted/lower-impact journal with the benefit of their recommendations. Sometimes the editor of the next journal will assess the reviewers' reports from the first journal as well and may even short cut the review process.

Make a file for correspondence on each paper, particularly noting submission and response dates, so that you can review its progress easily.

Once your paper has been accepted for publication, gather together the documentation that demonstrates the history of its development and shows that it was independently refereed, and file it away safely. You may need to verify the paper's background for audit purposes or for some matter regarding IP at some time following its publication. It can be very time consuming looking for this information a long time after acceptance. Take the time now while you know where everything is!

Authorship and Acknowledgment Guidelines

Authorship of Papers

As discussed in Chapter 3.2 on Collaborations, it is preferable if matters relating to authorship and publication are resolved at the very beginning of the project or at the time any new collaborator joins along the way. It is important to understand if your research outcomes (including publications) will be placed in the public arena or a commercial arena. In either case, effective management of authorship/ownership is crucial, especially once you enter the public domain.

7 RESEARCH DISSEMINATION

If your outcomes are to be public, then you are mostly likely to proceed with joint publications. Increasingly, research is being conducted in teams, and publications resulting from this research have many authors. The inclusion and order of authors on a paper are often sources of discord in a team, so as part of your project plan you should develop a team policy to clarify how the author list is determined. This is highly dependent on the relevant culture of the discipline in question.

Authorship should be based on making a substantial contribution to the conception and planning of an article; acquisition, analysis, and interpretation of data; or drafting the publication, revising it critically, or giving final approval of the version to be published. Each author must take responsibility for the publication. Note that some journals have limitations on the number of authors.

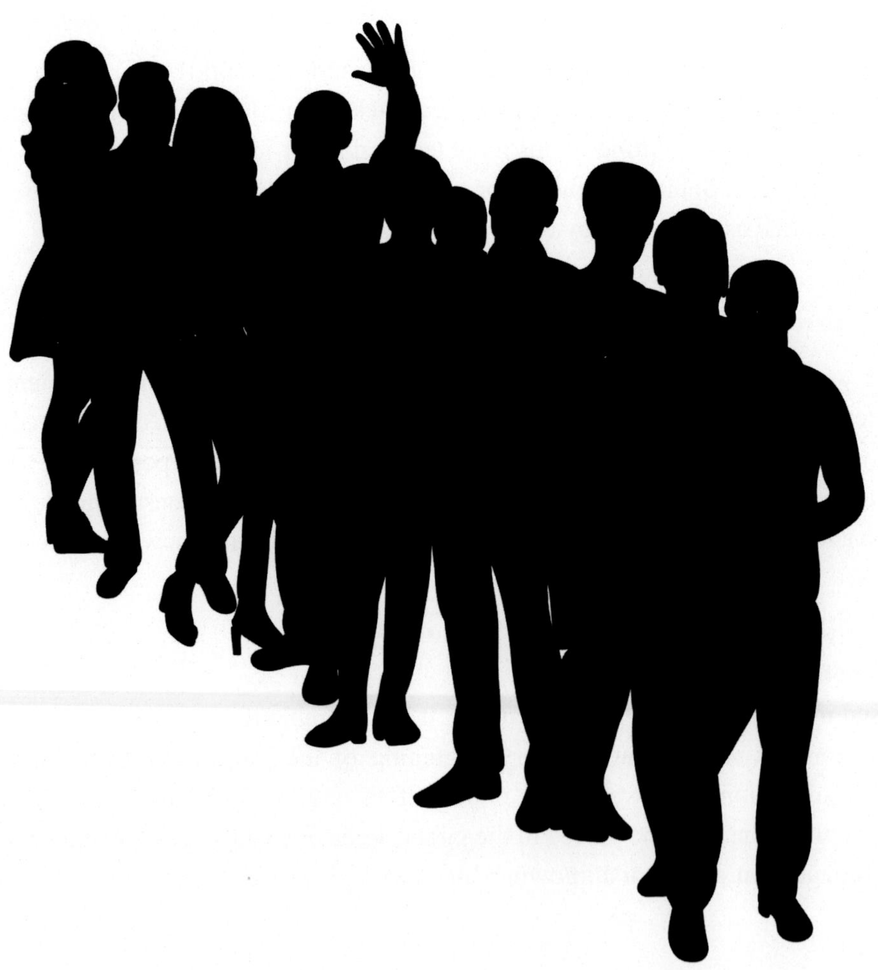

Image Credit: Silhouette of a queue by NadzeyaShanchuk/Shutterstock

In deciding who should be an author on a paper, the team leader must consider who has contributed to particular aspects of the work.

To make the selection process as fair as possible, all people who are involved in a project should be invited to express their expectations concerning authorship and credits on the resulting paper(s) and provide their rationale for being considered as an author.

Some guidelines to consider are as follows:

- You should only include someone as an author if you are able to determine that this project could not have been done without this person's conceptual or technical contribution.
- It is normally the person who is primarily responsible for the project who is named as the first author (This varies between fields; see further details about authorship order below).
- Rarely, two individuals may share that responsibility. Most journals permit a statement that indicates that the first two (or three) authors listed have contributed equally to the publication.
- It is unwise to make promises about authorship in advance. It is best to wait until you know how much each person has actually contributed before authorship is assigned.

Note that authorship policies should also apply to Web-based publications.

In summary, it is important that authorship
- is offered to *all* people who meet the above criteria,
- is *not* offered to people who do not meet the criteria, and
- those offered authorship must accept or decline in writing, and copies of the acceptances and refusals should be retained.

Your institution is likely to have a clear authorship policy which will help you develop and maintain criteria for authorship and prevent or manage authorship disputes. If you are stuck, refer to the research office for assistance.

The International Committee of Medical Journal Editors (ICMJE) [4] provides extensive guidance for managing authorship.

Authorship Order

Authorship order is another potential sticking point. In some disciplines, the order of authors carries meaning. In the sciences, the first and last author positions are the most important, with the student or postdoc who "did the work" usually named as first author, while the group leader is usually named as the last author. If you are conducting interdisciplinary research, it is worthwhile checking the usual practices for author order in the disciplines of your colleagues.

First authorship is often used as a promotion or general career assessment criterion. When deciding on author order, remember that your success as a researcher depends on the success of your team, and that a happy, well-rewarded team is generally the most productive.

While guidelines such as the Vancouver Protocol developed by the ICMJE describe what contributions warrant authorship, they do not provide guidance on determining author order. Various models have been established to assist researchers determine author order on their publications, including those by Beveridge and Morris [5] and Winston [6].

Acknowledgments

Where individuals have made a significant contribution to the project, but do not meet criteria for authorship, then they may be listed as a contributor. Contributors generally have more input than those listed in the acknowledgments.

You should acknowledge funding agencies in your article or report. Acknowledgments can also include those who critically reviewed the drafts but who are not authors, as well as administrative staff who contributed to significant data entry or the preparation of other support material.

Do your very best to avoid authorship disputes. As mentioned in Chapter 3.2 on Collaborations, collaborating researchers should agree on the process of authorship and author order determinations at an early stage in the research project. This process should also be discussed with anyone who joins the group at a later date. So there can be no doubt about it, you should keep a record of these discussions for later reference.

References—Step by Step Guide to the Publication Process

[1] Zinkernagel, R.M., Doherty, P.C., 1973. Journal of Experimental Medicine 138, 1266–1269.
[2] Diedrich, C., 2017. Collaboration in Scientific Writing: One Researcher's Thoughts. http://www.aje.com/en/arc/my-experience-with-scientific-collaboration/.
[3] Committee on Publication Ethics (COPE). https://publicationethics.org/.
[4] International Committee of Medical Journal Editors (ICMJE). http://www.icmje.org/.
[5] Beveridge, C.A., Morris, S.E., 2007. Order of merit. Nature 448, 508.
[6] Winston, R.B., 1985. A suggested procedure for determining order of authorship in research publications. Journal of Counseling and Development 63, 515–518.

Further Reading

American Journal Experts, an academic author services company, provides open access interesting articles about publication. http://www.aje.com/us/.

Bass, E., October 8, 2015. They won a Nobel for what? Why Good Science Communication Counts. The Conversation. http://theconversation.com/they-won-a-nobel-for-what-why-good-science-communication-counts-48722.

Brown, M. J., January 15, 2016. How not to Write about Science. The Conversation. http://theconversation.com/how-not-to-write-about-science-52202.

Chittaranjan, A., April–June 2011. How to write a good abstract for a scientific paper or conference presentation. Indian Journal of Psychiatry, 53 (2): 172–175.

Conte, S. Choosing the Right Journal for your Research. http://www.aje.com/en/arc/choosing-right-journal-your-research/.

Grigston, J., State of Authorship Report: Time and Costs Involved in Publishing Research. http://www.aje.com/en/arc/state-of-authorship-report/.

Jenkins, R., December 11, 2016. Why I Don't Edit Their Rough Drafts. The Chronicle of Higher Education. http://www.chronicle.com/article/Why-I-Don-t-Edit-Their-Rough/238618.

Menachemi, N. and Ginter, P. The Anatomy of an Empirical Research Manuscript Suitable for the Peer-Reviewed Health Administration Literature. http://www.ache.org/pubs/JHM/56-1/ResourceGuide-forAuthors.pdf.

7.3 Next Steps—Promoting Your Publication—and Planning More

> *Get people talking using social media to promote your research….your citation index will rise as a result of tweeting about your journal articles. Look at the journal in a couple of days and you'll see you'll have way more views than the people who haven't used social media.*
>
> **Lupton [1]**

Checklist

(Tick when completed)

- ☐ Sing from the rooftops when your paper comes out
- ☐ Make a media plan with your media office
- ☐ Mention your paper on social media, all channels
- ☐ Update your web profile, including your CV
- ☐ Update the project website
- ☐ Load the paper onto ResearchGate or other academic social platforms
- ☐ Make a presentation plan
- ☐ On to the next paper

When your paper is finally accepted, and it is published, please don't leave it at that, thinking the job is done. Now is the time to cry from the rooftops! This is so important—and so under recognized—it has a chapter on its own.

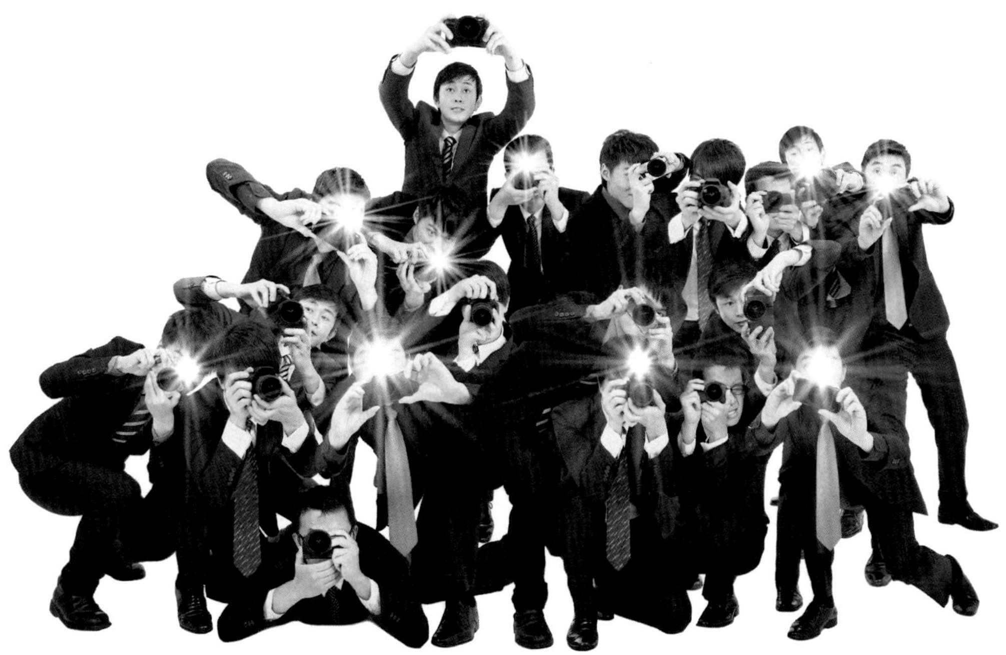

Image Credit: Many photographers by Tom Wang/Shutterstock

Consider the points of interest to the various sectors of your target audience(s). There may be several audiences—your peers, the general public, your stakeholder groups. It is likely they need different messaging. Use Form 7.3.1 Publication Promotion Template on page 371 to help you think through the interests of the different groups.

As a first step, let your institute's media department know the paper is due and the approximate date it will be released. It is their job to promote your work, and they will be glad to be provided with some subject matter, even if it is a nerdy topic. With your help, they will find the correct audience. Take the time to explain the subject to them, what is new and why it matters. Work with them to identify potential internal and external media opportunities. Remember to let them know if there are any restrictions (such as date of embargo) and, important (!) if there is likely to be any form of public outcry.

Together, draft a short press release written in everyday language focusing on newsworthy aspects of your research project. Remember to acknowledge your funding sources, collaborators, and stakeholder relationships (even though this may not be reported or included in any story—at least you have tried).

Later, plan the release strategy with the media office, and identify a point of contact so a quick reaction is possible. There will often be an embargo date for your publication; the media office will want to release the story as soon as it can.

If you expect this story to attract media attention, which might involve you, try to attend media or communication training. It is probably available through your institution. Doing media interviews can be difficult and can go horribly wrong; training will help you prepare properly for the unexpected.

Further Promotion

Advise your funding agency about your publication, and send them a copy. If the media department has prepared a media release then send that to them too, otherwise include a lay summary. They are always glad to see evidence of outcomes from their investments.

Promote on Social Media

There are great opportunities for growing your reputation when you promote your paper on social media.

- Mention it on Twitter, including your institution's Twitter handle so they pick it up and share it.
- You are restricted with characters on Twitter, so mention it again, this time including your collaborating institutions' Twitter handles and a third time with your individual authors so they all pick it up and share it.
- Upload the paper, or its abstract, onto LinkedIn. Tag the individuals and institutions and share.
- Upload it onto SlideShare, remembering the keywords.
- Post it onto Facebook and include a link. Tag the authors and their institutions and share.
- Write about it on your blog, then tweet about the blog to get cross-fertilization.

You will be amazed how many "reads" and "likes" you have had when you get to the end of this process.

Promote Online

Don't forget to put your paper, or its abstract, onto your personal Web profile and on the project website and, of course, add it to your CV (including the electronic version on your Web profile).

Upload it onto ResearchGate, Academia.edu and other academic social platforms where you have a profile.

Email Your Colleagues

Let your colleagues know too. Email your colleagues from previous institutions, and your mentors, past and present, including a link to the paper on your personal profile page, project website, at its home journal or on an academic social platform. This is all about promoting you, so work out which best enhances your reputation!

Share Your Results

Create an opportunity to present internally or include this work in external presentations. Now that you have published, you should make a plan for providing your stakeholder and end-user groups with access to—and appropriate explanation of—the results. If the audience is scientific, you might consider organizing a seminar or lecture. If your stakeholders are members of the general public, explain your results in a newsletter and distribute it promptly.

Present at Scientific Meetings

Scientific meetings are, of course, a valuable way to disseminate and publish findings. Seek opportunities to present to your peers internally and at conferences within your field.

Open Access and Your Institutional Repository

It is becoming more and more common for funding agencies to require that you make publications resulting from projects that they have funded available with "OA"; likewise, there is often an obligation to make your data available.

Consequently, institutions have created institutional repositories which have developed beyond collections of the university's peer-reviewed journal articles and conference proceedings to become collections of all the digital outputs of the university including research data, monographs, and books.

If you are required to, or wish to make your publications OA, and you haven't published in an OA journal, there are some steps available, which can help you meet your obligations. You can either purchase the copyright from a non-OA journal so it can be placed in a public repository, or you can place the final draft version of your non-OA paper in your institutional repository. (Note that sometimes you will not be able to do this until six months post-publication.) Alternatively, you may be able fulfill your obligations by publishing just the abstract and a link to the journal in an OA environment.

This is a field that is complicated and changing rapidly. It is recommended that you seek the advice of your institutional librarian to determine the best way forward.

If you are not restricted, it is a good idea (or may even be compulsory) to also lodge all relevant raw data in an appropriate database such as Genbank, and/or in your institutional repository.

Planning More Publications

When you have submitted your paper, you might be tempted to relax for a while and wait for a response. Try not to do that—it is much better to start the next paper immediately. Many prolific researchers have multiple papers on the go, all the time.

Note that while this is sound advice, you need each paper to stand on its own. You must avoid the problem journal editors see as "salami slicing," the breaking up of a body of work into smaller parts to be published, with the objective of inflating the authors' publication records.

Keep a list of your publication ideas prominently displayed in your workspace so that you are regularly reminded of what you want to achieve this year. When you think of a new idea for a paper, add it to the list.

References—Next Steps—Promoting Your Publication—and Planning More

[1] D. Lupton, University of Sydney research impact: research communication, using social media to promote research. http://libguides.library.usyd.edu.au/c.php?g=508217&p=3475813.

Associated Documents—Next Steps—Promoting Your Publication—and Planning More

7.3.1 Publication Promotion Template

Citation (Authors; Title; Journal; Vol; Issue; Page Numbers OR Authors; Title; Publication Details) (Include URL where possible): Click here to enter text.

What is the background to this publication? Click here to enter text.

What is the purpose of this publication? Click here to enter text.

Abstract: Click here to enter text.

Lay description: Click here to enter text.

Best Contact for this publication: Click here to enter text.

Target Audiences	Do They Care?	Why Should They Care?	What can they do and what can be done to help them to that?	By Whom?	Date Carried Out
Smokers	*Some Yes; Most Ambivalent; Some No.*	*The study shows that smokers are worse off physically, mentally and socially than non-smokers*	*Encourage smokers to join quit support programs, discuss with their GPs – Email abstract to Quitline and other quit-smoking campaigns.*	*Freddy*	*29/03/2012*
GPs	*Most Yes; Some No (too busy)*	*Further evidence to encourage patients to stop smoking – which we assume they are already doing.*	*GPs can be notified of findings – we should email the Abstract to College of GP suggesting circulation to members. Email should include HELPLINE Number.*	*Freddy*	*15/03/2012*

Please supply one sentence quotes or summaries of findings (as many as are suitable): Click here to enter text.

What were the outcomes/impact of this publication (including media, social media, policy change, collaborations, Institute action)? Click here to enter text.

7.4 Documenting Your Research Impact

The software "Publish or Perish" is so named for a very good reason. The adage holds true in all areas of research. Unless you publish, and have a readership, you will soon find you don't have a paid research position.

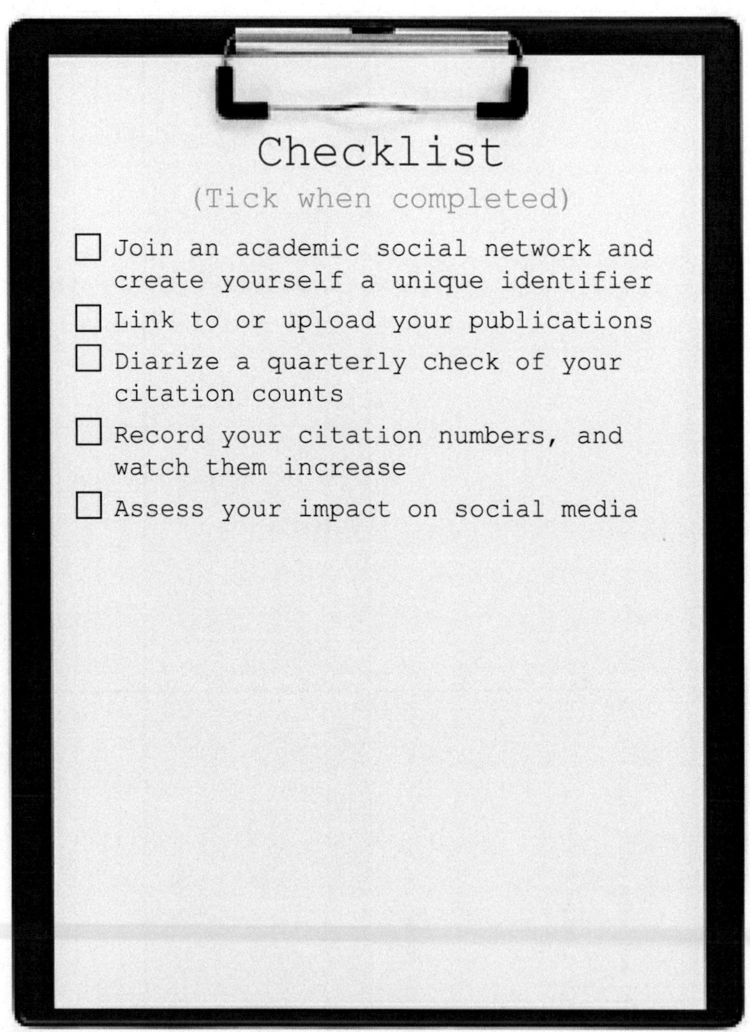

Thinking About Your Research Impact

Research impact is defined by UK Economic and Social Research Council (ESRC) [1] as "the demonstrable contribution that excellent research makes to society and the economy." This can involve "academic impact," "economic and societal impact," or both. ESRC explains that academic impact is "the demonstrable contribution that excellent research makes in shifting understanding and advancing scientific, method, theory and application across and within disciplines." Economic and societal impact is "the demonstrable contribution that excellent research makes to society and the economy, and its benefits to individuals, organizations and/or nations." These are complicated words, but this impact is likely to be what your research career is all about.

Most researchers are good at keeping their CV and list of publications up to date, but there are some who feel that keeping track of citations, or otherwise noting the effects of their research, can be a chore.

Nevertheless, you should be doing it! It is in your interests to document the scholarly impact of your research, to know who is citing your work, and to keep an eye on the consequences of your research. Understanding your impact helps you confirm you are making the impact you want to be making and will allow you to demonstrate it to others.

Be aware that your research impact is wider than your count of citations. Or it should be. While you aim for publications, and for those publications to be read and then cited, the impact of your research will be felt beyond those publications as it adds to knowledge in your field, and/or influences changes in practice.

Your research findings will be presented at your internal meetings, at conference presentations, both spoken and on a poster. Your Web presence, your project newsletters, and your social media posts all make a contribution to the exposure of your research, as do media releases and mentions in publications of either your institution or your funding body. Last, but far from least, is the impact you have when speaking to a lay audience at a fund-raiser or other community gathering. You never know who is reading or listening or how they are going to respond to what you have to say. Don't under-estimate their importance. Keep a note of all these audiences, to both make sure you have covered all bases and to remind you of different promotional avenues for next time.

Processes for evaluating impact are changing very rapidly, indeed. Examples are given on following pages, but you should be able to get the best current advice from your institutional librarians or websites of the larger universities.

Demonstrate Your Scholarly Impact

Until recently, practically no one continuously monitored citations of their work, as it can be very time consuming. This was done only for promotion, new job applications, or for funding bodies that obviously have an interest in the consequences of the research they have paid for.

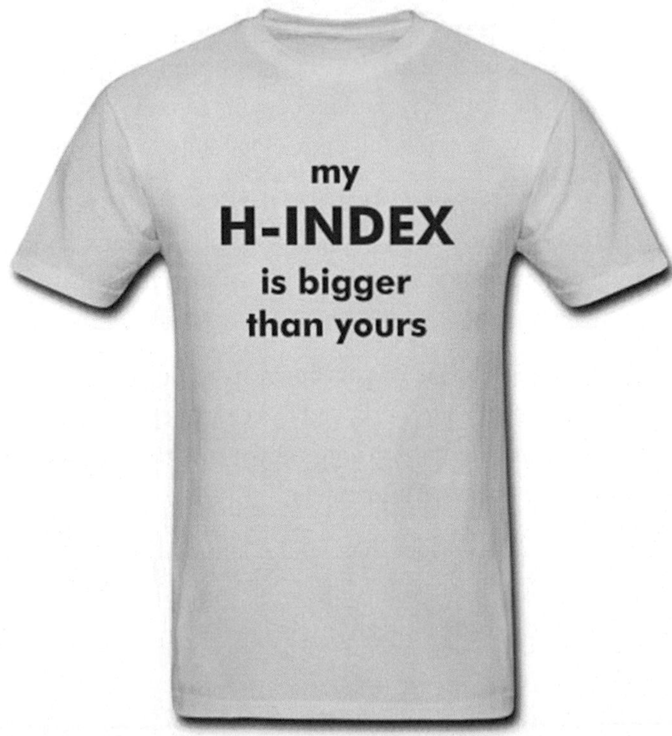

Image Credit: T-shirt available from BitesizeBio.com

Work Out Your h-Index

Now, there are a number of academic social networks including ResearchGate [2], Mendeley [3], and Academia.edu [4] which are dedicated to science and research and allow you to connect, collaborate, and discover scientific publications, jobs, and conferences. They are services, some free, some by subscription, which claim to have many millions of authors. They can provide you with in-depth statistics on who has been reading and citing your work.

You can demonstrate your scholarly impact by working out your "h-index," essentially a measure of "whole career" citation volume, which provides a measure of a person's research impact. The h-index is increasingly being used by universities as a measure of researcher impact, and increases in h-index are being used in assessments for promotion.

Counts of citations and papers have limited meaning unless they can be put into some kind of context. You can use a variety of citation analysis tools for calculating your h-index including Web of Science [5], Google Scholar [6], and Scopus [7] in the context relevant to you.

- Web of Science provides good coverage of both science and non-science subject areas. It is good for finding citations to books (using Cited Reference Search) and collects some citations to non-journal publications such as books, artworks, and newspaper articles.
- Scopus is the largest abstract and citation database of peer-reviewed literature: scientific journals, books, and conference proceedings.
- Google Scholar also tracks citations, but across a much wider range of documents, including books, working papers, and reports, giving you a different perspective on your impact. You can set up a Google Scholar profile for an individual or a group and link this from a website or include the link in an email.

Be warned that these sources index different journals and may give you a very different h-index. For this reason, it is important to always quote your source database.

Another tool is "Publish or Perish" [8], a free software package that generates many impact statistics including h-index, g-index, total cites, average cites, etc.

Manage Your Identity

When you are looking for information about your impact, rather than just using your name, which may be the same or similar to another's, you can create a unique identifier.

Searching for a name can be a hugely important problem, especially for Chinese and Korean authors where there is a limited number of surnames. One particular combination of Chinese family and given name has been seen to generate about 1100 citations in a single year, but the name represented numerous different authors in different fields.

The problem is not restricted to Asian names. It is all too easy for computer-generated systems to create incorrect attributions to people with moderately common names working in a complete different field of study.

The unique identifiers are referred to differently for the different tools: Web of Science has "researcherID," Scopus refers to "author identifier," and ORCID iD is an identifier provided by non-profit organization, ORCID [9], and is used by many journals and granting bodies. You should link your papers to the special identifier, which refers only to you in whichever of these tools you use.

Your institutional librarians are experts in referencing and likely to be able to assist you with learning to document your impact.

Increasing Your Citation Count

University of Leicester [10] identifies additional ways you can use to help maximize your citation count. Some have been mentioned previously, but these are so often overlooked by researchers who depend on them that here they are again. They matter!

Choose Your Title Carefully: It Is the Key to People Finding Your Paper

Longer, more descriptive article titles generally attract more citations. Title (and abstract) words are heavily weighted by search engines, and a keyword-rich title will push your article toward the top. Many people also search using title words, and a good title helps people to make rapid relevance judgments in the few minutes they spend online.

Make Sure You Include Your Institutional Address in the Correct Form

Citation databases extract address information automatically from a paper, indexing each corporate author. You should always cite your address the way your university does, e.g., "University of X, Department of Y," otherwise your paper may be invisible to the league table compilers. Credit has been lost for hundreds of good papers in the past.

Don't Be Too Frugal With Your References

A number of carefully controlled studies have found that papers with longer lists of reference tend to be cited more often. This may seem strange, but there are reasons. People are more likely to notice papers that have cited them and perhaps they reciprocate; and in today's extensively cross-linked digital libraries, the more work you cite, the higher the visibility of your article (most services now have clickable "Cited by" and "Related articles" links).

Submit to a Journal That Is Indexed by the Major Citation Service

Citation services (Web of Science, Scopus, and Google Scholar) are big information factories that index millions of articles each year. They work from lists of "source" journals, only counting citations to these titles. However good your paper, you will not get any citation credit if you publish in a journal that is not one of their sources.

Don't Sell Yourself Short: Go for the Highest Impact Journal You Can

Publishing in a high-impact journal does not of itself guarantee citations, but there is a strong halo effect. Researchers, faced with information overload, increasingly rely on impact factors to filter what they read; papers in high-impact titles tend to attract more citations and sooner. Visibility is key (however see page 354 for another view).

Consider Publishing Your Article in an Open Access Journal

OA is a means of disseminating scholarly research that breaks from the traditional model.

Readers with a Web browser and an internet connection can access the publisher's website without payment or even a library membership. OA translates into more downloads, greater use, and more citations.

Your research funder may insist you make your work OA.

Include a Link in Your Paper to Your Underlying Research Data and Materials

As well as making your paper available to everyone, why not provide details of where your research data are available, allowing other researchers to re-use and build on it—and cite you—in the process? You will be saving them time and effort, so your paper will be very attractive to them.

Deposit a Copy of Your Manuscript in a Digital Repository

Most publishers allow you to archive your submitted manuscript in a subject repository (such as arXiv, RePEC) or an institutional repository. This raises the digital visibility of your paper, increasing the chances that your work will be cited. Many universities mandate you do this, and many funders are now insisting that you do so as a condition of your grant.

Don't Be Shy: Work at Marketing and Promoting Your Paper

Although the research project may be over, the life of your paper has only just begun and there are lots of ways you can help it on its way. Actively promoting and marketing your work will pay big dividends in terms of building your networks of contact and influence: and extra citations! (see Chapter 7.3).

Use Social Media to Build Your Network of Influence

A good tip is to use social media tools to communicate to an international audience of potential authors through your blog, Twitter, or Mendeley account. Evidence is accumulating that all forms of social media power downloads and citations, especially when a direct link to your paper is included.

Reclaim Any Misspelled Citations, Why Lose Credit?

Authors sometimes make errors when compiling their list of references. If they misspell your name, you may lose a citation. If propagated by other researchers, you lose even more. The Web of Science offers a feedback service that allows you to reclaim any misspelled citations.

Manage Your Online Identity and Get Personal Credit for Your Work

As mentioned above, there are millions of journal authors around the world, many with similar names to yours. The major citation services have developed unique researcher IDs to deal with this problem and to ensure that someone searching for your publications finds all of them in one place—and no one else's. You need to actively manage your online identity or risk losing credit for your research.

A Note About Self-citation

Self-citation is sometimes necessary and unavoidable, but also can be exploited in an unethical way, both by authors and shady editors. Some systems distinguish between self-citations and citations by others because of this problem of inflated impact factor due to self-citation.

Some journal editors have been caught out commissioning multiple review papers for publication in their journal, which cited every paper published in their journal. This practice grossly inflated the citation impact of their journal. These journals have been banned from the Thomson Reuters impact factor calculations as a result. Impact factors can be "gamed" by authors and editors.

Demonstrating Wider Impacts

As mentioned earlier in this chapter, your research impact is more than a count of your citations. Demonstrating wider research impacts, those outside academic journals is becoming increasingly important, and new tools are emerging to help you show just that.

"Altmetrics" is an umbrella term for new metrics based on social media engagement. You can report the number of times your paper has been tweeted, mentioned in a blog, or socially bookmarked by using a tool in academic social networks such as Mendeley.

Altimetric [11] is the current market leader in this field. A free bookmarklet that collects statistics on interest in each article from Twitter, Facebook, science blogs, mainstream news outlets, and many more sources, Altimetric points out that knowing who's talking about your research and what they're saying is crucial in today's increasingly online world. Ensuring your work is being accurately represented and interpreted, as well as getting to the right people at the right time, are important factors in broadening its impact.

References—Documenting Your Impact

[1] Economic and Social Research Council, 2017. What is Impact? http://www.esrc.ac.uk/research/impact-toolkit/what-is-impact/.
[2] ResearchGate. https://www.researchgate.net/.
[3] Mendeley. https://www.mendeley.com.

[4] Academia.edu. https://www.academia.edu/.
[5] Web of Science. https://www.webofknowledge.com.
[6] Google Scholar. https://scholar.google.com/.
[7] Scopus. https://www.elsevier.com/solutions/scopus.
[8] Publish or Perish. http://www.harzing.com/resources/publish-or-perish.
[9] ORCID. https://orcid.org.
[10] University of Leicester Library Research Services, Twelve simple ways to maximize citation count. https://www2.le.ac.uk/library/downloads/research-services/maximise-your-citations.
[11] Altimetric. https://www.altmetric.com/audience/researchers/.

7.5 Facilitating Translation—Helping Your Research Move Into Practice

Johnny conducted a thorough systematic review into patient outcomes following a particular type of surgery practiced in the health service where he worked. There was clear evidence that method (b) was much better for the patients than methods (a) or (c) and that this should be followed up.

What did he do about it? Effectively nothing. He wrote a report published in the in-house journal and moved on to the next topic. There weren't any outcomes because no one read it. No one read it because no one knew about it. What a waste!

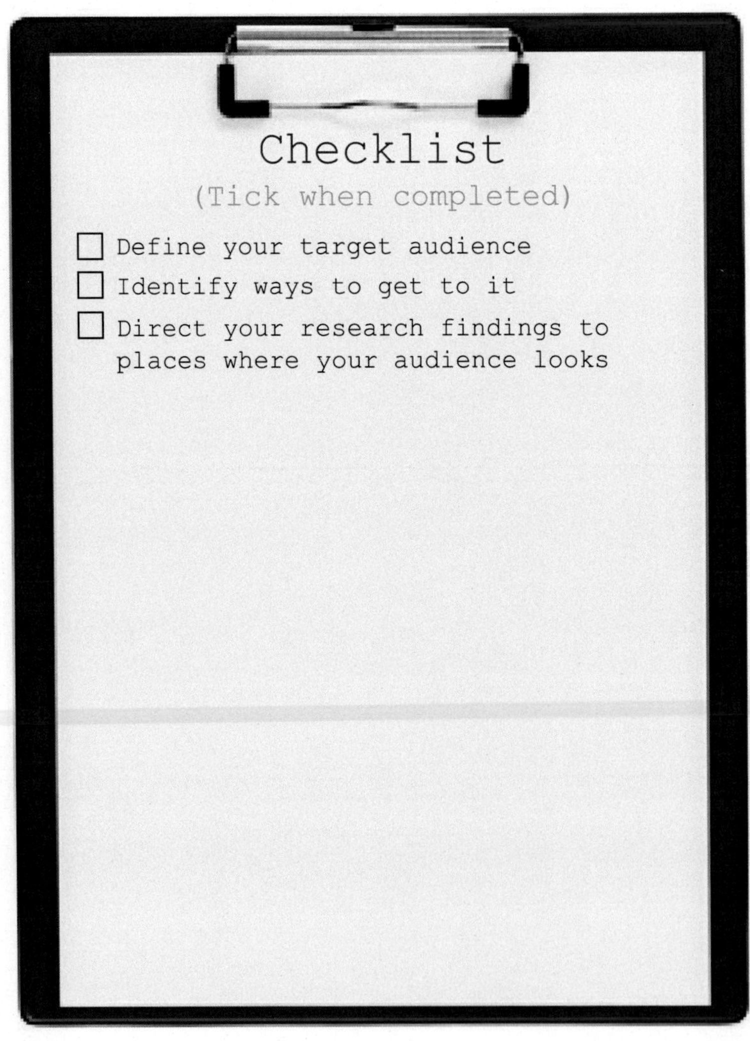

It is more than likely that you are doing the research because you want to find a newer or better way to do something, or you want to understand a mechanism that no one understands yet. You want to make a difference.

Let's assume you have found an answer to your questions. The number one aim is usually to get your work published, but it doesn't, or shouldn't, stop there.

This comes back to the advice expressed elsewhere in Define Your Target Audience, Research Dissemination and Communication. Every time the message is the same: you need to communicate, communicate, and again communicate.

If you want someone to know about it, tell them. Seek them out and get them to listen. Sell the story about *how* and *why* your research—your methodology, your machine, your plan—should be translated into practice. It takes a bit of effort to change someone from doing what they have always done to a new way. If the reasons are explained well, and the benefits are pointed out clearly, you will get their attention.

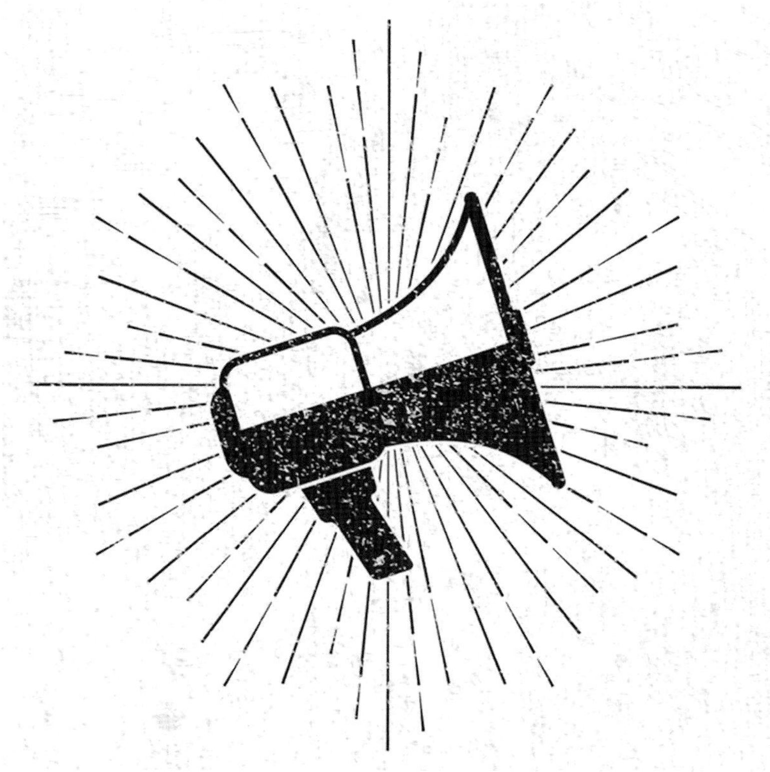

Image Credit: Vintage megaphone by mhatzapa/Shutterstock

7 RESEARCH DISSEMINATION

Direct your story to the listener's perspective, not yours. They will be interested in the following:

- Credibility
- Cost-effectiveness
- Time-effectiveness
- Efficiency and efficacy
- Evidence

In addition to publication in appropriate journals, think of the following:

- Writing an opinion piece
- Presenting at internal research meetings
- Presenting at conferences
- Drawing attention via general media

Think of the places where you dream about seeing your findings either presented, or in practice—and do something about it. It is you who is in the driver's seat here. This is <u>your</u> subject.

7.6 Commercializing Your Research Findings

Bessie and her team made a discovery that led to changing the process for manufacturing a new drug. Unfortunately, she presented some of her findings at a conference before she applied to patent her invention. The patent application was rejected. The drug could still be developed using her process, but she and her institution lost its ownership and control of usage—and potential royalties.

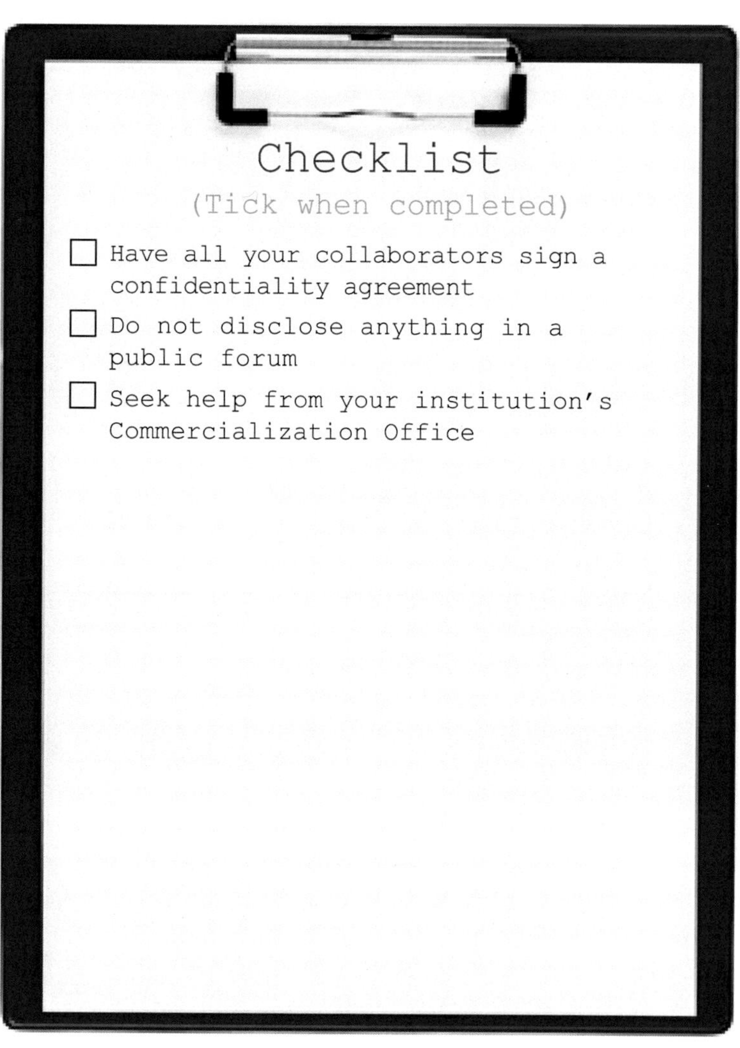

7 RESEARCH DISSEMINATION

Commercializing your research finding is a big step and you need to start planning early. It is easy to make a mistake which could accidentally make it impossible for you to patent your invention.

Commercialization is the process of managing the transfer of research knowledge to the place where it becomes an application in the broad marketplace. The knowledge might be a research outcome or a skill; it might result in the development of a product, a technology, service or business, a community development program, or consulting activities. With any luck, commercialization will result in economic returns (perhaps sufficient to fund your continued research) or translation of your research into real products. Universities will aim for commercialization that benefits the common good.

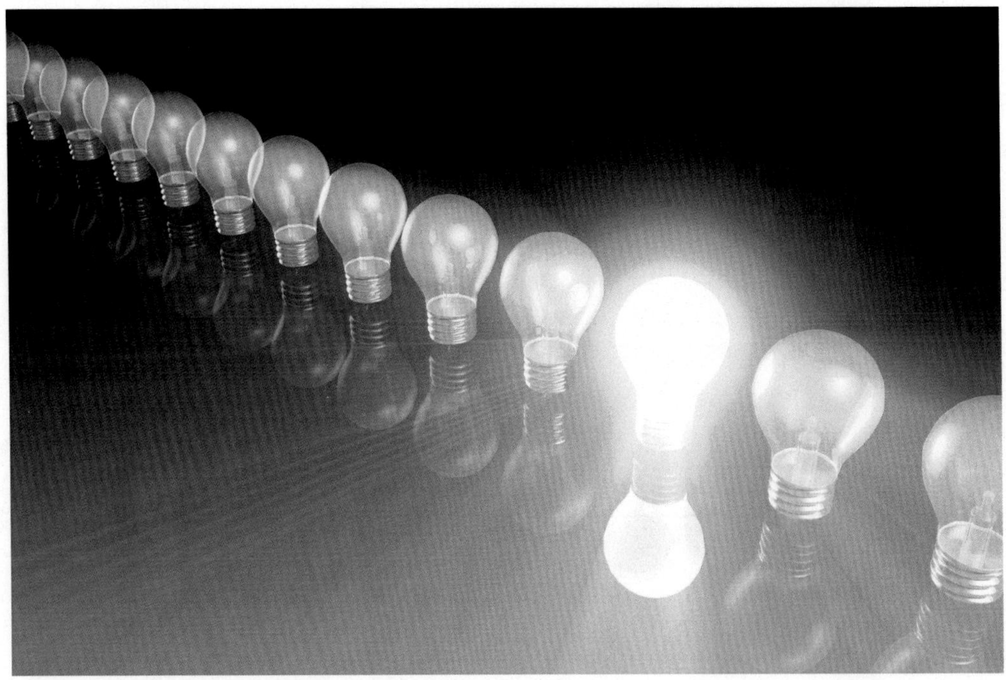

Image Credit: Original Idea by Kentoh/Shutterstock

Commercialization is not easy though; the process is almost always difficult. Very few innovations go on to become a major commercial success. In their book *Research Technology Management (1997)* Stevens and Burley [1] estimate that there will be only one successful business outcome for every 3000 raw ideas. About 300 are disclosed to a commercialization office. From these, about 125 or less are taken forward to be commercialized and result in nine early-stage developments. These lead to four major developments, about two product launches, and ultimately just one successful business.

You will definitely need the help of experts at your institution for commercialization, but you must have taken the first steps yourself. You will need evidence that this is your idea and your invention. If you have followed the practices outlined in this book, you should have all you need to be able to patent your work.

As mentioned in Chapter 4.3 on Agreements, if you are intending to lodge a patent application *you must not disclose the invention publicly before lodging the application*. Public demonstration, sale, or public discussion of the invention may well invalidate the patent application. Any discussions with your colleagues or partners must be on a confidential basis, and they must have signed a confidentiality agreement.

Detailed assistance with commercialization is beyond the scope of this book, but it should be noted that commercialization and/or patent protection can take a very long time. It can also take a lot of money. There are many stages of the commercialization process once research and discovery has led you to what appears to be a viable product.

The evaluation stage is the first big hurdle, and you should think about these questions before taking the idea to the University Commercialization Office. Evaluation involves assessment of the following:

- Can the IP be protected?
- Who are the competitors?
- Who are the end users?
- What is the size of the market?
- What is the time to market?
- How much funding is required?

Some Ways Your Intellectual Property Can Be Protected

Some ways to protect your IP for commercialization might include the following types of registrations. These descriptions, modified from those of the Future Leaders Research Program [2] are somewhat technical but provide a brief explanation or background for expressions you might expect to hear.

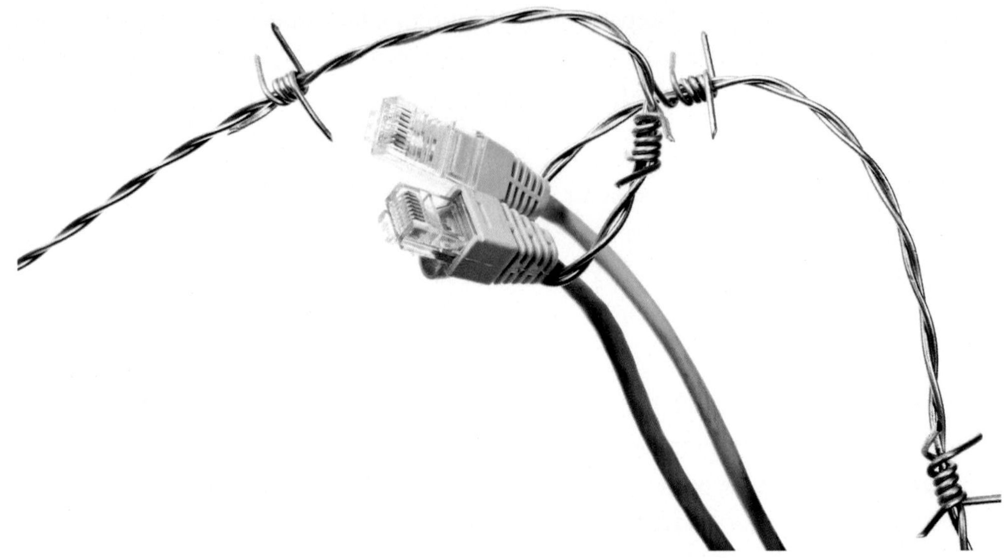

Image Credit: Ethernet cable with barbed wire by 1001nights/iStock

Design Registration

Design registration protects a design of manufactured goods which has not previously been known or applied. Design registration might be registration of the shape, configuration, pattern, and/or ornamentation which give the goods a unique appearance; however, it does not include the feel of the product, the materials it is constructed from or its function.

Registered Trademark

Trademarks can be an identifying word, picture, logo, sound, or smell (or a combination of these) used to distinguish the goods and services of a trader from others. Trademarks are used to associate a certain quality and image with goods and services. Consequently, a trademark can become an important means of maintaining goodwill. Once a trademark is registered, the owner has the exclusive right to use it within the country where it is registered and for the goods and services for which it is registered. Note that it is not strictly necessary to register a trademark, as a trademark can be established merely by using it and becoming well known.

Copyright Law

Copyright law provides incentives for creators to invest their time, talent, and other resources in creating material from which society benefits. In return for the creation of material, creators are granted limited monopolies to exploit and control their work.

Copyright protects against the unauthorized reproduction of original artistic, literary, musical, or dramatic work. It protects the expression of the ideas of the author, not the ideas themselves. It should be noted that copyright applies to computer software, and that copyright initially vests in the creator of the code, Ownership may also be covered by other agreements, such as employment contracts or research contracts.

Plant Breeders' Rights

Plant Breeders' Rights (PBRs) are used to protect new varieties of plants that are distinguishable, uniform, and stable. A PBR is legally enforceable and gives you, the owner, exclusive rights to commercially use it, sell it, direct the production, sale, and distribution of it, and receive royalties from the sale of plants.

In many countries PBR lasts for up to 25 years for trees and vines and 20 years for other species. To be eligible for protection, the new variety must be shown to be distinct, uniform, and stable. In a comparative trial the variety must be clearly distinguishable from any other variety, the existence of which is a matter of common knowledge.

In Australia, for example, a new variety may be sold for up to 12 months in Australia, and 4 years overseas, yet still remain eligible for PBRs. These times may be different in other countries. The rights do not cover the use of a grower's crop (the grower does not have to pay a royalty on the crop produced) nor do they extend to retention by growers of seed for the production of another crop or the use of the variety in plant breeding.

Circuit Layout Rights

Circuit layout rights automatically protect original layout designs for integrated circuits and computer chips for a defined period up to 15 or 20 years, depending on your country's legislation. These rights are based on copyright law principles but are a separate, unique form of protection. The owner of an original circuit layout has exclusive right to do the following:

- Copy or authorize the copying of the layout in a material form
- Make integrated circuits from the layout
- Exploit it commercially

Commercial exploitation may occur by importation, sale, hire, or distribution of a layout or an integrated circuit made according to the layout.

References—Commercialization

[1] Stevens, G.A., Burley, J., 1997. Research Technology Management 40 (3), 16–27.
[2] Future Research Leaders Program. http://www.frlp.edu.au/.

8 RESEARCH INTEGRITY AND RESPONSIBLE CONDUCT OF RESEARCH

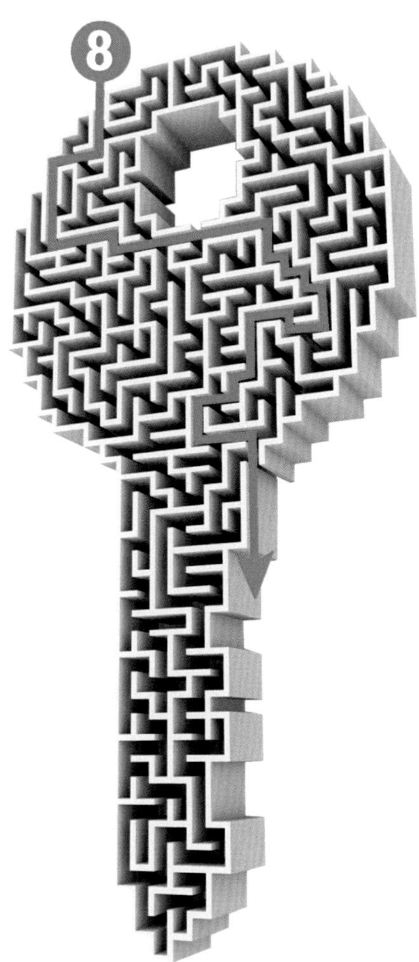

8.1 Introduction to Research Ethics

High-profile cases of research misconduct include the following:

- *Jon Sudbø—who created 900 fictitious patients*
- *Luk Van Parijs—who falsified data in a paper, several unpublished manuscripts and in grant applications*
- *Geoffrey Chang—whose faulty software led to incorrect results*

You don't want to be joining the list!

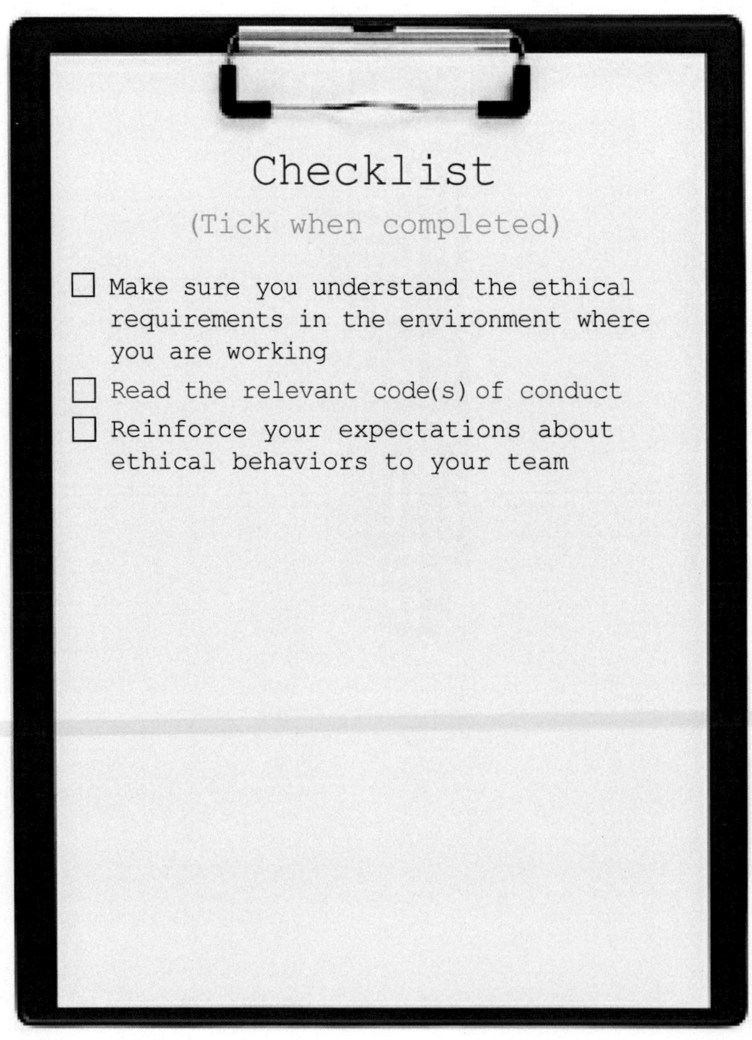

The broad area of research ethics covers the behaviors of researchers toward their research subjects, one another, their funding bodies and, indeed, the general public.

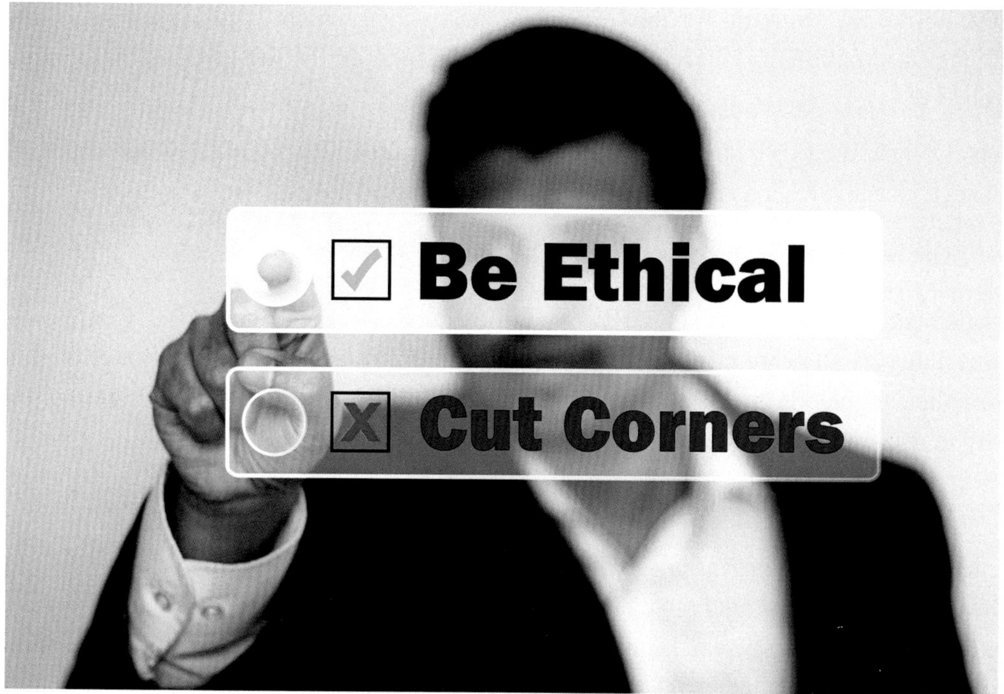

Image Credit: Choosing to be ethical instead of cutting corners by Harish Marnad/Shutterstock

With respect to people and animals in research, good ethical behavior ensures that the people and animals are treated appropriately. This includes maintaining privacy and confidentiality and avoiding distress.

With respect to other members of the research community, we need to consider ethics as it applies to the following:

- Authorship
- Content ownership
- Conflict of interest

and work to prevent the following:

- Plagiarism
- Research fraud
- Submission of the same research to more than one publication

8 RESEARCH INTEGRITY AND RESPONSIBLE CONDUCT OF RESEARCH

It is not surprising that approaches to responsible research and research ethics differ around the world. This can lead to difficulties and misunderstandings in international collaborations, where you must aim to maintain the standards of the more vigilant country. To make it more difficult, unlike the situation for intellectual property (IP), which is governed by a range of agreements internationally, there are no comparable treaties for the responsible conduct of research.

Fortunately, there are two bodies of work that aim to make researchers and governments conduct and manage research responsibly, both locally and on a global basis:

- The Singapore Statement on Research Integrity [1].

This statement was developed in 2010 by participants at the second World Conference on Research Integrity. It represents the first international effort to encourage the development of unified policies, guidelines, and codes of conduct, with the long-range goal of fostering greater integrity in research worldwide.

- The OECD Guide [2].

This international document was produced in 2009 by the Organization for Economic Cooperation and Development (OECD) Global Science Forum. This OECD guide describes the core principles that should underpin any research misconduct investigation and includes agreed definitions of research misconduct and a practical guide for conducting investigations into research misconduct in international collaborative research projects.

This guide recommends that any agreement for collaborative research involving people from more than one country should include mention of good practice in research and describe the principles, standards, and procedures for any investigation of allegations of research misconduct within the project. It recommends that the collaborative agreement for the project should name appropriate experienced individuals who would be responsible for implementing these requirements, should they be needed.

8.2 Ethics Requirements in Human and Animal Research

An engineering study investigating the success, or otherwise, of a new type of machinery experienced a substantial delay when it was found that the necessary ethics approvals had not been obtained. How could research about machinery have ethics implications? The investigators were asking employees about the new machine, but data collection included collecting their names and duration of their employment in the factory (personal information).

Collecting personal information = approval required.

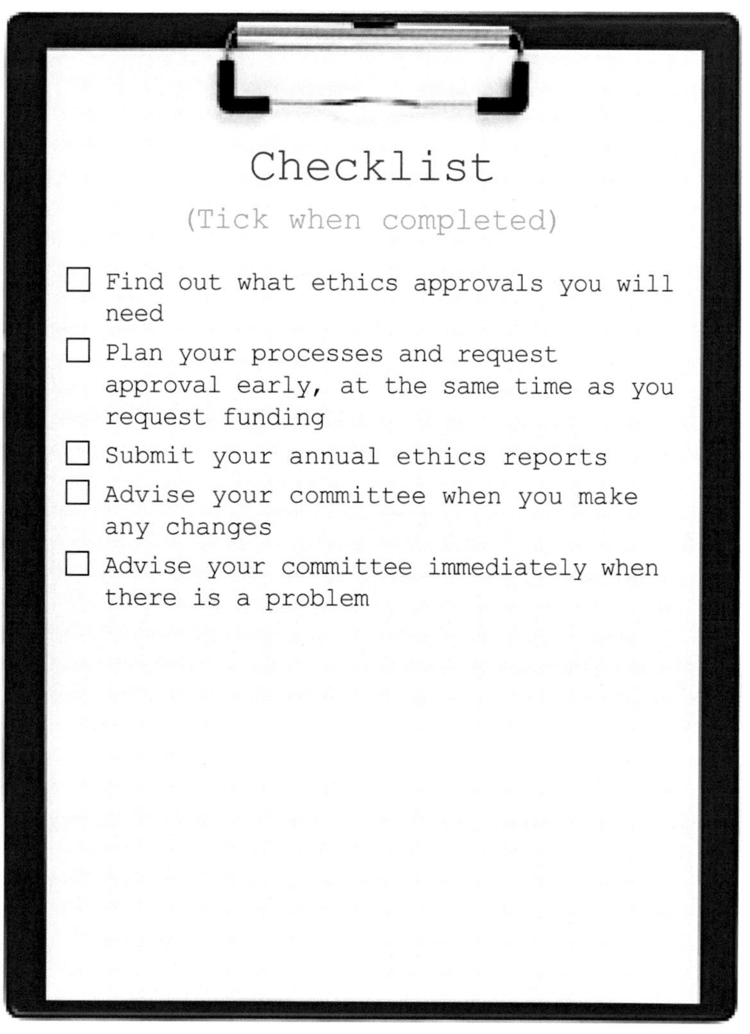

8 RESEARCH INTEGRITY AND RESPONSIBLE CONDUCT OF RESEARCH

Sound ethics and good research practice go hand in hand.

There are no exceptions for needing research ethics approval for projects involving humans or animals: if you haven't got appropriate approvals for your research, it shouldn't start. If it does, you will find that you won't be able to publish your research.

It is alarmingly common for researchers to overlook their need for ethics approval. Perhaps they think ethics approval is only for health research. They are genuinely surprised that approval is necessary <u>any time</u> personal information is to be collected.

Society now regulates interactions between researchers and people because, quite simply, people and animals have been unduly harmed by research in the past.

Research involving human subjects—whether gathering information, administering tests; collecting tissue, blood, or other body fluids; or using archived material where the subject is identified—requires appropriate demonstration of respect for the people involved. The ethical principles underlying this are now well described and accepted, but historically, they follow in the wake of a record of failure which no modern day researcher of integrity could support.

In most countries, researchers must also consider and comply with the regulations regarding the use of animals in research and the appropriate use of chemical and biological agents.

All institutions that receive funding from governments are likely to be required to follow statutory codes of practice for the use of human subjects and the use of animals in research. They must also set up, or at least have a formal relationship with, appropriately constituted ethics committees that review all research at their institutions before it starts, while it is underway, and at the end of the project.

Best practice research requires you to include working toward ethics approval in your research planning. You must be able to identify any potential risks involved in your planned research and have in place mechanisms to protect research subjects and your research colleagues for any project that involves the following:

- Human subjects
- The use of animals
- The use of chemical or biological agents, which could affect humans or the environment
- Importation of plant materials

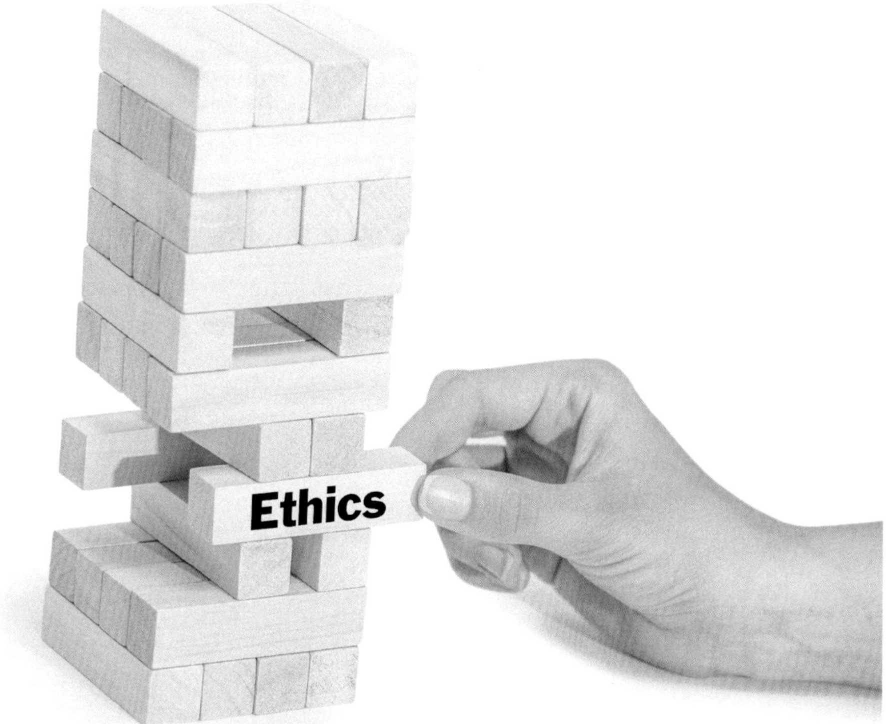

Image Credit: Ethics plus tower from wooden blocks by Ruslan Ivantsov/Shutterstock

Ethics Approvals Take Time—Plan for Delays

Ethical and biosafety review committees usually have a high workload, and each application needs to be carefully considered. It should be no surprise, then, that you can take a long time to obtain ethics or biosafety approval; this can lead to a delay of the start of your project.

Try to avoid delays by lodging your application for ethics or biosafety clearance at the same time as you submit your grant application. If you do this, and receive your approval, you will not only be able to make a start on preliminary work, but you will also be able to begin your project as soon as the funding agreement has been signed.

If your research is going to use human subjects, you must meet the requirements of the ethics committee or institutional review board (IRB) for protection of your participants' rights and well-being. Your research must meet the ethics/IRB guidelines in your state or country. You must have processes for obtaining and appropriately documenting participant consent, comply with the rules for protecting your participants' privacy, and obtain the IRB's approval for your research before you begin your research.

If you don't get your ethics right, you will get nowhere. The ethics committee has, quite justifiably, enormous power over you, so you need to keep them happy. Get it right, and keep it right.

If you are having a difficulty getting something approved by the ethics committee, ask to attend their meeting. There is nothing like a face-to-face conversation for sorting out problems.

During the life of your project you may be required to maintain documentation on your research processes and outcomes for the IRB's inspection, and you may need to present an annual report.

You might feel that all of this is slowing your progress, but failure to comply can shut down your research program, and that delay will be costly to both your project and your reputation.

The best advice is to keep the ethics committee on side. It's easy really. In summary:

- Submit your applications in plenty of time, and make sure they are complete
- Always advise the committee when you plan to make a change
- Remember to provide your annual reports, and on time
- *Never* let your approvals expire

Ethical Research for Indigenous Peoples

All Indigenous peoples have inherent rights, including the right to self-determination. Treat them as you would do the rest of us, but aim to tread even more carefully as there may often be pitfalls where you weren't expecting them. Your principles for ethical research involving Indigenous peoples should be founded on the respect for those rights we should all be afforded, including rights to full and fair participation in any processes, projects and activities that impact on them, and the right to control and maintain their culture and heritage.

It is essential that Indigenous people are full participants in research projects that concern them, share an understanding of the aims and methods of the research, and share the results of this work.

At every stage, research with and about Indigenous peoples must be founded on a process of meaningful engagement and reciprocity between the researcher and the Indigenous people. It should also be recognized that there is no sharp distinction between researchers and Indigenous people. Indigenous people are also researchers, and all participants must be regarded as equal partners in a research engagement.

There will often be special ethics requirements and even special ethics committees for research involving Indigenous people. See Chapter 4.12 for information about recruitment of Indigenous people. Again, see Chapter 4.12 for further information.

Ethical Research in Culturally and Linguistically Diverse Communities

The same principles and courtesies as for research for Indigenous people should apply to any research specifically within culturally and linguistically diverse populations.

8.3 Breaches of Ethics and Research Misconduct

A high-profile international example of research misconduct that continues to jeopardize the reputation of research is the case of Andrew Wakefield and the measles, mumps, and rubella (MMR) vaccine. In 1998, Wakefield et al. [3] published an article that implied there is a link between the MMR vaccine and a "new syndrome" of autism and bowel disease.

In the decade following the paper's release, subsequent studies found no evidence of a link between the MMR vaccine and autism. Following claims that the data reported in the 1998 paper were falsified, several subsequent investigations proved the data to be false. The paper was retracted in 2010. Despite the retraction, the fear of a potential link between the MMR vaccine and autism rapidly spread around the world; the ramifications of this paper continue and parents still question the risks of vaccinating their children against MMR today.

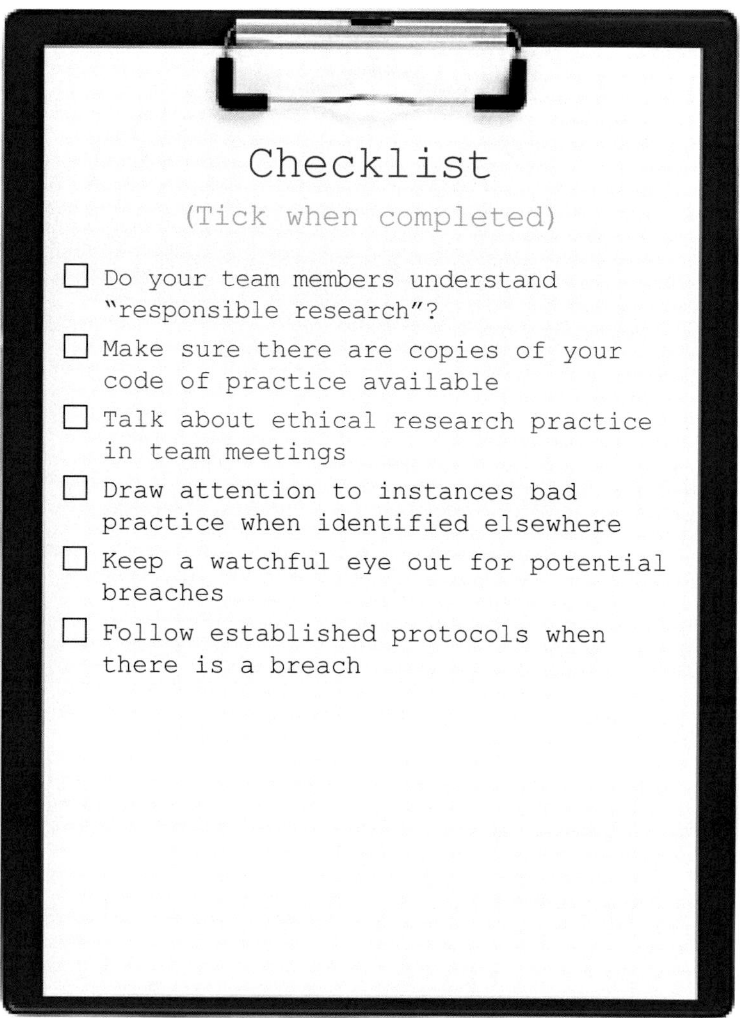
Checklist
(Tick when completed)
☐ Do your team members understand "responsible research"?
☐ Make sure there are copies of your code of practice available
☐ Talk about ethical research practice in team meetings
☐ Draw attention to instances bad practice when identified elsewhere
☐ Keep a watchful eye out for potential breaches
☐ Follow established protocols when there is a breach

8 RESEARCH INTEGRITY AND RESPONSIBLE CONDUCT OF RESEARCH

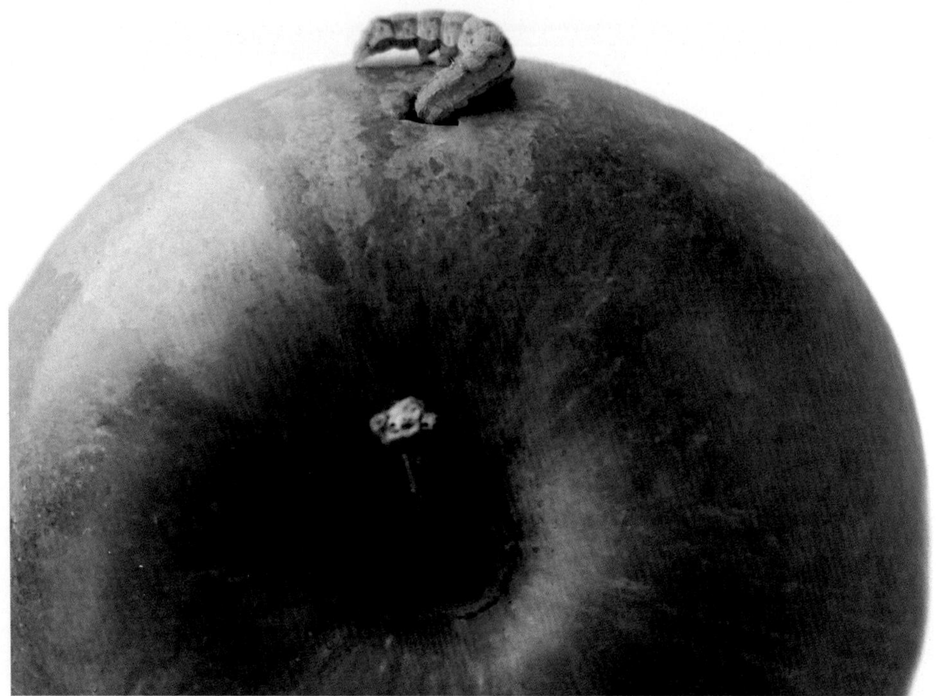

Image Credit: Caterpillar on Red Apple by AlexD75/iStock

Maintaining high research standards is a shared responsibility for research institutions, researchers, and funding agencies. Institutions have the primary responsibility for managing concerns or complaints about the conduct of research for which they are responsible and for investigating concerns, complaints, or allegations of breaches of research standards. They are required to do the following:

- Promote a culture that encourages and rewards responsible research practice
- Develop, implement, and review processes that comply with their research standards
- Establish processes to allow people to submit formal complaints, knowing that their complaints will be treated confidentially and sensitively, and without adverse consequences
- Regularly review their processes

It is not all up to the institutions. All researchers should ensure that their research conduct and practice reflects their institution's principles.

Breaches of Research Standards

A "breach" is defined as behavior by a researcher or researchers that fails to meet the principles or responsibilities of the research standards, or fails to comply with relevant policies or legislation, and may refer to a single breach or multiple breaches.

Some examples of breaches of research standards are as follows:

- Not meeting required general research standards
  - Conducting human or animal research without ethics approval
  - Not conducting the research in the manner that had been approved
  - Conducting research without the approvals, permits, or licenses that were required
  - Misusing research funds
- Risking the safety of human participants or the well-being of animals or the environment
- Fabrication, falsification, or plagiarism
  - Fabricating research data or source material
  - Willfully concealing or falsifying research data or source material
  - Plagiarizing someone else's work
  - Publishing the same results in more than one place without acknowledging that you have done so
  - Using false information or misrepresentation to obtain funding
  - Concealing or assisting with breaches of the standards by others
- Record keeping
  - Failing to keep research records, and/or inappropriately destroying research records, research data, or source material
- Supervision
  - Failing to provide adequate guidance or mentorship for researchers or research trainees under your supervision

- Authorship
  - Failing to fairly acknowledge the contributions of others
  - Misleading allocation of authorship, including failing to offer authorship to those who qualify, or awarding authorship to those who do not meet the requirements
- Conflicts of interest
  - Failing to disclose and manage conflicts of interest

A breach of research ethics is serious, sometimes very serious. There needs to be a protocol for dealing with the situation. In cases of a serious breach, the head of department will need to be called in immediately and advised of this potential reputational risk to the institution.

Breaches occur on a spectrum, from minor to major. Major breaches would typically require investigation; some minor breaches can be addressed more informally. The minor end of the spectrum includes, for example, administrative errors and clerical errors or oversights due to careless practice. At the major end of the spectrum are practices of a more serious nature, such as falsification, fabrication, and plagiarism, widely referred to in codes as "research misconduct."

Whether minor or major, breaches of research standards must be acknowledged and fixed. This is particularly so if inaccurate data have been published and are contributing wrong information to the body of knowledge in a field.

Unfortunately there is not one universally agreed definition of research misconduct. Some international research codes refer only to breaches or behaviors that are not in line with good research practice. International research codes of conduct stress that misconduct does not include either differences of opinion or honest differences in judgment in management of the research project.

Research Misconduct

Allegations of misconduct in research are made from time to time. A prompt and effective response is required in each case. All affected parties must be treated fairly and the situation remedied, and appropriate steps should be taken to maintain public confidence in research. In many cases, minor matters are handled entirely within institutions.

The 2011 version of the Australian Code for Responsible Conduct of Research [4] noted that more serious matters have been treated in a variety of ways, lacking consistency and public acceptance. Studies in Australia, the United States, and the United Kingdom [5–7], indicate a higher rate of unreported offenses than you might expect. Commentators have suggested that there is an increasing number of serious offenses as the result of commercial and other pressures for success, particularly in areas such as biotechnology and medicine.

A complaint that a researcher has acted irresponsibly requires a response that may include the following steps:

- A discreet investigation
- A formal inquiry
- The imposition of a sanction or penalty
- Actions to remedy the situation
- Advice to expert groups and public statements as appropriate

In most cases the response will not require all these steps, for example, when the complaint cannot be sustained or when the researcher concedes. However, an allegation of serious misconduct that may attract a significant penalty, if proven, will require all the steps and great care in handling.

The process outlined above resembles the process for almost all complaints of misconduct. However, research is complex and requires great care to get it right because of the number of interested parties and the extent to which a serious offense may lead to collateral damage. Interested parties range from the employing institution to professional journals and funding bodies; those affected by the offense range from colleagues and students to the professions and public confidence in research.

The number of serious misconduct cases may be increasing, but it is still small, and so is the number of people with experience in managing such cases. Therefore, it is important that processes are consistent and that there is a repository of experiences and advice to guide future cases.

References—Responsible Conduct of Research and Research Integrity

[1] Singapore Statement on Research Integrity. http://www.singaporestatement.org.
[2] OECD, 2009. Facilitating International Research Misconduct Investigations in International Collaborative Research Projects: A Practical Guide. http://www.oecd.org/dataoecd/42/34/42770261.pdf.

[3] Wakefield, A.J., Murch, S.H., Anthony, A., Linnell, J., Casson, D.M., Malik, M., Berelowitz, M., Dhillon, A.P., Thomson, M.A., Harvey, P., Valentine, A., Davies, S.E., Walker-Smith, J.A., 1998. Ileallymphoidnodular hyperplasia, nonspecific colitis, and pervasive developmental disorder in children. The Lancet 351, 637641 (since retracted).
[4] Australian Code for the Responsible Conduct of Research, 2007. https://www.nhmrc.gov.au/_files_nhmrc/file/research/research-integrity/r39_australian_code_responsible_conduct_research_150811.pdf.
[5] Geggie, D., 2001. A survey of newly appointed consultants' attitudes towards research fraud. Journal of Medical Ethics 27 (5), 344–346.
[6] Henry, D.A., Kerridge, I.H., Hill, S.R., McNeill, P.M., Doran, E., Newby, D.A., Henderson, K.M., Maguire, J., Stokes, B.J., Macdonald, G.J., Day, R.O., 2005. Medical specialists and pharmaceutical industry sponsored research: a survey of the Australian experience. Medical Journal of Australia 182, 557.
[7] Martinson, B.C., Anderson, M.S., de Vries, R., 2005. Scientists behaving badly. Nature 435, 737–738.

Further Reading

From Integrity in Scientific Research: Creating an Environment That Promotes Responsible Conduct (2002) a Report of the US National Academies (p. 5). http://www.nap.edu/books/0309084792/html/.

Guidelines for Ethical Research in Australian Indigenous Studies 2012. http://aiatsis.gov.au/sites/default/files/docs/research-and-guides/ethics/GERAIS.pdf.

National Reference Center for Bioethics Literature. https://bioethics.georgetown.edu/.

Office for Human Research Protections, Department of Health and Human Services (DHHS). http://www.hhs.gov/ohrp.

U.S. Food and Drug Administration (FDA): Clinical Trials and Human Subject Protection. https://www.fda.gov/ScienceResearch/SpecialTopics/RunningClinicalTrials/default.htm.

The European Science Foundation's European Code of Conduct for Research Integrity (2017) can be found at: http://www.allea.org/wp-content/uploads/2017/03/ALLEA-European-Code-of-Conduct-for-Research-Integrity-2017-1.pdf.

The International Committee of Medical Journal Editors (http://www.icmje.org/) and Committee on Publication Ethics (COPE) (http://publicationethics.org/) also have a range of resources for researchers interested in publication ethics.

The Office of Research Integrity (ORI) in the US Department of Health and Human Services has a number of downloadable resources for responsible conduct of research. https://ori.hhs.gov/.

There are many books, articles, and commentaries on contemporary research ethics and integrity in the governance of research. Other references include the following:

Brown, M.J.I., 2017. How to Quickly Spot Dodgy Science. The Conversation. https://theconversation.com/how-to-quickly-spot-dodgy-science-65160.

Chong, S. and Normile, D., 2006. Stem cells. How young Korean researchers helped unearth a scandal. Science, 311: 2225.

Gerber, P., 2006. What can we learn from the Hwang and Sudbo affairs? Medical Journal of Australia, 184: 632, 635. http://www.mja.com.au/public/issues/184_12_190606/ger10184_fm.html.

Maher, B., 2010. Sabotage! Nature, 467: 516, 518.

Martinson, B. C., Anderson M. S. and de Vries, R., 2005. Scientists behaving badly. Nature, 435: 737, 738.

Miller, G., 2006. A Scientist's Nightmare: Software problems lead to five retractions. Science, 314: 18, 561, 857.

8.4 Handling an Adverse Event

A mailing went out to all participants from a study investigating coronary heart disease. The letter was received by the widow of Mr. Brown, a man who had recently died, and Mrs. Brown was very upset that "…you are still harassing him. Don't you know he is dead?"

This is an example of a real-life situation. The study managers must be quick to update their records and to apologize to Mrs. Brown to prevent further damage.

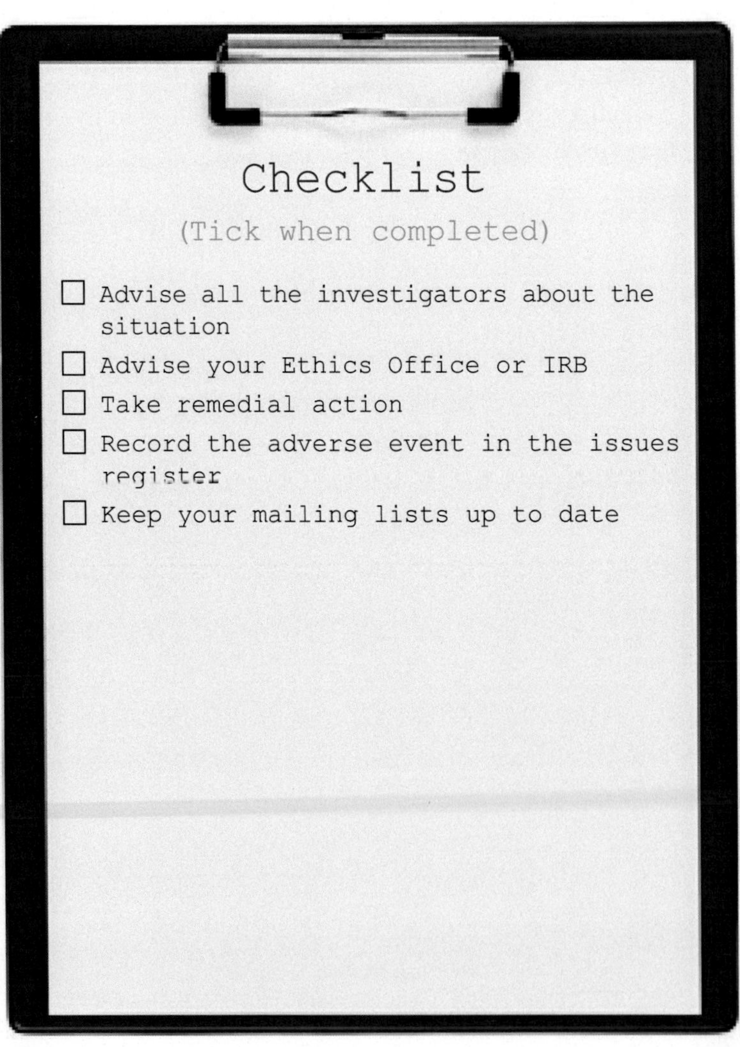

Your project is planned, and you have all the necessary approvals. Now your research is underway. Unfortunately, in spite of all your good planning, things can still go wrong. You might experience an "adverse event."

Note that this section is not about serious adverse events as they apply to clinical trials. An adverse event in research is a situation where something has happened, which has caused distress to a human or animal. This event will usually be unexpected, and, one would hope, inadvertent. It is an event that is contrary to the intention of the human or animal ethics approval for the project.

Adverse events in health care are defined as unintended and sometimes harmful incidents in which harm resulted to a person receiving health care. They include infections, falls resulting in injuries, or occurrences associated with the use of a medicine, vaccine or medical device (collectively known as therapeutic goods).

If you have an adverse event, it must be reported and recorded appropriately, and you must do your best to rectify the situation.

You should have a protocol in place for handling an adverse event so that all team members know what to do.

Steps will include the following:

- Advise all the investigators about the situation
- Advise your ethics office or IRB
- Take remedial action
- Record the adverse event in the issues register

Where the adverse event involved a human study participant, the adequate response should be personal and as prompt as possible. It should be undertaken by a senior person. The response might be a phone call or a letter, and should offer an explanation for the event, and steps that have been taken to rectify the situation. You should allow the aggrieved person to explain their cause(s) of concern and listen politely. When the opportunity arises, try to explain the background.

The most important thing here is the quick response. A grievance left to fester can quickly get out of control and become a much bigger problem than it should be. This can cause reputational risk to the investigators, the project, the institution, and even the funding body.

Your ethics authority may require further action, which again must be take place as soon as possible.

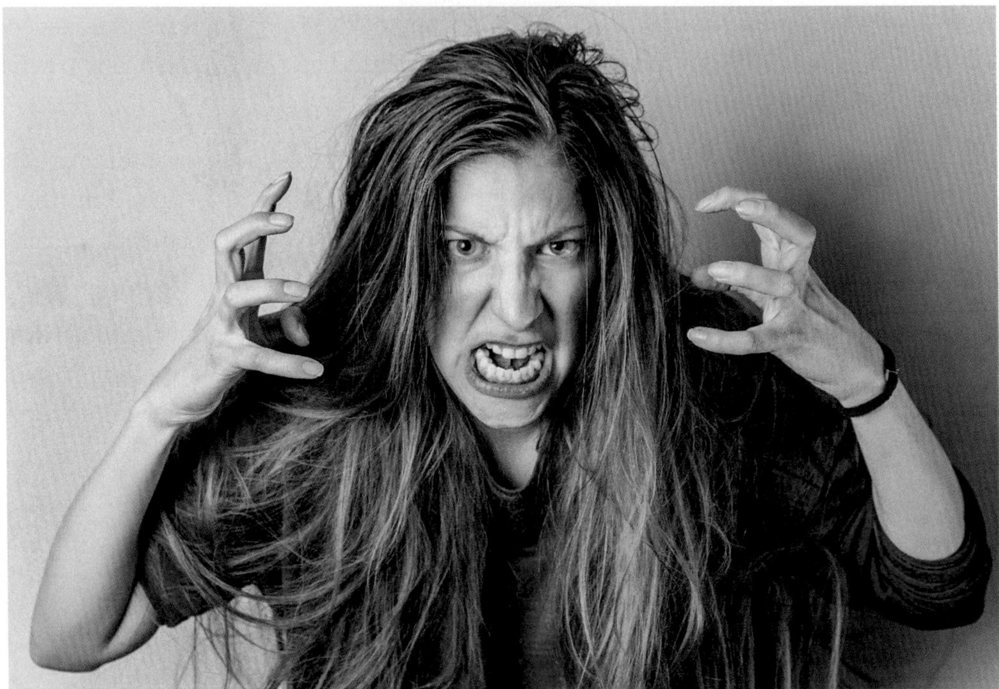

Image Credit: Angry woman yelling by TeodorLazarev/Shutterstock

Dealing With a Distressed Participant

The case study at the beginning of this chapter is a situation that happens all too often in medical research. Although your view might be that the widow is being unreasonable, particularly as you haven't been advised that Mr. Brown is dead, and you wonder how a letter can hurt her, she is truly upset. Apologize on the phone, write a letter and take steps to ensure that no more letters go to Mr. Brown. In your letter, thank Mrs. Brown for the contribution she and her husband have made to better understanding this disease, and point to the outcomes that will benefit people in the future. This might bring Mrs. Brown around.

This second case study gives a variation on the theme:

A mailing went to people known to have cancer, inviting them to take part in a research project. Names on the list had been provided by the cancer registry, so there was confidence that all would be well. There is the potential for four things (at least) to go wrong here:

- *A person on the list might have died*
- *The person might not have been told he has cancer*

- *As the recipient is likely to be unwell, someone else might open the letter. They might not know he has cancer, thus a confidentiality is broken*
- *A name might be on the list incorrectly*

Again, receipt of this letter has the potential to cause serious upset. In addition, to the steps outlined above for Mrs. Brown, in any of these cases a senior investigator would need to liaise with the cancer registry to find out what went wrong in the processes and to amend them so the situation does not arise again.

It is possible that, as in the cases noted above, you could find yourself in a situation when a study participant, or the family member of a potential study participant, is caused distress by the processes of your research project. This is particularly so when you are working in health, and where the disease or condition you are investigating commonly causes severe ill health or death. As noted above, you might inadvertently cause distress by doing the following:

- Sending mail to someone who has died or who is terminally ill
- Asking questions of a personal nature which cause offense, or
- Sending mail to someone when other family members don't know about their condition

If you do find yourself dealing with a distressed participant, listen carefully to everything the person has to say, keep notes of the conversation, and do your best to provide reassurance. You may be able to provide a satisfactory explanation, although this is sometimes better done by a letter or other written communication, which will be read when the person is calmer.

It is probably best not to admit guilt, and certainly best not to pass the blame onto someone else.

If the person requires you to take some further action, undertake to follow up on that request and report back. Follow up accordingly. Ignore a member of the public at your peril!

A situation nipped in the bud quickly is much better than one left to grow its own personality.

Where appropriate, report this situation to your ethics committee/IRB or a higher authority within your institution, as this is the sort of situation that can cause a lot of reputational damage.

In all cases of this nature, ensure you keep a record of the call or the written complaint in your study records, as well as your follow-up actions.

Some steps you can take to avoid these situations are spelled out below.

Keep Your Lists Up-to-Date

Make sure you update your contact lists. Update your records promptly if mail is returned, or marked "do not contact." If they have taken the trouble to return the mail, then they mean they don't want to be contacted.

If you obtain your lists from third parties, update them regularly.

Review Your Questions With Consumers

It is wise to test your questions with real people from outside your research environment. You will be surprised at the different perspectives lay people have from you. When you work in medical research, you get inured to conversations about topics "normal" people don't cover in their conversations.

Keep the Mail Private

If there is a chance that this a matter your participant might prefer to keep confidential, give consideration to sending your project mail in plain envelopes, marked only with the postal address.

8.5 Privacy and Confidentiality in Research

Billy was a research assistant tasked with recruiting patients to a study in a hospital. She collected names and contact information and a brief personal history on a paper questionnaire. Unfortunately, she attracted unwelcome attention by both interviewing the patients in an open waiting room, then leaving the completed forms lying about for anyone to see.

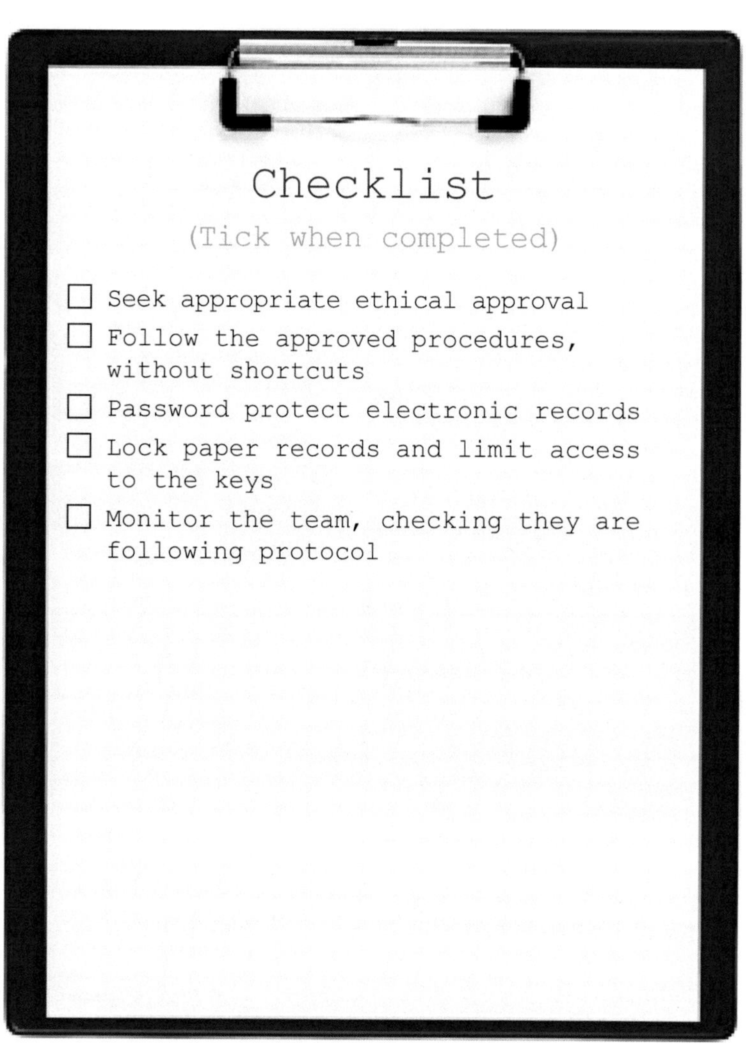

Your obligation to preserve confidentiality comes from the principle of respect for people. As a researcher, you are required to do the following:

- Keep in confidence all data obtained from study subjects where an assurance of confidentiality has been given.
- Ensure your practices for storage and maintenance allow for the privacy of individuals and the confidentiality of research materials.
- Maintain confidentiality in all communications (oral and written) about your research.

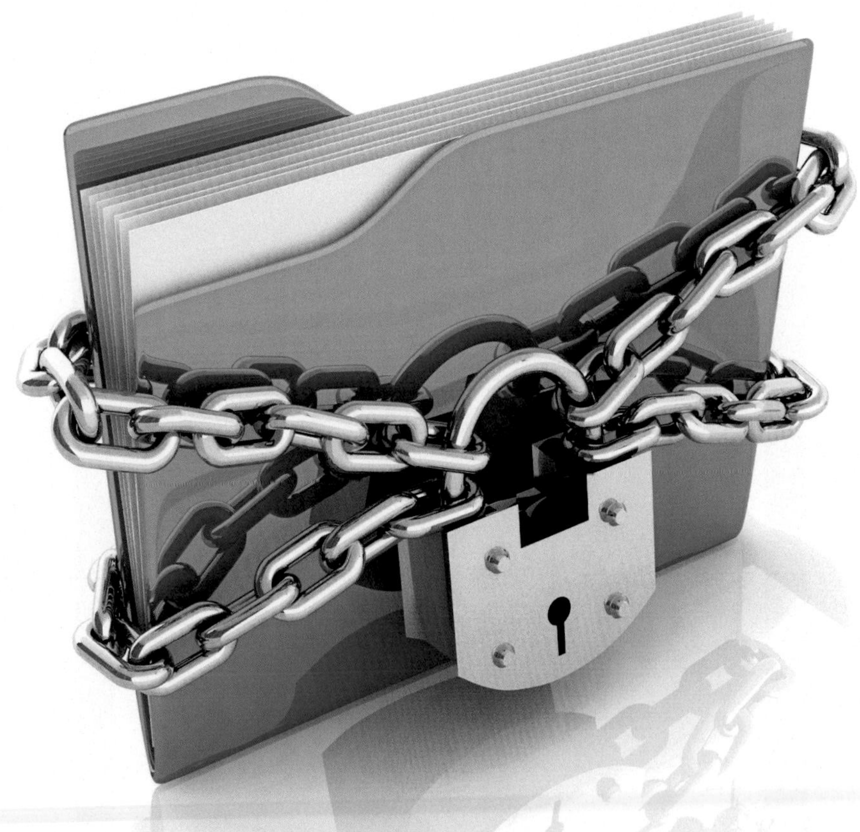

Image Credit: Folder locked by chains by Valentin Drull/Shutterstock

See the section on confidentiality agreements in Chapter 4.3 on Agreements. These agreements for your staff and/or your collaborators should be developed in consultation with your institution.

What is the Difference Between Private Information and Confidential Information?

Essentially, privacy is about people. Confidentiality is about data.

In more detail:

Privacy is your control over the extent, timing, and circumstances of sharing oneself (physically, behaviorally, or intellectually) with others. For example, a person may not want to be seen entering a place that might stigmatize them, such as a drug counseling center, which is clearly identified by signs on the front of the building.

In research, the evaluation of privacy also involves consideration of how the researcher accesses information from, or about, potential participants in the recruitment process. Ethics committees consider strategies to protect the privacy of potential participants and access to their private information.

Privacy is
- about people,
- a sense of being in control of access that others have to information about ourselves,
- a right to be protected, and
- in the eye of the participant, not of the researcher or the ethics committee.

Confidentiality relates to the treatment of information that an individual has disclosed in a relationship of trust. There is an expectation that the information will not be divulged to others without permission, or in ways that are inconsistent with the understanding of the original disclosure.

During the informed consent process, if applicable, subjects must be informed of the precautions that will be taken to protect the confidentiality of the data. They must also be informed of the parties who will or may have access (for example, the research team, or in the United States, say, the FDA, or OHRP). This process will allow the subjects to decide about the adequacy of the protections and the acceptability of the possible release of private information to the interested parties.

Confidentiality is
- about identifiable data,
- an extension of privacy, and
- about the maintenance of identifiable data and who has access to it.

What Do Researchers Need to Understand?

Ethics committees or IRBs are there to decide, on a project-by-project basis, whether the proposed projects have built in adequate provisions to protect the privacy of study subjects and to maintain the confidentiality of their identifiable data. They will be concerned about each segment of the research, from recruitment to long-term storage of the data.

When they make their assessments, they need your ethics application to include information on how you are going to manage both privacy and confidentiality.

With regard to privacy, they will consider the following:

- The needs of the proposed subject population. The cultural norms of the proposed subject population are relevant, as some cultures are more private than others.
- The ages of the proposed subject population. There may be differences in privacy preferences for people of different ages (e.g., teenagers may be less inclined to share than older adults).
- Your proposed methods for both identification and contact of research subjects:
    - Acceptable recruitment methods include the following:
        - Advertisements, notices, and/or media
        - An introductory letter requesting colleagues to distribute to eligible individuals; interested individuals are invited to contact the researcher
        - Direct contact of qualifying patients by primary care staff to determine interest
    - Unacceptable methods for recruitment include the following:
        - Searching through medical records or an existing database for qualified subjects; then having a researcher who has had no previous contact with the potential subjects try to recruit them. This method violates the individual's privacy.
        - Recruiting subjects immediately prior to a sensitive or invasive procedure (e.g., in pre-op room).
        - Retaining sensitive information for possible future studies without the consent of those who either failed to qualify for the current study, or who refused to participate.
- The sensitivity of the information being collected. The greater the sensitivity, the greater the need for privacy.

- The method of data collection (e.g., focus group, individual interview, covert observation). They will consider whether subjects will feel comfortable providing the information by your proposed method.
- Whether the individual would have an expectation of privacy (e.g., in a chat room for patients with breast cancer), if you plan passive observation of the subjects.
- Whether you will collect private information from someone about a third party (e.g., in the case of mental illness, or if there has been substance abuse in a family). Here, they will consider whether informed consent should be obtained from the third party.

As already mentioned, privacy is in the eye of the participant, not the researcher or the IRB.

Maintaining Confidentiality

Your protocols should always be designed to minimize the need to collect and retain identifiable information about your research subjects. If possible, you should collect your data anonymously, or else remove any potential identifiers as soon as possible. Furthermore, you should only grant anyone access to your research data when they really "need to know," then make that access a "minimum necessary" standard.

Where it is necessary to collect and maintain identifiable data, your ethics committee or IRB will ensure that your protocol includes the necessary safeguards to maintain both the confidentiality of identifiable data and the data security, at a level appropriate to the degree of risk from disclosure.

Bottom line: If you are going to collect confidential data, or if release of the data has the potential to cause harm, you should incorporate measures to maintain confidentiality into your protocol.

8.6 Other Ethical Considerations

Chief investigator A accepted a long-term position in China. He wrote to say that the project would continue under the supervision of another researcher who had not been named on the initial grant. This was not acceptable to the funding institution. The request was declined and the funding withdrawn.

Chief investigator B planned six months' maternity leave. She wrote to request that the project should continue under her remote management, with an occasional visit and the guidance of her own supervisor. This was acceptable to the funding institution because it remained her project and would continue under her management.

Checklist

(Tick when completed)

- ☐ Check with your institution before accepting funding from an organization which could pose an ethical dilemma or conflict of interest
- ☐ Make sure you have followed ethical publishing guidelines
- ☐ Make sure you haven't asked for the same funding from multiple sources without disclosure
- ☐ Advise your funding body if you want to make changes to your objectives
- ☐ Diarize your reporting requirements
- ☐ Have you applied for all the permits you need?
- ☐ Do you have the correct arrangements for disposal of hazardous waste?

Ethical Funding

While it is usually very hard work attracting sufficient funding, there could be occasions when you might be better off turning down funds which could be made available to you. It would be clear to most, for example, that people working in cancer research should not accept funding from the tobacco industry. The matter might be more difficult to decide upon if the potential donor made its profits from gambling or alcohol or fast food. You will need to weigh up the benefits of accepting against the disadvantages.

Public funding for research comes with an expectation that it will make a contribution to society, while, equally, research sponsored and funded by private or corporate interests can come with the expectations of fulfilling sponsor or industry goals. If you were to be offered funding from, say, a pharmaceutical company with an interest in the outcomes of your research, this could lead you to a situation where there might be conflict of interest, either real or perceived. Here you have to be very careful of the terms under which you would proceed. Funding from a company selling armaments could also cause a problem, and might be contrary to the policies of your institution.

There are, of course, occasions where these situations could be perfectly acceptable, and there are ways in which you can ensure that your research is entirely independent. As a researcher, you should be aware of the circumstances under which the funding would be accepted so that you can make an informed decision. You should be aware of any funding sources, which are judged by society and/or your university to be inappropriate.

Ethical Obligations in Publishing

Your publications demonstrate your research activities and allow your peers and potential funders to evaluate your contribution to your discipline. They can also attract other researchers to investigate your work, either as peers and colleagues, or as potential new recruits. In many respects you have the freedom to publish however, and whatever you see fit, but you must pay attention to the ethical responsibilities of publication, for which there are both institutional and individual responsibilities.

The Australian Code of Practice [1], which provides a good example of principles common in the developed world, specifies that your institution is responsible for the following:

- Promoting the responsible publication and dissemination of research findings
- Protecting confidentiality and managing IP
- Supporting communication of research findings to the wider public

As has been mentioned in the previous chapters in this section on research ethics, you, as a researcher should do the following:

- Disseminate all your research findings
- Ensure the accuracy of reporting of your results
- Cite other authors' publications appropriately and accurately
- Disclose multiple submissions of research findings
- Obtain permission for republishing
- Disclose your research support accurately
- Register your clinical trials
- Manage confidentiality appropriately
- Responsibly communicate your research findings to the wider public after
    - findings have been tested through peer review;
    - you have informed those directly impacted by the research; and
    - outcomes of research with a strong commercial element have been presented to a stock exchange or financial body before any public release.

You also need to ensure that all contributors to your project have sufficient access to the results so that they can judge whether the results are accurate and your interpretation is not biased.

You can see that many of these responsibilities are shared between researchers and their institutions.

The Obligations of a Grant Recipient

When you accept funding for your project, that funding comes with a set of obligations to your funding body and your institution.

It is generally accepted that you will not seek or receive funds for the same research project from multiple sources, unless this forms part of the award, or has been agreed in writing at the award stage. If you are offered funding for the same work from two bodies, you must disclose this. It is most likely that you will have to relinquish one grant, but with open communication with both parties, it might be possible to negotiate a reallocation of funds which could allow you to extend the aims of your project.

Likewise, you may modify the aims and objectives of your approved research project with appropriate reasons and approvals from your funding body, provided you remain within budget, but you have an obligation not to use any amount of your grant for purposes not related to the research project.

Funding is usually awarded for a specific research project and nominated personnel. If at any time during the term of funding a named chief investigator changes institution or ceases to contribute to the funded work, your institution and the funding sponsor should be notified. This, of course, applies to you as well, and is something that must be thought about carefully before you consider changing institution.

There is an expectation that personnel be appointed at the correct level and that personnel costs are expected to have the first call on research funds.

You will be expected to meet any reporting requirements specific to your grant program.

You must acknowledge your funding support wherever possible, in publications and presentations. You should refer to the funding agreement for your project to ascertain the correct format for acknowledging the funding source.

You should also advise your funding body about any significant delays to your project. A common, and unavoidable, delay is the consequence of parental leave taken by key team members. Even though it is unavoidable, the funding body should be informed.

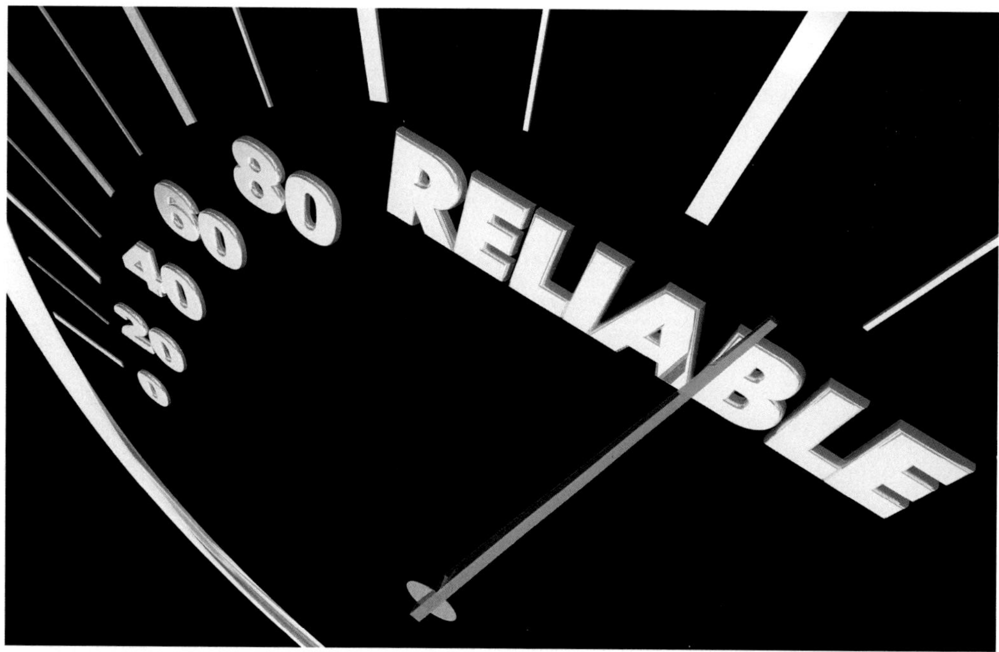

Image Credit: Reliable illustration by IQoncept/Shutterstock

Legal Requirements in Research

Requirements for ethical practices for research with humans or animals have been discussed (see Chapter 8.2); however, you must also be aware of the need for legal compliance in research.

You will need to be sure to be following appropriate practices and procedures for a wide range of areas including the following:

- Importation or exportation of biological material
- Use of, or creation of, genetically modified material
- Research involving radiation, including ionizing and non-ionizing radiation, such as radioisotopes, X-rays, UV light, and lasers
- Use of hazardous materials, such as dangerous chemicals

Importantly, if you or your team members disregard compliance procedures you may risk the safety of human participants, or the well-being of animals or the environment. This would be viewed as research misconduct.

Matters relating to employment law are also of great consequence. Not only must your staff be employed legally (no special "off-the-record" deals) and then treated fairly, (something, no doubt, managed via your Human Resources Department), but you must ensure that staff from other countries or international colleagues, who have come to work short-term on your project, hold appropriate visas for their stay.

References—Other Ethical Considerations

[1] Australian Code for the Responsible Conduct of Research. , 2007. https://www.nhmrc.gov.au/_files_nhmrc/file/research/research-integrity/r39_australian_code_responsible_conduct_research_150811.pdf.

8.7 Conflicts of Interest

Poor Management of Perceived Conflict

A man was employed in the organization of which his wife was Chairman. Whether or not there was access to inside information or special treatment, there was definitely a perception among the staff that there was at least a potential conflict of interest.

The leadership of the organization, though of course aware of the situation, chose not to manage it. In the end, the potential conflict became a reality, and resulted in significant distress and substantial reputational damage to the organization.

Good Management of Potential Conflict

A committee made up of ten senior researchers meets to decide collectively on the allocation of grant funding for the coming year. The individuals must be careful to declare a conflict of interest with anyone who might be from their same institution, or who is a collaborator or works with a collaborator. This necessitates the conflicted committee member(s) to absent themselves from the room for the individual discussion on each application for which they are conflicted.

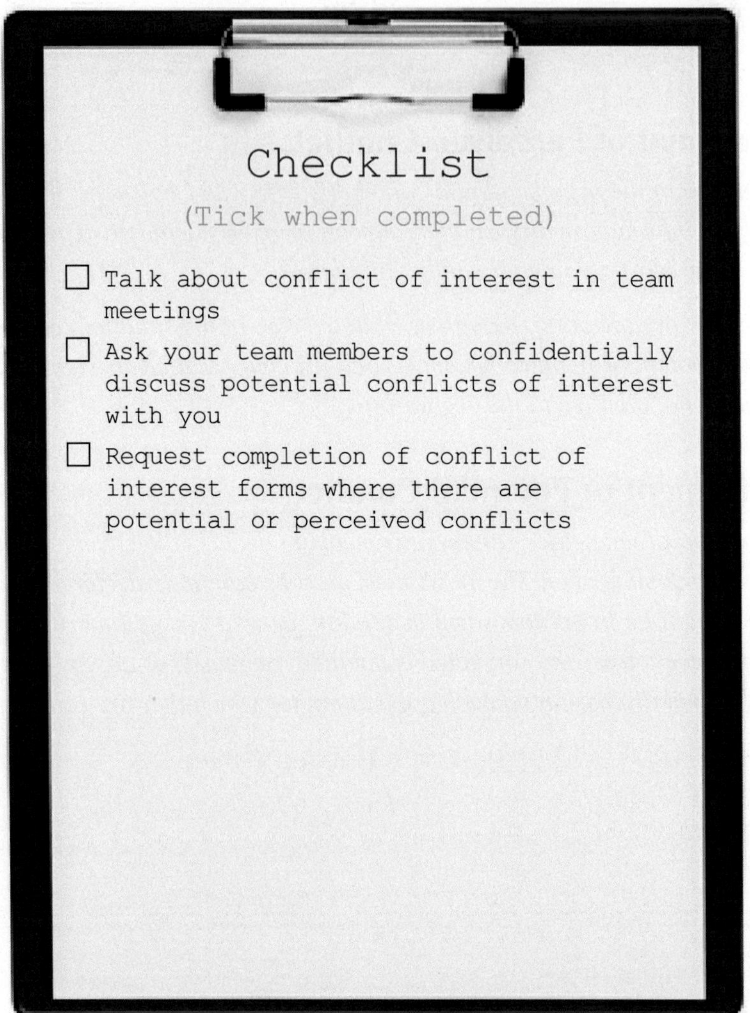
Checklist
(Tick when completed)
☐ Talk about conflict of interest in team meetings
☐ Ask your team members to confidentially discuss potential conflicts of interest with you
☐ Request completion of conflict of interest forms where there are potential or perceived conflicts

A conflict of interest in research occurs when the private interests of a researcher interfere, or appear to interfere, with the performance of their work. As described in many guidelines, conflicts of interest can be actual, perceived, or potential:

- An *actual* conflict of interest involves a direct conflict between a [researcher's] current duties and responsibilities and existing private interests.
- A *perceived* or apparent conflict of interest can exist where it could be perceived, or appears, that a [researcher's] private interests could improperly influence the performance of their duties—whether or not this is in fact the case.
- A *potential* conflict of interest arises where a [researcher] has private interests that could conflict with their official duties in the future.

To a certain extent, conflicts of interest can be obviated by an appropriate declaration.

Financial conflicts of interest are typically the foremost in the public mind, but other conflicts of interest also occur in research, including personal, professional, and institutional advantages. You must avoid any financial or other interest that could compromise, or be perceived to influence, the impartial performance of your duties. Conflicts of interest that lead to biased decision-making may constitute corrupt conduct.

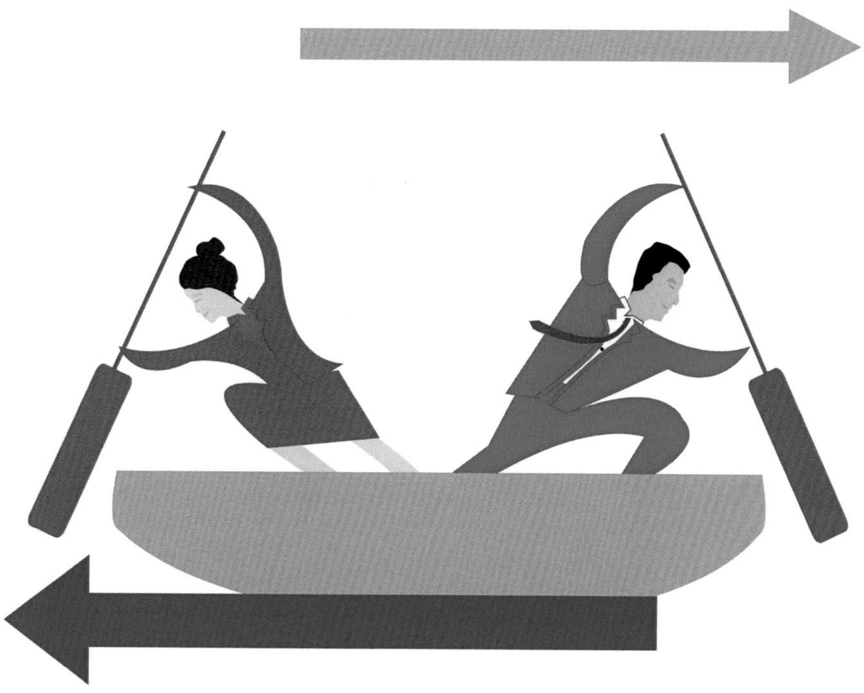

Image Credit: Rowing In Different Directions by Gabor Miklos/Shutterstock

Conflicts of interest in the research area are common. Decision-making processes in research often need expert advice, and the pool of experts in a field can be so small that all the experts have some link in the matter under decision. An individual researcher should expect to be conflicted from time to time, and be ready to acknowledge the conflict and make appropriate disclosures and withdraw themselves from the conflicted position. Conflicts should be managed to limit their potential to compromise judgments and decisions that should be made impartially. Compromised judgments could undermine community trust in research.

Outside the research-related area, conflicts of interest may occur where you (or a member of your team and, at times, your/their family)

- Have financial interests in the outcomes of your research
- Have access to information that could be used for personal gain
- Have made any promises or commitments in relation to the research outcomes
- Hold personal beliefs or attitudes that influence your impartiality
- Have personal relationships with people involved in your research or connected with the funding body, which go beyond the level of a professional working relationship
- Are involved in secondary employment, business, commercial, or other activities outside the workplace, which impact on your work
- Stand to benefit in any way that could cast doubts on my objectivity regarding reporting the project's findings

There are many instances of husband and wife teams working within the same research institution. While these teams are often highly productive and a credit to their institution, this provides an example of a potential conflict of interest. Some major research institutions choose to forbid husband and wife teams on the staff as a matter of policy.

It is your responsibility to disclose any potential or actual conflict of interest of this nature to your institution. They will assist you in resolving the conflict through solutions such as divestment of the interest, withdrawing from the conflict situation, and declaring or documenting the interest.

It is usual to disclose any conflicts of interest that relate to a research project when submitting your research results for publication.

Associated Documents—Conflicts of Interest

8.7.1 Conflict of Interest Registration Form

Complete this form to register a potential conflict of interest pertaining to research.

Applicant Details

Name:	Click here to enter text.
Position	Click here to enter text.
Notification Date	Click here to enter text.

Conflict Type

☐ Financial

☐ Non financial

Details

Detail of Potential Conflict
Click here to enter text.

Approvals

Confirmation that Conflict has been noted and approved:

Signature ____________________

Position and Name: ____________________

Date: ____________________

Remedial action to be taken (if appropriate)	Click here to enter text.
Date to be rectified	Click here to enter text.
Date Completed	Click here to enter text.

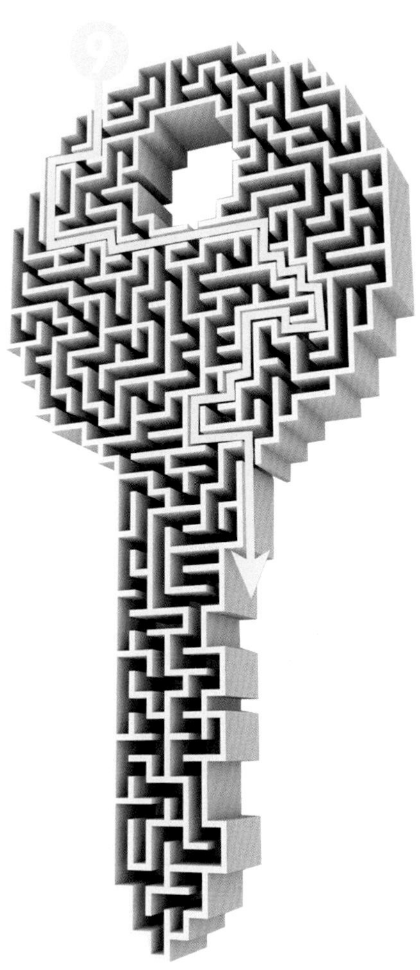

Checklist

(Tick when completed)

- ☐ Take a breath and time to reflect
- ☐ Talk to your mentor
- ☐ Try to focus on solutions to the problems and avoid getting caught up in your emotions
- ☐ Find someone who can help you!
- ☐ Go straight to the chapters following and start fixing things!

9.1 Introduction—Potential Challenges in Your Research

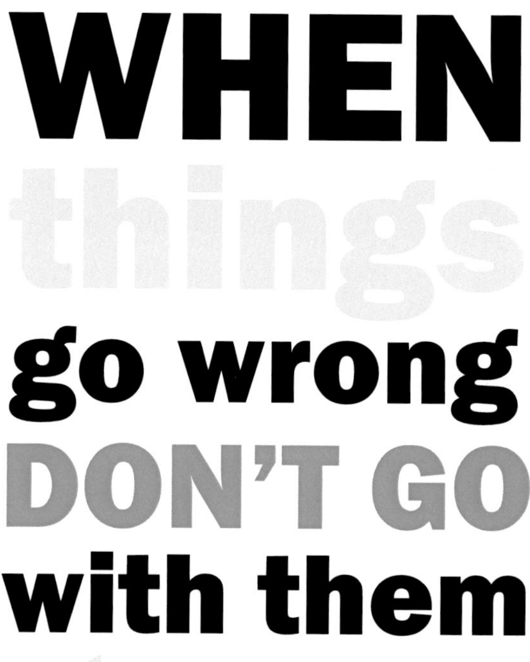

Image Credit: When things go wrong don't go with them by Letter Be/Shutterstock

9 WHEN THINGS GO WRONG

There are many things that can go wrong during the life of a research project, or indeed a of researcher. Most of them can be avoided with careful planning, and then sticking to the plan. Some are the result of matters outside your control, but you still have to deal with them.

Common problems include the following:

- Failure to keep proper records
- Loss of data
- Getting distracted by other projects
- Starting new tasks before the first ones are quite finished
- Project creep—adding tasks or objectives so timelines get pushed out
- Changes to project design that result in time-wasting and then delay
- Poor team selection, so knowledge gaps appear
- Slow study recruitment
- Under-estimation of time required to perform tasks
- Under-estimation of money required
- Ineffective delegation, especially the chief investigator's failure to insist on completion of tasks by others
- Leader is too busy to meet with the team, and therefore does not see that the project is, or some team members are, off course
- Equipment failure or unavailability
- Inconsistent practices or processes, usually a result of failure to document methodologys
- Failure to document methodology, leading to inconsistent practices or processe
- Cost blowouts as a result of unexpected rise in prices, or an unplanned need to repeat a costly experiment

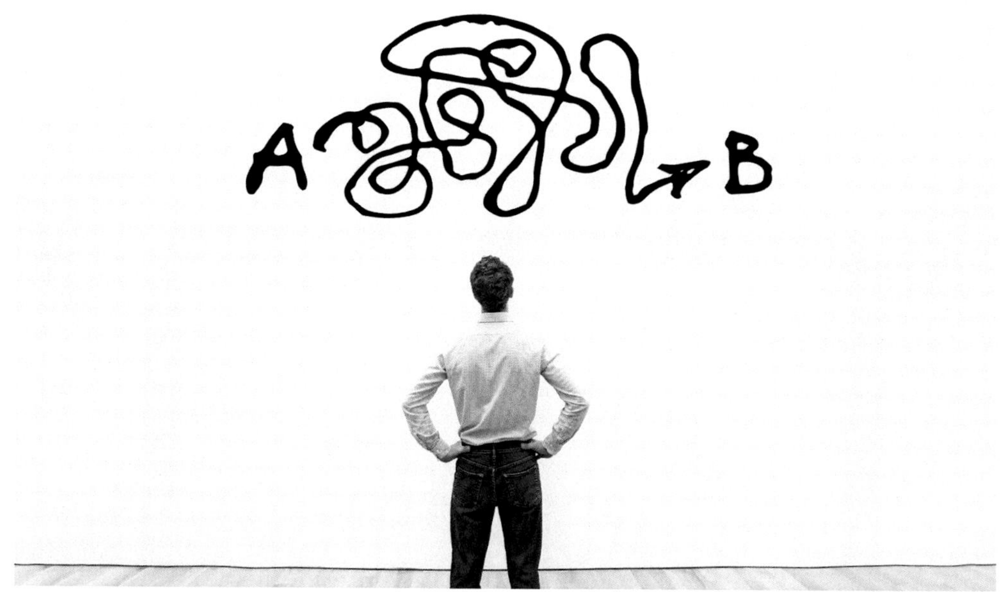

Image Credit: Problem solving, complicated solution by Ditty_about_summer/Shutterstock

Add to this all the other things that can go wrong in life with balancing your work and your family, trying to have a social life, and times of poor health. Lots and lots of things can conspire to catch you out!

Even if things are stacking up against you, please don't give up. Read the following chapters and, with any luck, they might lead you to some solutions.

9.2 Managing Work and Family Commitments

It's hard work in any career to balance the demands from work and the needs of a personal life. Sadly, it is probably as difficult as it gets in a research career because demands are compounded by the struggle to sustain funding and the uncertainty of outcomes, which is the hallmark of research. Many, many good people have been lost to research because it is just all too hard.

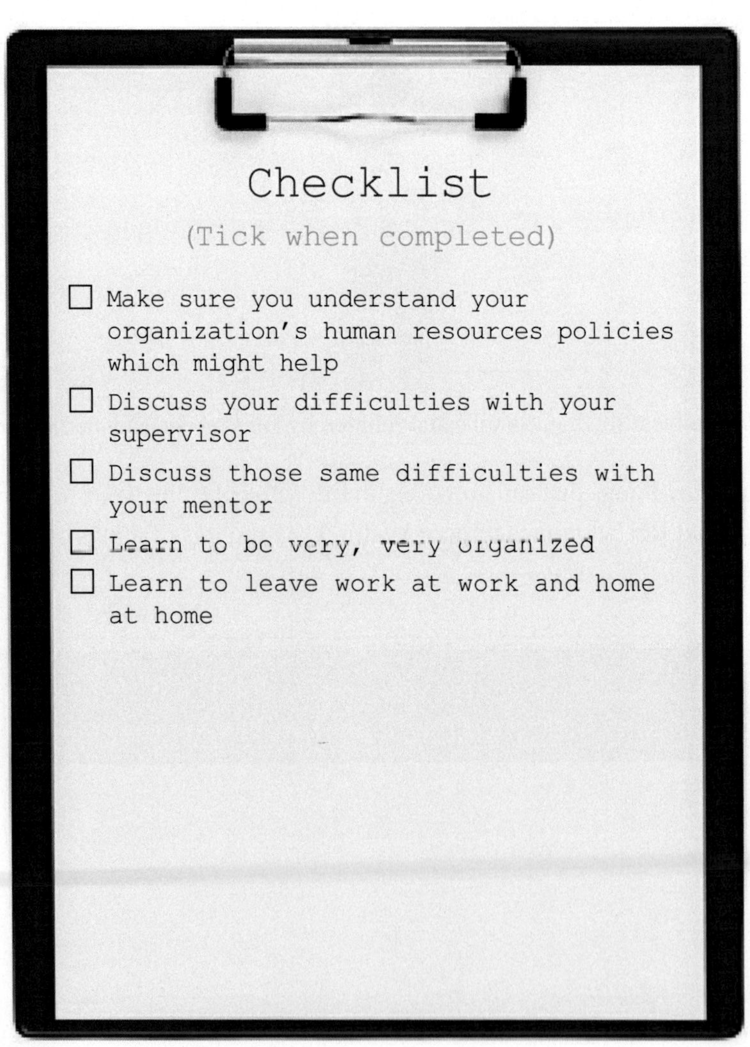

Many a young researcher has had to balance the impossible load of pursuing their unfolding research career with the pressure of family commitments. This is particularly the case for young mothers, when they need to take maternity leave (which comes with its own difficulties), then return to work and worry about the baby. What was already a very busy life before you had a partner or a child takes on many new dimensions when you add these (time-consuming) joys to your life. There are substantial commitments of time, money, and distraction that come with them and which eat into what was previously unimpeded work space.

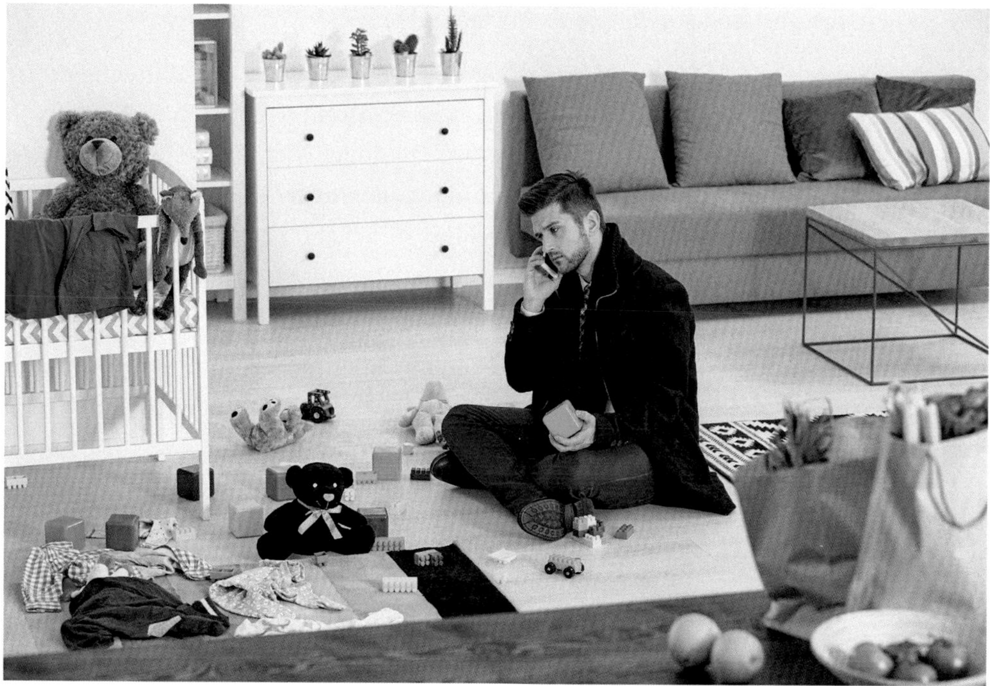

Image Credit: Dad sitting on floor by Photographee.eu/Shutterstock

When you are feeling that it is all too hard, try to remember that you are not alone! Thousands of other people are trying to do the same impossible tasks all over the world.

Parental Leave

While women in many parts of the world are now able to take maternity leave and return to their career without question, the time off still causes major disruption. In some countries the break is only three months, whereas in others it might be a year or more. In all cases, it is a career disruption, and the people who do not take parental leave can have an advantage over you.

If you are going to take maternity leave, see if you can negotiate the continuation of your projects under the guidance of your own supervisor, rather than putting them on hold. If you are able to check in regularly, this might well be possible. A next best, or additional option could be to focus on writing up and/or writing new grant applications while you are away. You will be greatly helped in this task if your institute allows you to access your work files from home during your period of leave. If not, things will have to wait until you get back. Tidy up as best you can, make sure you have excellent records of where you were up to, and don't stress about the things you can't do anything about. You may be interested to read about Moira Sheehan's preparation for maternity leave in her post-doc journal pieces in Nature [1].

Although many new parents find parental leave time a pleasure, if exhausting, it is definitely not so for everyone. Many people much prefer to go back to work. Don't worry, don't feel guilty. Make some suitable arrangements for your baby, and go back to doing what feels right for you. Again, Moira Sheehan [2,3] explains first her surprise at finding how many of her colleagues were also parents of young children, and then shares her feelings of isolation and her longing to get back to work. She also prepares other young mothers for the critical comments about "why I'd had children if I hadn't planned on raising them."

The difficulties of dealing with work and family responsibilities are a perfect topic for discussion with an appropriate mentor. There is nothing like sharing the problem with someone who has done it all herself to help you sort out your difficulties.

When You're Back at Work

Melissa Hayes, aka "postdocexperience," writes about her experiences in the lab after she has returned to work. This will really convince you that there is someone out there just like you! In her post "Sick Baby and Lost Work (Worth)" [4], she refers to the stresses of having to catch up. In particular, she says "Our companies and institutions are all very clear in that sick days are part of our benefits package. They all want to be seen as family friendly, striving to help achieve work/life balance for their employees. It all looks great on paper. But when you start to cash in and use those benefits (not abusing them at all), there seems to be some unspoken repercussions. Certainly my output and achievements will be affected and this will be reflected negatively upon review." Likewise, the trials of managing work and family that she describes in The Juggling Act [5] will be all too familiar to many.

The moral of the story is that you can only do what you can do. Do your best to deliver, but there is no question, it is going to be a balancing act.

Often there are opportunities to claim recognition for "career disruption" to your track record when you are applying for funding. Make sure you make use of this if you have taken maternity leave, returned to work part-time, or taken significant amounts of leave to care for a family member. When you mention it, provide as much detail as the space allows. "Took time off to have children" isn't enough.

References—Managing Work and Family Commitments

[1] Sheehan, M., June 28, 2007. Nature. 447. https://www.nature.com/naturejobs/2007/070628/pdf/nj7148-1140c.pdf.

[2] Sheehan, M., May 24, 2007. Nature. 447. https://www.nature.com/naturejobs/2007/070726/pdf/nj7152-508c.pdf.

[3] Sheehan, M., May 24, 2007. Nature. 448. https://www.nature.com/naturejobs/2007/070524/pdf/nj7143-504c.pdf.

[4] Hayes, M., 2013. Postdoc Experience. Sick Baby and Lost Work (Worth). http://postdocexperience.scienceblog.com/2013/02/13/sick-baby-and-lost-work-worth/.

[5] Hayes, M., August 01, 2013. Postdoc Experience Juggling Act. http://postdocexperience.scienceblog.com/2013/01/08/juggling-act/.

9.3 Gender Bias in the Workplace

Emma Johnston [1] is a marine ecologist and ecotoxicologist. She is a professor and pro-vice-chancellor, and she has spent her entire research and working life with male bosses or supervisors. She has never reported to a woman. She thinks the world would be a better place if this imbalance were addressed.

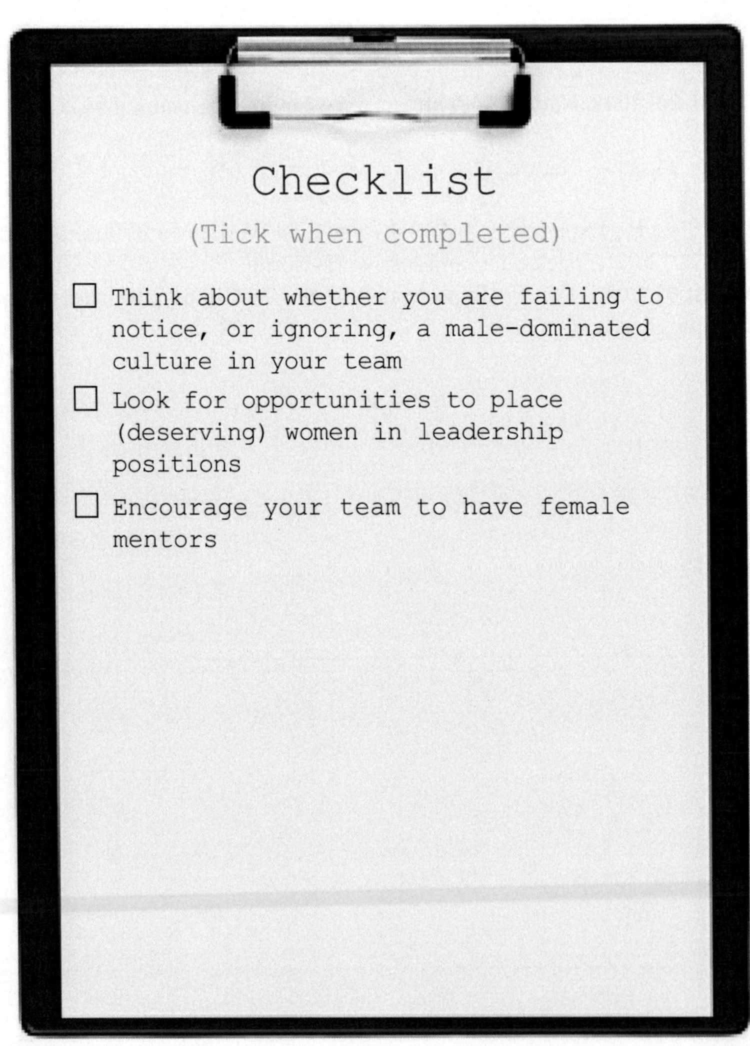

Gender bias in the workplace is still with us and is a very real limitation for many women across the world, particularly those working in science, engineering, mathematics, technology, and medicine. Whether you're a man or a woman, we all need to work to reduce it.

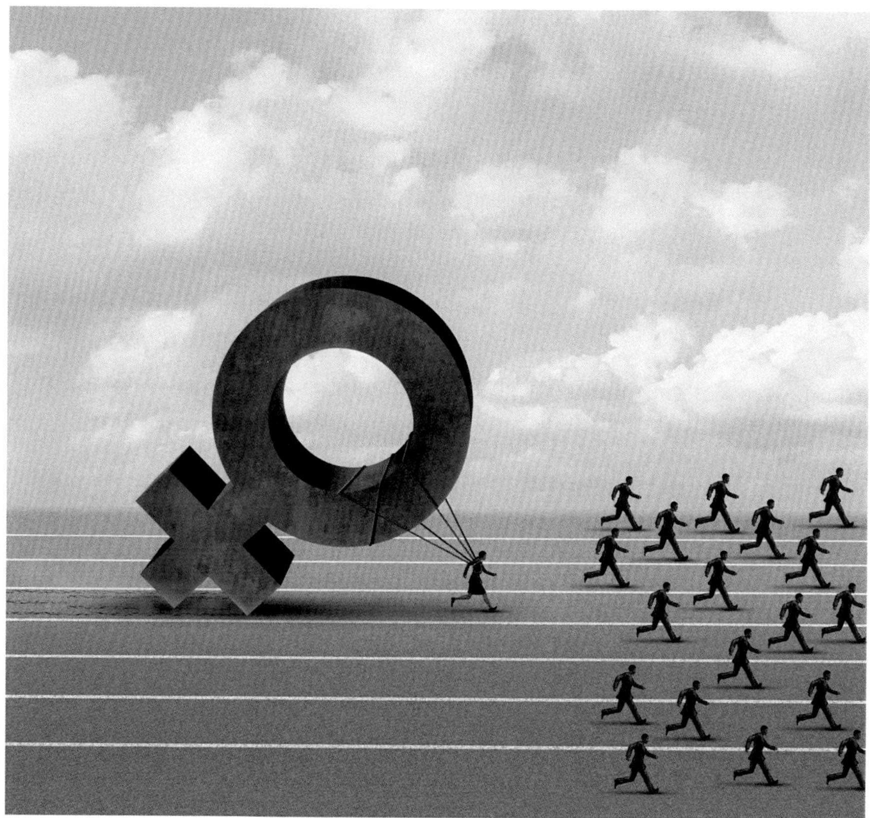

Image Credit: Sexism descrimination concept by Lightspring/Shutterstock

Johnston [1] looks first at the bigger picture. She cites a range of experts (Holter [2], Sandnes [3], Vafaei [4], Miller [5], McKinsey [6]) concluding that gender equality lifts us all. Johnston holds that men and women must work together to bring gender equity into the mainstream (UN Women [7]) by building gender equality into every practice and process so that it becomes the new norm. These are big steps to take in the male-dominated sciences.

Johnston suggests that, whether you are male or female, you should aim to surround yourself with female mentors and colleagues so that you can gain from their perspectives. She says

"Women will have diverse experiences and attitudes towards the gendered workplace. If you surround yourself with women, you can help recalibrate the world view and break down stereotypes."

Your whole team will benefit if you are able to work proactively to put systems and practices in place that reduce bias and promote equality and diversity.

These same principles apply, of course, to racial diversity or any other type of discrimination.

References—Gender Bias in the Workplace

[1] Johnston, E., 2016. The Conversation. How Men and Women Can Help Reduce Gender Bias in the Workplace. https://theconversation.com/how-men-and-women-can-help-reduce-gender-bias-in-the-workplace-62041.

[2] Holter, Ø.G., 2014. "What's in it for Men?" Old question, new data. Men and Masculinities. 17 (5), 515–548. http://journals.sagepub.com/doi/pdf/10.1177/1097184X14558237.

[3] Sandnes, H.E., 2012. Gender Equality Reduces Violence. http://sciencenordic.com/gender-equality-reduces-violence.

[4] Khadem, N., 2016. Quoting "board diversity and financial performance in the top 500 Australian firms Australian accounting review". Vafaei. http://www.smh.com.au/business/workplace-relations/asx-500-companies-that-employ-more-women-make-more-profit-study-shows-20160307-gnccnz.html.

[5] Miller, T., del Carmen Triana, M., July 2009. Demographic diversity in the boardroom: mediators of the board diversity – firm performance relationship. Journal of Management Studies. 46 (5), 755–786. https://ssrn.com/abstract=1410337.

[6] McKinsey Global Institute. The Power of Parity: how advancing women's equality can add $12 trillion to global growth. http://www.mckinsey.com/global-themes/employment-and-growth/how-advancing-womens-equality-can-add-12-trillion-to-global-growth.

[7] Supporting Gender Mainstreaming the Work of the Office of the Special Adviser on Gender Issues and Advancement of Women. http://www.un.org/womenwatch/osagi/gendermainstreaming.htm.

9.4 Retrieving a Project Which Has Gone Wrong

There are times when it seems just everything has gone wrong. The time has run out, the money has run out, the study staff have left, and the records are lost. Is there anything right? All that time and effort and money is wasted. It's very tempting to throw up your hands in horror and go to the pub to drown your sorrows.

Well, that is not a good idea. Yes, you have invested all that time and trouble. All that work has been done. Adjust your mindset and get on with some re-building. Start with this checklist.

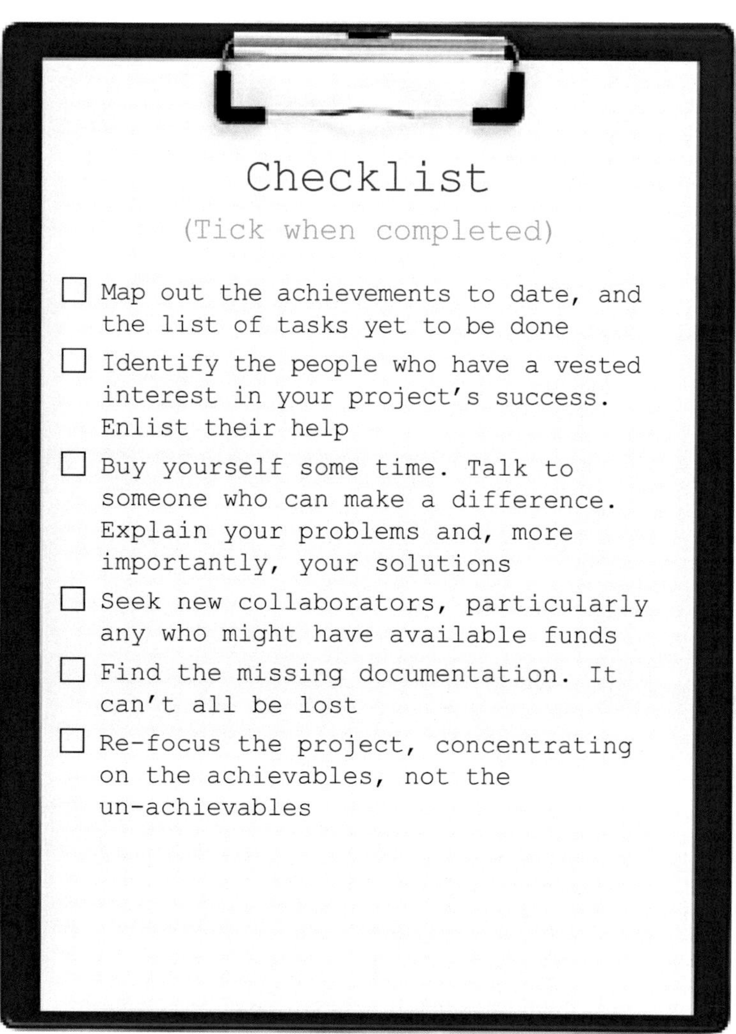

Do all these things as soon as possible. Delays will only make it worse.

Yet again, the secret to success is communication. If you can clearly and succinctly explain your difficulties, and then your planned resolutions, you stand a good chance of having someone help you with time, money, labor, and/or content.

Your project may have been re-organized, but it might also be re-born.

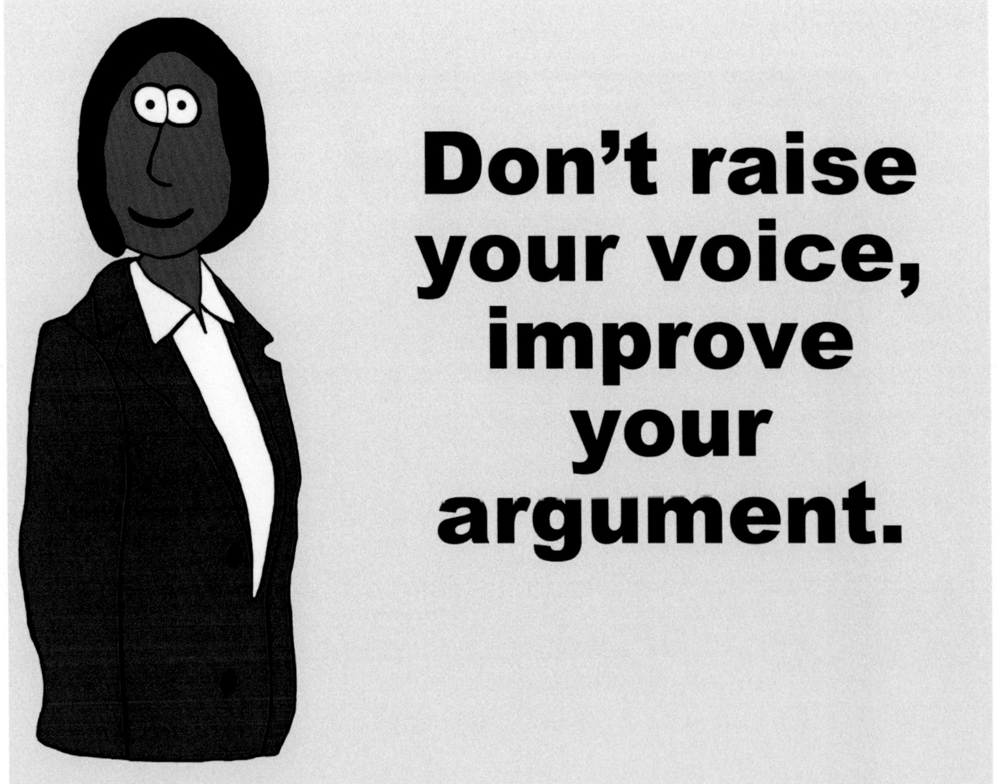

Image Credit: Don't raise your voice, just improve your argument by Cartoon Resource/Shutterstock

Resolving Conflict in Your Project

Resolving conflict and dealing with difficult people and situations in the workplace are realities of life. You'd like to brush them under the carpet, or pass them to someone else to deal with, but sometimes you have to tackle them head on.

It is useful to develop conflict resolution skills that enable you to bypass personal differences and to open up to possibilities. A useful resource is the CRN (Conflict Resolution Network) website [1] that offers background reading on 12 conflict resolution skills.

See Chapters 5.2 and 5.4 for more about dealing with conflict in your team.

Mending a Broken Collaboration

It happens. Sometimes it just doesn't work out the way it should have. Unlike a marriage, you can't just divorce. While collaborations are usually undertaken in good faith, and with the best of intentions, conflict may arise where you may not have predicted it.

If you want to keep that funding, you are going to have to find a way to resolve your problems.

The best ways forward are talking, talking, and more talking. With any luck you will be able to all talk to one another, and reach a resolution, although sometimes that isn't possible.

When the situation is dire, don't ignore the problem, but ask someone to help you. You could try to seek assistance from someone further up the line in one or both institutions, or from a third party with no vested interest. Resolve your problems one step at a time.

There are whole books written on this topic, and endless courses are offered. When you are trying to resolve someone else's conflict, remember that there will always be two sides to every story. Find out what has caused the problem—from both sides. Listen carefully. Tread gently.

In a nutshell, for all cases of conflict, resolution will come from communication, communication and then a bit more communication, and willingness to compromise.

Reference—Retrieving a Project Which Has Gone Wrong

[1] Conflict Resolution Network offers numerous resources for dealing with conflict. http://www.crnhq.org.

9.5 Some Traps for the Unwary

This is a quick summary of common problems that might arise during your career, most of which have been dealt with in other parts of the book.

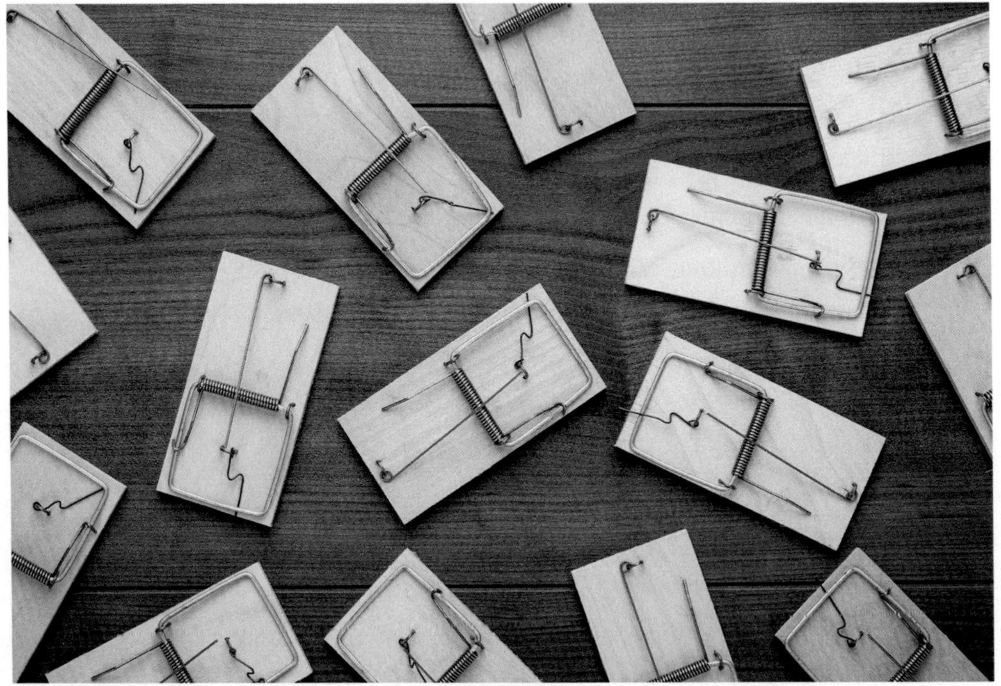

Image Credit: Many mousetraps by Ruslan Grumble/Shutterstock

Being Led Astray by Flattery

Having worked hard to enhance your reputation, take care to protect it. As a researcher, the integrity of your research output and practice helps to maintain not only your own reputation but also that of your colleagues, your research field, and your university.

Be careful not to be led into areas outside your particular research area by flattery. It is tempting when someone wants to work with you or be supervised by you. "Someone from somewhere wants *me* to supervise them. Oh yes, I've made it!" Guard your reputation carefully, and your time, and work within your space. Stepping outside your area of expertise, and making yourself look foolish, can leave your reputation in tatters.

The same applies to people, usually students, who want you to be named as an author on their paper. Don't do it if the paper isn't good enough. By all means help. Help them with their writing or their presentation, but ask them not to name you. Don't go to the opposite extreme and do it all for them or make them wait a year until you have time to review and re-write it properly.

University "Takes" Your Funding

Don't be taken by surprise if you find that the university is going to take 15% or 20% of your funding for "overheads" or some other generic reason. You can try to manage this by having sufficient funding in your initial budget request to cover this outgoing. See Chapter 1.6.

Your Grant Is Successful, but for a Reduced Budget

This situation was dealt with in Chapter 4.7 The bottom line is you should not try to do what you were going to do for \$x when you only have \$0.75x. Work out the best way to reduce the scope of your project, and liaise with your funder to reduce your objectives. If you are lucky, you might be able to attract further funding for the balance of the project on the basis of the early results.

You Budgeted in One Currency but Were Awarded in Another

See Chapter 1.5. Read the fine print!

You Can't Start Because You Don't Have Ethics Approval

You have your grant, you've employed your staff, but you can't begin because the ethics approval hasn't come through. Chapter 8.2 explains how you should aim to seek approval before you have funding. Staff costs are the greatest expense for the average project. It is very costly to be paying under-utilized staff.

Your Project Is Stopped for an Ethics Review

This can happen. It is very expensive, for time, money, and reputation. The best way to prevent it is to keep your ethics committee or institutional review board up to date with all the project developments, and do your best to comply with their requirements.

You Run Out of Time

First, this should never take you by surprise. If you have done your project planning properly at the beginning of the project, and if you review the project plan along the way, you will be aware of whether or not you are going to make your deadlines. Sometimes you won't, and, in fairness, it will sometimes be because of reasons out of your control. See Chapter 9.4 for suggestions about what to do.

You Run Out of Money

Similar to the point above, this shouldn't take you by surprise, but first, it simply shouldn't happen. Your project might be short of money for any number of reasons, but you only have the money you have, and your spending must stay within the allocated budget. If you spend more than your allocation you will be in trouble and will have to go begging to your director. This could be a career-limiting move. See Chapter 4.7 about managing project budgets.

You've Been Sidetracked—Scope Creep

When you decided on your project, you planned what it was to be about and then defined your objectives. You were planning to go from A to B by doing C, D, and E. You were going to investigate F and G. This is your project's scope. When you veer off to look at H and I, you have allowed "scope creep" into your project.

It is terribly easy to get distracted and to start following a new question. You must maintain control over your project's scope at all times, or you will find your project creeping into new areas, leading you to run out of time and money and possibly not achieving your original aims.

At the same time, though, you might well be coming up with clever or interesting, out-of-scope new ideas that you want to address. Don't dismiss them or lose sight of them. Keep a list of these ideas. They might be worthwhile to follow up if you find you do have time or money, or for the basis of a new grant application.

10 KEEPING AN EYE TO THE FUTURE

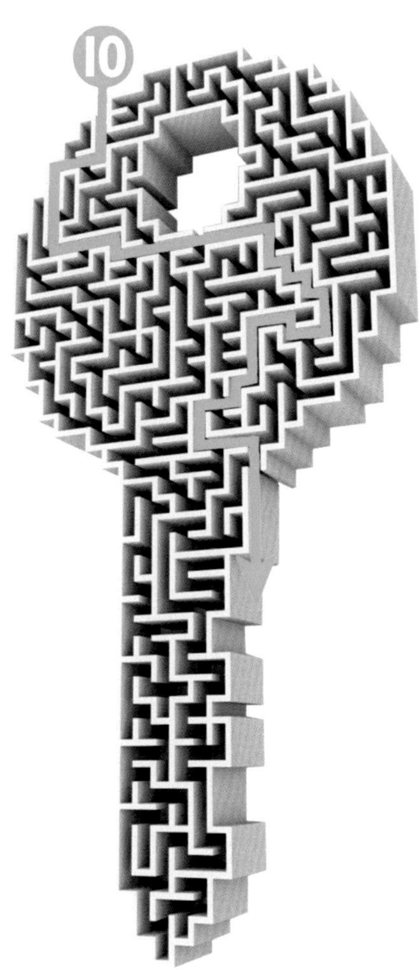

10.1 Career Management

Don't be Dumbo who never progresses. Really, there is more fun to be had (usually!) if you take the risk and aspire to the next rung on the ladder. Apart from anything else, you have learned lots along the way and now you can share the benefit of your knowledge with others.

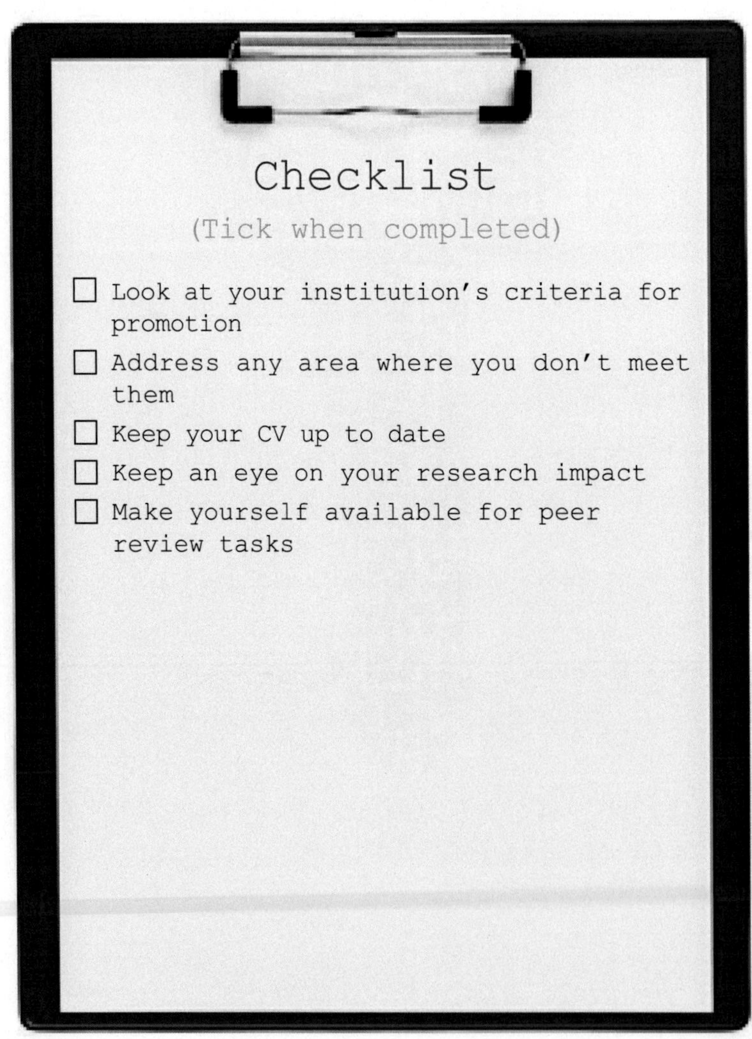

Career management is an ongoing priority—from the very first week in a new role, you should be thinking about your next steps!

From the beginning you must establish and then maintain and improve your track record because, in research, it is your track record by which you will be measured.

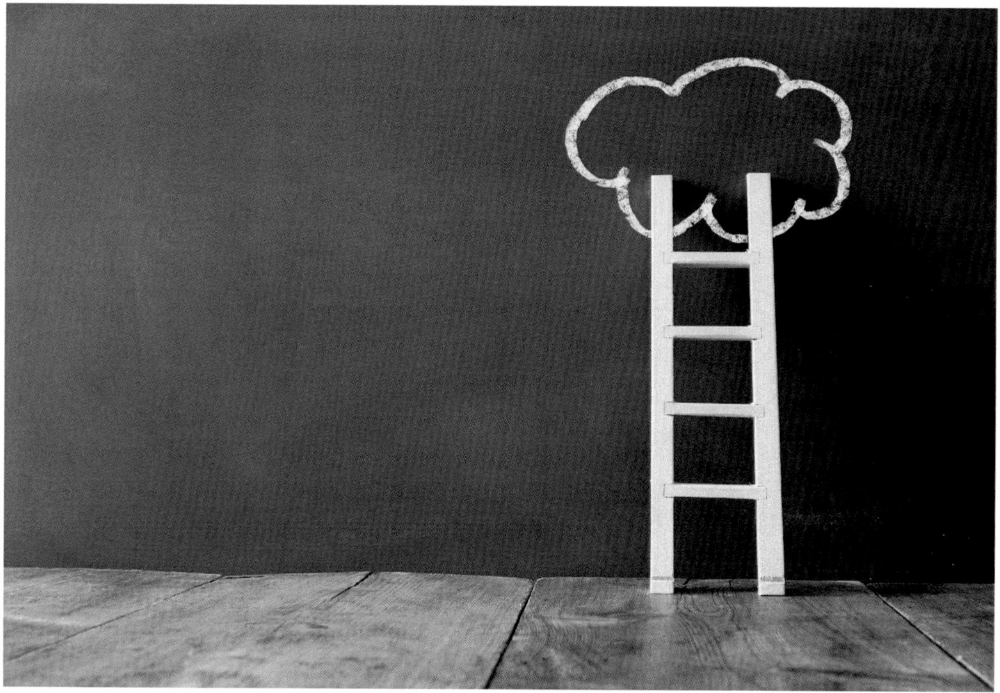

Image Credit: Wooden ladder and cloud by tomertu/Shutterstock

You should talk to your mentor (see Chapter 5.1) as a first step, to clarify what expectations are reasonable for you at the current stage of your career. Try to identify some successful role models, and review how and what they achieved in their research career—and when. Then map out your goals for the coming year, and, in less detail, for the years ahead.

As mentioned in Future Leaders Research Program [1], the typical goals for most researchers will relate to publications, research grants, supervision, and possibly research collaborations; however, you may have some other goals related to teaching, leadership, or project management. Your institution might have some standard expectations which you should treat as your starting point. Research is a competitive environment, so you should try to set higher goals than the minimum performance levels expected if you wish to fast track your career.

10 KEEPING AN EYE TO THE FUTURE

If you are working within a university, after a period of time you will want to be considered for promotion to the next academic level. Your university will have established guidelines for promotion, and you should familiarize yourself with the processes. You should familiarize yourself with these promotion guidelines, even if you are not within a university. They define sensible expectations for leadership, supervision, research community involvement and interactions with the public and will be applicable for your career progress, wherever you are working in research.

In addition to your track record in grants and publications, you might be assessed on the following:

- Favorable published reviews of your publications
- Awards by professional associations for outstanding research or creative work
- Invitations to positions, lectures, or demonstration at outstanding institutions or to leading professional conferences
- The value to industry of knowledge, processes, and products you have developed
- Research leadership, as evidenced by team achievements
- Breadth of expertise
- Any other clear evidence of exceptional contribution to your chosen field

You will also be assessed on service within and outside your institution:

- Academic "citizenship"
- Professional leadership within the university
- Community service and leadership

Once you have decided on your goals, make a list and refer to them in your planning, performance reviews, and ongoing activities. Monitor your progress. If you find you are falling behind, make the necessary adjustments.

At the end of each year you should be able to demonstrate high-level research outcomes, not just operational activities.

Keep Your Curriculam Vitae Up-to-Date

Part of the process of career management is keeping your CV up-to-date. Your list of appointments and publications is important, but don't undersell the "other" side of your career. There is increasing emphasis on community involvement, consumer involvement, and wider activities within your institution for people in research. Keep these records up-to-date, just as you will for your publications.

The same applies to student supervision. Include it on your CV, and remember to mention successful completions.

Make Yourself Available for Peer Review

Review Grant Applications

In every country where there is peer-reviewed funding available, there will be hard-working, unpaid reviewers who have offered their services on peer-review panels. There comes a time when you should do it too. While it makes for a very busy period in your life, being part of a peer-review panel comes with rewards. It provides a great way to keep up with the latest research in your field and also gives you exposure to the way others present their grant applications. You will learn a great deal from the comments of others on your panel and will come to understand much more clearly what makes a good application.

As will be perfectly obvious, the contents of the applications you review are to be treated confidentially; however, you can use your learnings to look up published work of researchers of interest to you, so increasing your knowledge for your field of interest.

Review Papers

Just as it is important to serve on grant review committees, you should take opportunities to review papers. Resist considering this as a nuisance. Reviewing papers from your field is a great way to keep up with developments in your field. It also provides you with exposure to the differences between a well-written paper and one which is not so well thought out. Importantly, it can help your reputation.

Take care with your review. Just as you expect your reviewers to take your work seriously, you should take the other person's work seriously. Make helpful clear comments and explain the reasons for them. The editors will see that you know your topic, and this in itself will enhance your reputation. In the fullness of time you may be invited to be an editor yourself.

Never hesitate to say no to reviewing a paper, which is outside your area of expertise. A poor review as a consequence of lack of knowledge will reflect badly on your reputation. It is much better to admit that this is out of your area and pass it back to someone else. On the other hand, if you find you have a conflict of interest, declare it immediately and return the paper to the editors with an appropriate explanation.

Just as with grant applications, you will be bound by confidentiality requirements for the papers you review. Do not allow the content knowledge acquired to creep into your own writing until the paper has been published.

Reference—Keeping an Eye to the Future

[1] Future Leaders Research Program. http://www.frlp.edu.au/.

Further Reading

These web articles provide some interesting perspectives on career management.

Andresen, K., LinkedIn Pulse, 2017. How to know when it's time to leave your job - and where to go next? https://www.linkedin.com/pulse/how-know-when-its-time-leave-your-job-where-go-next-katya-andresen?trk=v-feed&lipi=urn%3Ali%3Apage%3Ad_flagship3_profile_view_base_recent_activity_details_all%3BpZLIWTTCnwn60cBugnJUaQ%3D%3D.

Callier, V., Vitae Chronicle 2016. From Bench science to patent adviser: An Interview with Jeremiah Mitzelfelt. https://chroniclevitae.com/news/1632-from-bench-science-to-patent-manager-an-interview-with-jeremiah-mitzelfelt.

Castro F. W., 2016. Vitae Chronicle December 12 2016. Do you speak resume? https://chroniclevitae.com/news/1643-do-you-speak-resume.

10.2 What Comes Next?

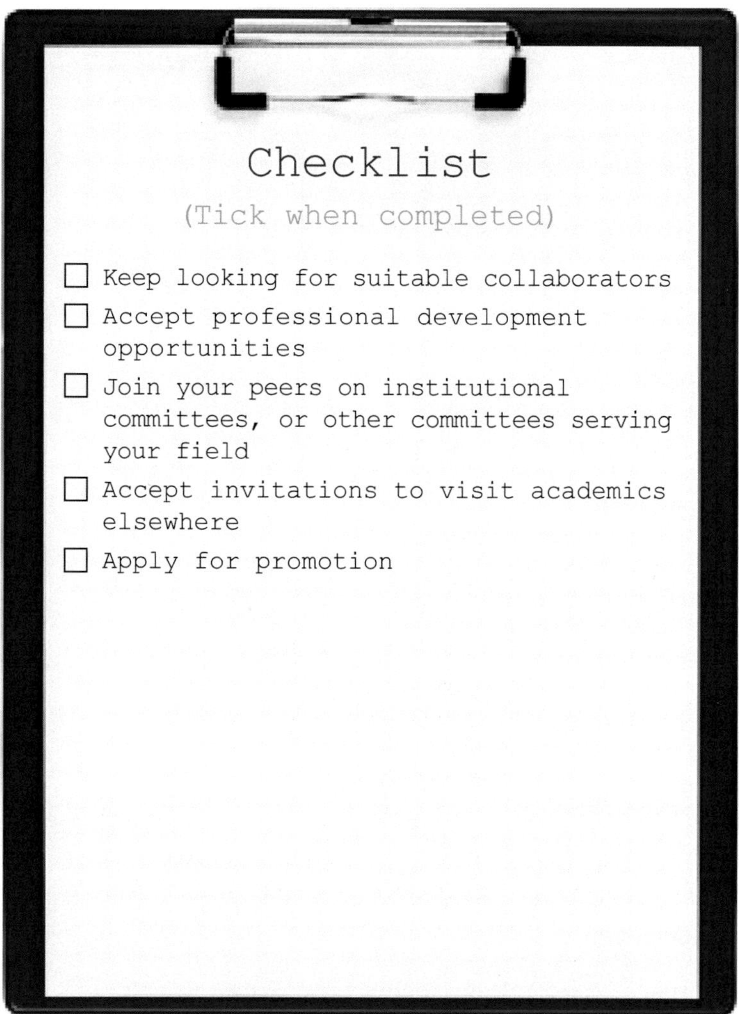

10 KEEPING AN EYE TO THE FUTURE

There are some relatively standard steps in the life of the researcher. While you might not choose, or be able, to follow these paths, a usual pattern from early-career researcher to mid-career researcher (MCR) and then to research leader is described below.

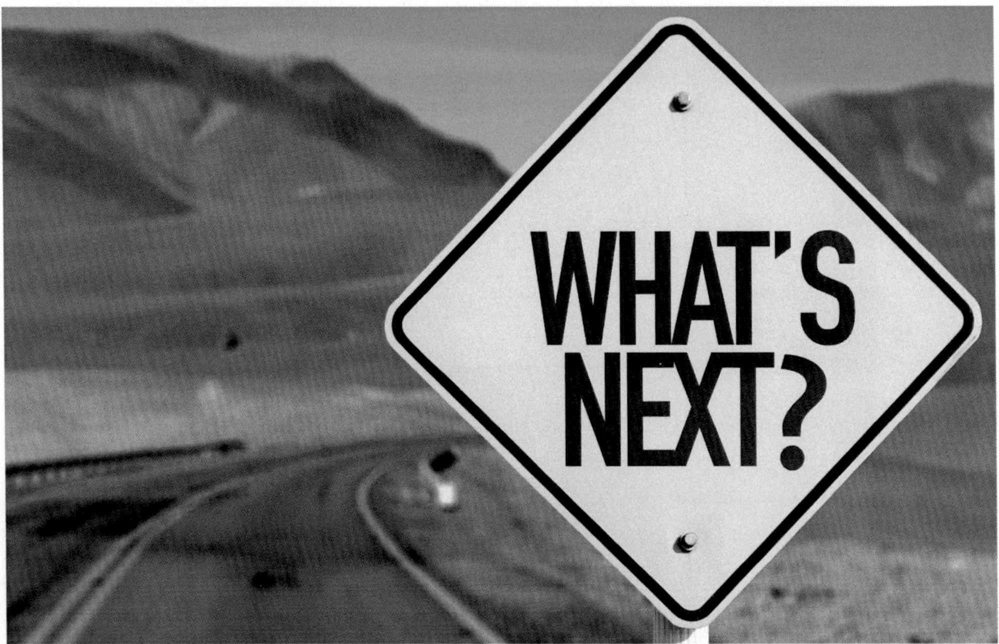

Image Credit: What's Next by Gustavo Frazao/Shutterstock

Mid-Career Researchers

MCRs are those who have established their track record, achieved grants, published papers, had successful postgraduate completions, and built a creditable profile. This stage might be reached about ten years post-doctoral.

MCRs commonly manage projects, teams, and areas of research activity. Sometimes they have large administrative responsibilities and work closely with their research leaders. They commonly supervise a number of staff and students and have multiple grants and publications underway. They might also have senior teaching responsibilities.

While the next step for an MCR will be research leader, MCRs will usually not have experience as the Principal Investigator on grants for a while. They Consequently, they will often still find themselves listed as second author, behind the research leader, on publications. It can be a very frustrating time. The researcher is keen to improve her track record and get to the next step, but hasn't quite got there.

When you find yourself in this position, it is time to take advice from your mentors about how to make the next move. This might mean you need to change your institution, or perhaps you just need to wait patiently for the right opportunity to arise.

The biggest challenge facing MCRs is usually lack of time to think and to plan their approach for coming years. It is hard to take the time to learn new skills. Researchers who now have management roles often find that they get caught up with management tasks which take them away from their research.

At this mid-time of your career, it is important to concentrate on the following:

- Building and strengthening collaborative research partnerships with colleagues, national and international partners, and industry
- Career management (particularly with respect to gaining increased profile and recognition)
- Project team leadership and management (particularly with respect to planning, financial management, and performance management of the research team)

This is also the time to work hard on your reputation within the university. Serving on committees or advisory bodies, building cross-disciplinary collaborations, networks, and developing knowledge of university processes all help you to build your network and enhance your reputation in your academic community.

Research Leaders

Established research leaders with high profiles and exemplary track records have an even more complicated program. Research leaders are normally well established in their fields, with a strong and sustained research profile and a secure group of researchers, students and collaborators who work in their research niche. They are generally secure in their ability to maintain their research reputation and attract additional research grants to fund their activities. By now they may also rely on consultancies and research contracts as well as grants to generate their funding base and maintain their teams. Balancing the demands of these grants and fellowships as well as the needs of their staff is challenging. Added to that, the established research leaders will have many external obligations and duties within the university.

By the time the research leader has reached this leadership position, she should have developed strong human resource management skills from her years of work with students, junior colleagues, and across larger research groups. These skills will have been built up from the time of supervision of the first honors or postgraduate student. As leader, she needs to have a strong understanding of how to recruit, select, manage, and develop other people, and an understanding of the policies and protocols of the institution.

As in all fields, the very best research leaders also recognize a need to continue developing their own interpersonal skills while continuing to focus on their objectives. They will also be planning for their handover to new leaders and their ultimate retirement.

If the research leader is also head of a research institution, that role will carry the great responsibility for the management of a facility, large budgets, multiple research programs, and relationship management with many stakeholders. She has the reputation of the institution in her hands and she must present its public face. It is difficult to manage all these leadership roles and still carry on her research program.

It is not surprising that many research leaders and heads of institutions eventually choose to "retire" to quietly pursue their research in an emeritus position.

10.3 Moving on Gracefully

Janie did her PhD with Professor Stern, but when the time came to look for a post-doc position, he made it clear it would be with him. He didn't want her results going anywhere. He had some funding, so she took the easy option and stayed where she was. She wasn't happy; therefore after a year or so, she started to plot her escape. Professor Stern caught wind of the plans and let her know he was not pleased.

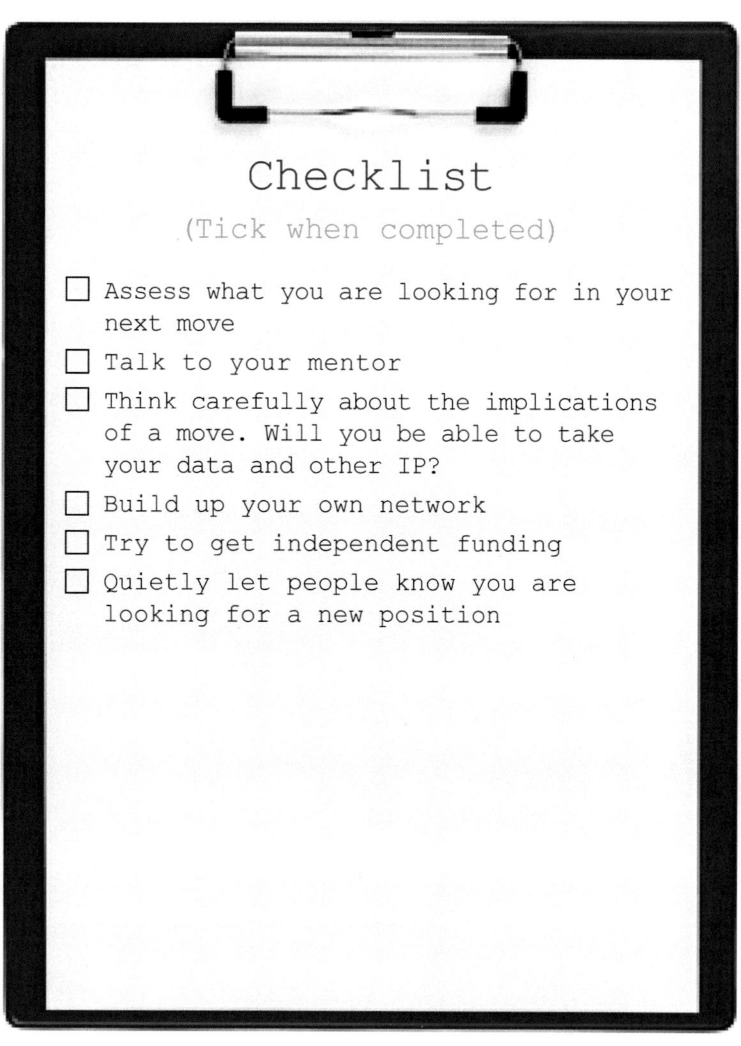

10 KEEPING AN EYE TO THE FUTURE

Something to consider when you are established in your first post-doc position, and indeed, before you take that first position, is how you will move away from your group leader and become an independent group leader yourself. It is not as easy as it might seem.

When assessing your opportunities, take the time to research how the careers of others who have been in that lab have progressed. Is the potential supervisor someone who appears to encourage success and independence for his/her team or someone who hangs on to them and their intellectual property? How many people have come out of that lab and established themselves in other institutions?

The break from the original group doesn't have to be painful, though sadly it often is. Like many a problem, this is one that can be made better by transparency and open communication. Discuss your plans with your group leader, and start those conversations well before you want to move. Discuss the plans with your mentor, for an independent view. Enlist the leader's help with your next steps, keeping the doors wide open for future collaboration, something of mutual benefit.

This is a bit different from changing jobs in the world outside research, where you would usually be quite justified in keeping your plans to yourself.

Once you have attained independence and your own group, remember the needs of your young team and encourage them to seek their own opportunities in the wide world.

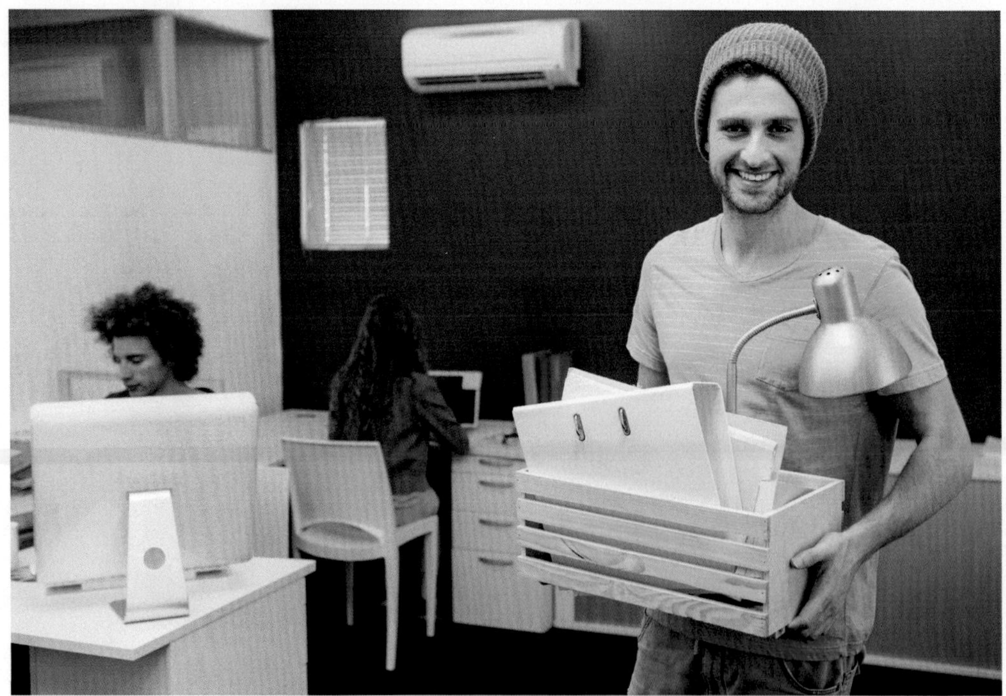

Image Credit: Man carrying his belongings in box by wavebreakmedia/Shutterstock

A variation of this theme is often found at the point where the Honors student wants to become the PhD student, (or the PhD student wants to take a postdoc role) but with a different supervisor in a different lab. If the student wants to be supervised by someone else, it can be difficult to break away. Understanding the perspectives of both sides is helpful here. The potential supervisors, though they will have to do work with the student, sees an extra pair of hands to do their bidding. They see results on projects they want carried out, and their names on the papers. The students, on the other hand, sees themselves tied into the same lab. They want to spread their wings and explore different options.

Whichever side of this story you are on, the best advice is to tread gently. Leave by all means, but take care not to leave an enemy behind you.

What to Do if Your Supervisor Won't Help

The best way to move away from a supervisor who doesn't want to let you go is to be offered (rather than applying for) an attractive position elsewhere. If this happens you obviously can't be criticized for disloyalty.

First, though, you need to increase your chances of receiving such an offer by growing your network. At the same time, do your best to enhance your reputation by promoting your work via your website and social media (see Chapter 1.9). Take opportunities to attend, and if possible, present at, conferences or otherwise meet with others in your field. Whenever you can, quietly let people know that you could be interested in a more senior position elsewhere, should one come up. This is important, because if people don't know you're looking to move they might not make an offer. Take care, though, not to openly criticize your current institution. People will be reluctant to employ someone who is seen to be disloyal.

You will also increase your chances of finding a new position if you are fortunate to have independent funding. This makes you attractive to a prospective employer who can see that the quality of work has been independently recognized. Further you come at least partially provided for, so you are cost-effective.

If things become very uncomfortable in your current position and your supervisor does everything to prevent you from leaving, you will have to stop talking about your plans with her. Continue to do your work properly, but, on the side, quietly pursue your search for another place. If an offer comes, it might be best to ask someone other than your supervisor, for example a former supervisor or your mentor, to provide you with a reference, in case your supervisor is tempted to (unethically) provide a deliberately poor reference. If you are lucky, your referee might tell your prospective supervisor that your current one is a bit difficult and doesn't want to let you go because of the quality of your work!

A Addendum—Some Tips About Biobanking

Protecting Your Biobank Samples

True story. A research institute in Johannesburg, a city known for its electrical storms, had its store of frozen blood samples in the −80°C freezer. Lightning struck on Good Friday night, the beginning of a 4-day weekend. Out went the power and the alarm, and there was no one there and no one coming back. On a "normal" night, or even a "normal" weekend, there could have been a chance of saving something. After a 4-day weekend it was just a smelly melted mess.

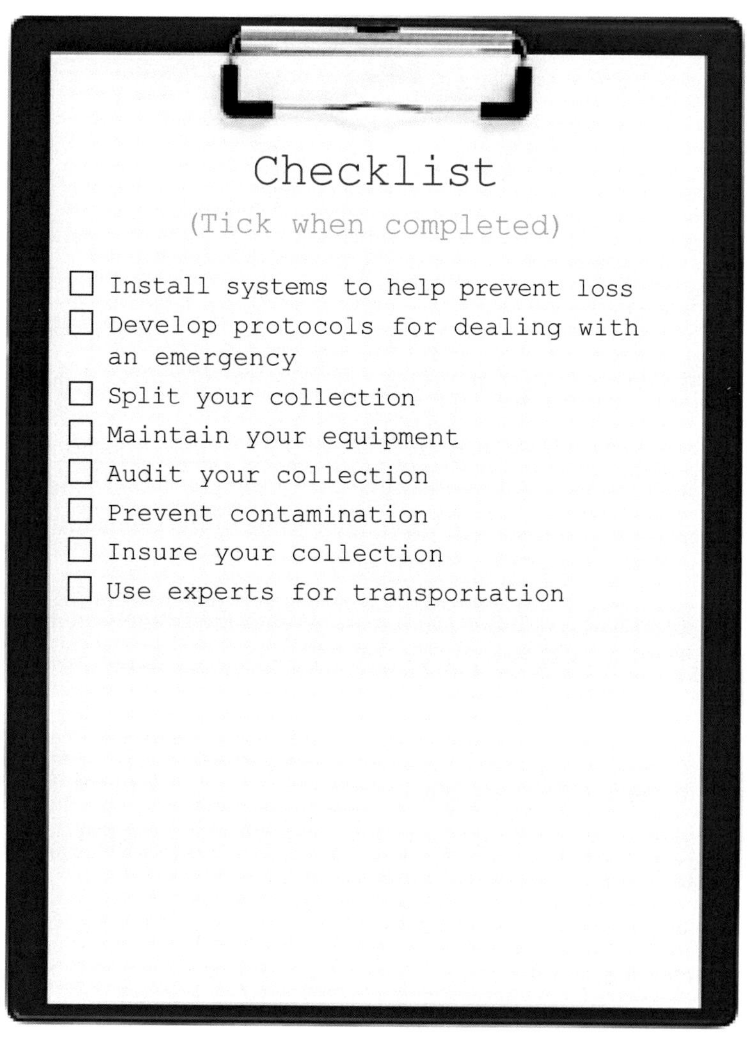

Everyone knows a tale of someone who has lost their whole biobank collection, usually as a result of loss of power. It can happen, does happen—and really, shouldn't happen. The cost of doing all that work again simply outweighs the costs of protection and good maintenance.

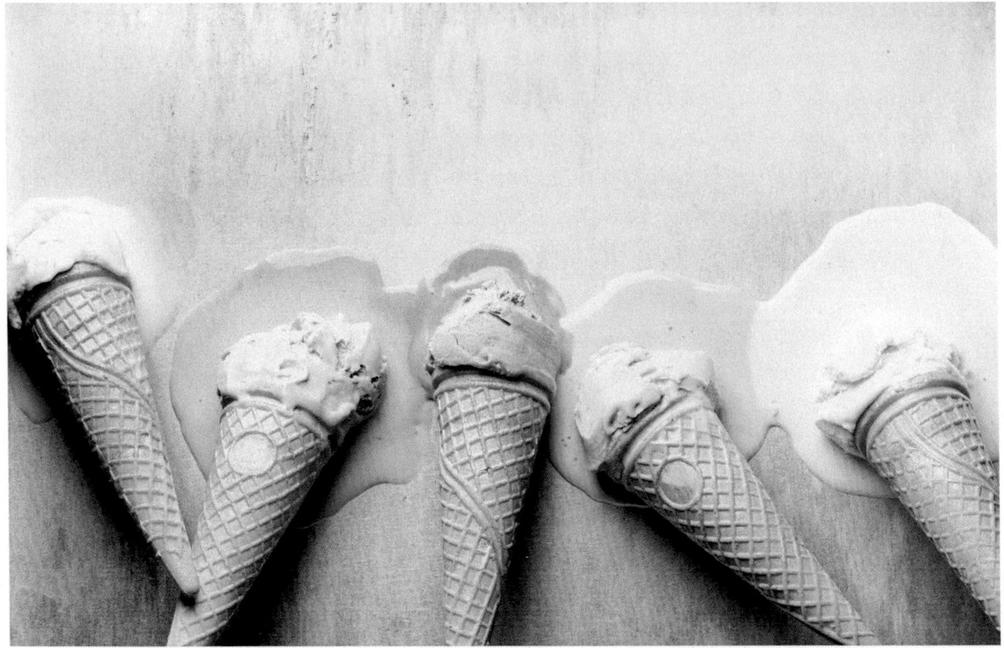

Image Credit: Colorful ice cream cones by Foxys Forest Manufacture/Shutterstock

There is one simple way to avoid total loss, and that is to split your collection. Work out a way to divide it, perhaps something as simple as dividing every sample in half, and storing the second collection in a different place. In the ideal world, this will not just be in a different freezer, but in a different building and on a different electricity grid.

For frozen samples, additional precautions should be taken if the budget can manage it. These can include an alarm to alert you of failure and CO_2 backups for your freezer to provide some hours of "breathing space."

Protect Your Sample Collections

If you are fortunate to have your own freezer(s) for your collection, it is not good enough to just turn it on, pop the samples in, and hope for the best.

The first thing to do is lock it. You don't want people from another lab either putting something in or taking your precious samples out.

Second, keep an eye on it. Draw up a roster for checking and recording the freezer temperature. Placing a graph on the freezer door for date and temperature is a usual practice.

Alarms and Emergency Procedures

You should develop a backup plan for the times when you have a freezer failure or power outage. If you have a −80°C freezer, a good start is the installation of a CO_2 bottle to connect with a backup cooling system, which will automatically give you about 9h extra time in the event of a power failure. In addition to this, you can do the following:

- Install a second freezer—although of course this only helps in the event of a freezer malfunction. It isn't useful in the case of a power outage.
- Buy some large polystyrene iceboxes to keep on hand, and source a provider of dry ice who can deliver promptly.
- Make an arrangement for emergency storage with someone with a freezer with capacity on the different electricity grid.
- Ensure you have contact numbers for key staff.
- Ensure those key staff have appropriate access to the building.
- Keep some standard spare parts for your freezer.

Write a protocol for emergency response and circulate it to the people involved. It is no good if you find out the power will be off for the next 24h if you don't have a plan for what you will do about it.

In an emergency, many people tend to panic and might do something silly. Minimize this possibility by providing a detailed protocol covering every step. Assume the alarm respondent knows nothing. This protocol should provide specific detail about the following subjects:

- Precise nature of the alarm calls which would be received and what each means
- Location of the freezers
- Access to the building
- Location of freezer keys
- Steps to take, one by one
- Location of equipment to be used
- Work health and safety precautions to be observed
- Supplier list—for maintenance, dry ice, spare freezer, extra gas bottle
- List of colleagues who might help

- Summary of causes of alarms
- Detail of time until the freezer is likely to reach dangerously high temperatures

Just as for building fire alarms, it is a good idea to regularly run through emergency procedures with all team members who might be required to respond.

Good Maintenance Procedures

You should also have a protocol for routine maintenance of your freezer and alarm system(s). When developing protocols for looking after your frozen collection, consider the following:

- Routine maintenance such as de-icing
- Conduct audits of your collection
- Routine alarm testing (monthly is suggested), both of the freezer's temperature alarm (if it has one) and of a power outage alarm (if you have one)
- Regular weighing of your spare CO_2 bottle to help you detect a gas leakage

Keep a record of the maintenance and testing.

Prevent Contamination

Contamination is another problem, which is all too real. In the past, many cell lines that were widely used for biomedical research had been contaminated and overgrown by other, more aggressive cells. The literature shows, for example, thyroid lines were actually melanoma cells, prostate tissue was actually bladder cancer, and normal uterine cultures were actually breast cancer [1]. You don't want to be part of this folly.

It is beyond the scope of this book to provide instruction of laboratory practices; however, it is suggested that novel cell lines should be proliferated and distributed and/or deposited at a safekeeping institution such as the ATCC as soon as possible after establishment, to minimize the odds that the line becomes spoiled by contamination. It is good practice to periodically check cell lines maintained under laboratory conditions (i.e., not placed in long-term storage) for contamination with HeLa or other common contaminants to ensure that their quality and integrity is maintained.

Don't keep your samples in a risky shared freezer. Think of the time and effort and money that has been put into collecting them. There are times when you just have to pay for something better.

Insurance for Your Samples

There is a common misconception that biobank samples cannot be insured because they do not have a commercial value. This is incorrect. They can be insured, and they should be as, after all, they are a valuable asset for your institute.

The "value" of your samples is the cost of replacement. Work out the cost of doing all the work again, divide it by the number of samples, and calculate the cost of each aliquot. You have your value. This cost might be very high if it involves recruitment all over again; it will be less if it is a matter of going back to ask again.

Quite reasonably, your insurance company will require you to take steps to protect the samples. The insurance premium will be reflected in your ability to offer that protection.

Use Experts for Transporting Your Samples

The first time you are required to send some samples offsite or bring some in from elsewhere you might well wonder what on earth to do. Will I have to go to collect them myself? No.

There are many specialist transport companies who have expertise in delivering research samples, whether room temperature, refrigerated, or frozen, across the country or across the world. It does take time to set up arrangements the first time, so don't leave it to the last minute. There are often approvals required.

You will need to be absolutely precise about the address at the receiving end and about making sure there is someone appropriate to take delivery. You want to avoid the last hours of the journey involving melting in the container at the airport!

References—Some Tips About Biobanking

[1] Neimark, J., 2015. Line of attack. Science. 347 (6225), 938–940. http://science.sciencemag.org/content/347/6225/938.full.

Acknowledgments

Two bodies of work informed a great deal of the background research for this book.

I particularly acknowledge:

The Future Research Leaders Program developed by the Group of Eight universities (Go8) in Australia.

and

"Making the Right Moves: A Practical Guide to Scientific Management for Postdocs and New Faculty" supported by the Burroughs Wellcome Fund and the Howard Hughes Medical Institute.

http://www.hhmi.org/developing-scientists/making-right-moves.

Each of these works provided me with a great number of ideas and helpful references.

In addition, I wish to thank the following people who went out of their way to assist me with this project:

- Dr. Matthew Brown
- Associate Professor Gillian Gould
- Emeritus Professor Adrian Lee
- Michael Milne
- Emeritus Professor Christopher Moran
- Sir Gustav Nossal, AC, CBE
- Associate Professor Clare Scott
- Associate Professor Freddy Sitas
- Dr. Daniel Speidel
- Robyn Williams, AM
- Associate Professor Wendy Wright
- The team at Cure Cancer Australia and many of the researchers we fund

I thank Mary Preap and Poulouse Joseph from Elsevier.

Very special thanks are due to my friend Stephen Treble, who has helped me at every stage in the creation and production of this book, and my tolerant husband, Richard, who patiently puts up with all my time-consuming schemes.

Glossary

Add-on costs	Costs incurred by an employer for an employee in addition to actual salary
CALD	Culturally and linguistically diverse
CV	Curriculum vitae
DUA	Data use agreement
ECR	Early career researcher
Ethics committee	Sometimes called institutional review board (IRB)
FTE	Full-time equivalent
H index	Author-level metric that attempts to measure both the productivity and citation impact of the publications of a scientist or scholar
HDR student	Higher degree by research student
HR	Human resources or personnel
IP	Intellectual Property
IRB	Institutional review board (sometimes called ethics committee)
Impact factor	Measure of impact of an academic journal
JIF	Journal impact factor
KPI	Key performance indicator
MCR	Midcareer researcher
MIA	Multiinstitutional agreement
MoU	Memorandum of understanding
MTA	Material transfer agreement
NDA	Nondisclosure agreement (or confidentiality agreement)
NIH	National Institutes of Health, USA
OA	Open access
PD	Position description (sometimes called JD—job description)
Pension	Sometimes called superannuation
SOP	Standard operating procedure
SWOT analysis	Strengths, weaknesses, opportunities, threats analysis
WBS	Work breakdown system
WH&S	Work, health, and safety

Index

'*Note*: Page numbers followed by "f" indicate figures and "t" indicate tables.'

INDEX

D

E

F

G

M

N

INDEX

Q

R

S

INDEX

T

U

V

W

Y

Printed in the United States
By Bookmasters